THE OHIO STATE UNIVERSITY

# VETERINARY PARASITOLOGY



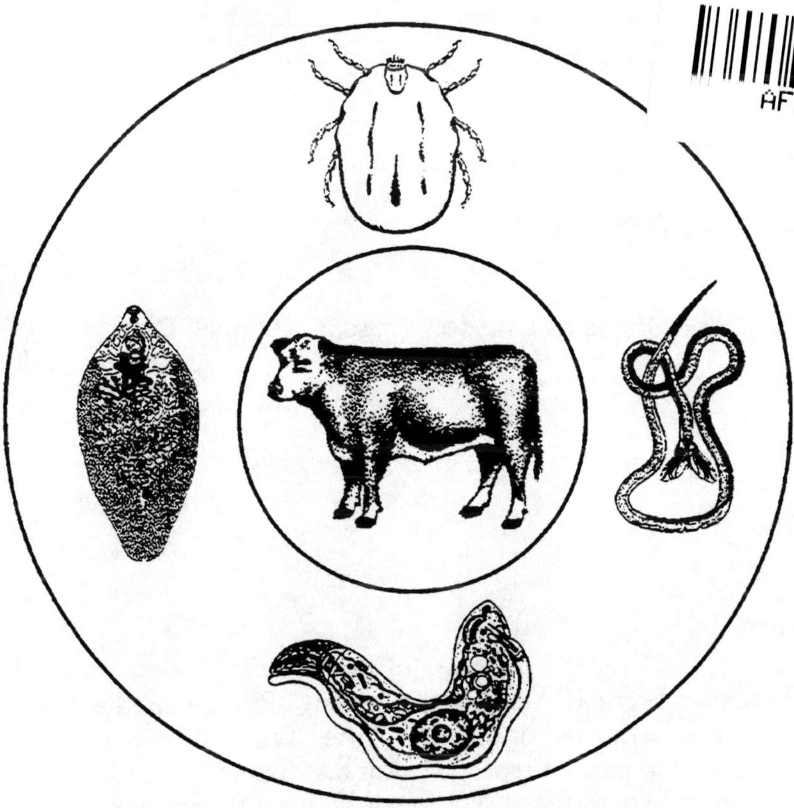

BY OMAR O. BARRIGA, DVM, PhD
Department of Veterinary Preventive Medicine

COLLEGE OF VETERINARY MEDICINE

Manufactured in the United States by Greyden Press, Columbus, Ohio

Veterinary Parasitology



ISBN 1-57074-242-1

Printer/ Binder: Greyden Press, Columbus, Ohio.

This book is dedicated:

To A. Neghme, N. D. Levine, and E. J. L. (Lord) Soulsby, who made it possible;

To my past, present, and future students, who made it worthwhile;

To Inés, Omar Jr., and Alvaro, who made it meaningful.

## Foreword

This text is the incomplete prepublication draft of a book of Veterinary Parasitology under preparation. It contains information that you have to learn in this course, in other courses of your veterinary curriculum, and during your future practice. It also contains references that you may need occasionally in your professional life, and basic information that will enable you to think parasitic problems logically.

You will have to find the information relevant to this course by yourself. This is not an oversight. A considerable part of your professional life will be spent looking for specific data among a mountain of information. We want you to become skillful at it *before* you are in front of your client. This is an opportunity to start sharpening your skills. To help you, I have prepared a syllabus (pages v to xix) that list my expectations for this course. Use it! It is meant to give you a clear view of what you are expected to learn.

**Objectives of the course**

The general objectives of this course are:

1. To help you learn to recognize the common parasites of veterinary or public health importance that exist in the United States, with emphasis on those present in Ohio.

2. To help you learn the life cycles of these parasites inside and outside the host. This information is essential for you to understand, in later courses, the clinical manifestations, diagnosis, treatment, epidemiology, and control of the corresponding infections.

3. To help you learn the mechanisms of the diseases caused by these parasites. This information is essential for you to understand, in later courses, the probable evolution, prognosis, and treatment of the condition.

The particular objectives of each lecture are listed in the syllabus.

**Sources of information**

The lectures will provide guidance and the skeleton of the knowledge that you are expected to acquire. You are expected to supplement this information with readings from your book and recommended bibliography, discussions with your classmates, and reasoned reflection on the factual information gathered. Do not overlook the formation of study groups. You will be surprised how much you can learn by simply talking about the subject.

**Exam questions**

To the extent possible, the exam questions will ask for applications of the knowledge acquired rather than for regurgitation of memorized data. Keep this advice in mind when you study and try to imagine the circumstances in which you might use the information you are learning in your professional life.

**Instructor availability**

You may talk to the instructor at any time. No prior appointment is necessary. I can be found at 301 Sisson (office), 316 Sisson (laboratory), or reached at 292-1206. I prefer not to answer long or personal questions at the end of the lectures. This rightfully upsets the next instructor who is waiting to start his/her lecture.

# VMC.550.02. BIOLOGY OF DISEASES
# SECTION VETERINARY PARASITOLOGY
**Instructor: Omar O. Barriga, DVM, PhD**

## SYLLABUS OF THE COURSE

**LECTURE 1**. Introduction to Veterinary Parasitology (pages 1 to 8)

**A. Contents**:

1) Importance of parasitism
2) Association between species
3) Types of parasites
4) Types of hosts
5) Types of host-parasite associations
6) Principles of systematics

**B. At the end of this lecture you should be able to**:

1) List three areas in which parasitology is important and provide an example in each case,
2) Describe four classes of association between different species, explain their identifying characteristics, and provide an example in each case.
3) List six types of parasites, explain their identifying characteristics, and provide an example in each case.
4) List three types of hosts, explain their identifying characteristics, and provide an example in each case.
5) Mention three types of host-parasite associations, explain their identifying characteristics, and provide an example in each case
6) Name the taxonomic categories in order and provide the complete classification of one parasite.
7) Explain why it is important to a veterinarian to know the general characteristics of the family to which a parasite belongs.

**C. Example of a test question applicable to this lecture**:

Which of the following situations involves a paratenic host?:

a) Microfilaria of *Dirofilaria immitis* in a mosquito
b) *Haemonchus contortus* in the stomach of a sheep
c) *Cryptosporidium* oocysts in he stomach of a domestic fly
d) Larvae of *Toxocara canis* in a mouse
e) Larvae of *Dipylidium caninum* in a flea

NOTE: This question assumes that you have attended the entire course already. At this time, you may need search in your book for information regarding the parasites mentioned.

**LECTURE 2**. General concepts regarding arthropods (pages 9 to 19)

**A. Contents**:

1) External morphology
2) Identification and classification
3) Biology

**B. At the end of this lecture you should be able to**:

1) Label the parts of an insects as seen from the outside
2) Name four subphyla of arthropods, explain their identifying characteristics, explain which are the two most important subphyla, and provide an example in each of these last cases
3) Describe three types of reproduction that exist among insects and give examples
4) Describe the types of development that exist among insects, contrast them, explain their importance for a veterinarian, and give examples.
5) Define what diapause is and explain its importance for the insect and the veterinarian
6) Define what arthropod hormones or pheromones are and describe their possible use in insect control.
7) Describe five methods of arthropod control and give examples
8) Use Key 2.I to classify an ectoparasite

**C. Example of a test question applicable to this lecture**:

Which of the following statements explains best that one application every two weeks of an appropriate insecticide on a dog (for a total of 2 applications) are more effective to eliminate lice than fleas?

a) Fleas are much more resistant to insecticides than other insects
b) Lice are much more susceptible to insecticides than other insects
c) Fleas are hematophagous
d) Not all lice are hematophagous
e) Lice have an incomplete but fleas have a complete metamorphosis

**LECTURE 3**. Orders Mallophaga, Anoplura, and Siphonaptera (pages 26 to 47)

**A) Contents**:

Morphology, identification, classification, biology, and medical importance of the:

a. Mallophaga,
b. Anoplura,
c. Siphonaptera,

**B. At the end of this lecture you should be able to**:

1) Distinguish between a chewing louse, a sucking lice, and a flea by their morphology
2) Give an example of each of the 3 groups (Mallophaga, Anoplura, and Siphonaptera) using the scientific and common names, and indicate the respective host
3) Describe and contrast their respective biologies.
4) Describe and contrast their respective medical importance.
5) Use Plates II, III, and IV to classify specimens of the respective groups.

**C. Example of a test question applicable to this lecture**:

Which of the following pathogenesis or pathologies is NOT attributable to fleas?

a) Production of skin allergy in carnivores
b) Production of ulcers in the head of chickens
c) Transmission of the cestode *Dipylidium caninum*
d) Transmission of the filaria *Dirofilaria immitis*
e) Transmission of the bacterium *Yersinia pestis* (plague)

**LECTURE 4**. Diptera: Nematocera, Brachycera and Cyclorrhapha (pages 49 to 77)

**A. Contents**:

1. Identification, biology, and medical importance of the:
    - a) Nematocera (as a group)
    - b) Simuliidae
    - c) Ceratopogonidae
    - d) Culicidae
    - e) Brachycera
    - f) Cyclorrhapha (as a group)
    - g) non-biting Muscidae (the face fly as an example)
    - h) biting Muscidae (the stable fly as an example)
    - i) Calliphoridae
    - j) Sarcophagidae
    - k) Oestridae (the horse bots as an example)

**B. At the end of this lecture you should be able to**:

1) Identify a Diptera and recognize whether it is a Nematocera, a Brachycera, or a Cyclorrhapha
2) Identify a Nematocera and recognize whether it is a Simuliidae, Ceratopogonidae, or Culicidae
3) Describe and contrast the biology of Simuliidae, Ceratopogonidae, and Culicidae
4) Describe and contrast the medical importance of Simuliidae, Ceratopogonidae, and Culicidae
5) Describe the biology and medical importance of the horse flies
6) Recognize Muscidae, Calliphoridae, Sarcophagidae, and Oestridae adult flies.
7) Describe the general biology of the Cyclorrhapha and describe and contrast the biology of Muscidae, Calliphoridae, Sarcophagidae, and Oestridae.
8) List the morphological features that are important for the identification of adult or larval stages of flies.
9) Name four ways that the Cyclorrhapha may cause damage to their hosts and give appropriate examples.
10) Use Plate VI to identify a fly larva.

**C. Example of a test question applicable to this lecture**:

Because the conduct of the veterinarian in front of an accidental myiasis may be quite different from his/her conduct before an obligatory myiasis, he/she may be interested in identifying fly larvae found in the skin of food animals. The easiest way to distinguish between larvae of *Lucilia* (syn. *Phoenicia*) or *Cochliomyia*, for example, is to:

a) Examine the cephaloskeleton of the hooks
b) Examine the respiratory openings
c) Compare the size of the larvae
d) Examine the feminine genital organs
e) Evaluate the lesion produced in the host

**LECTURE 5**. The Order Acarina: Ticks and Mites (pages 78 to 104)

**A. Contents**:

1) Morphology and classification of the acarina
2) Classification, general biology, and medical importance of the hard ticks
3) Identification, biology, and medical importance of the:
    a. Mesostigmata mites
    b. Sarcoptiformes mites
    c. Trombidiformes mites

**B. At the end of this lecture you should be able to**:

1) Identify and differentiate a hard tick, a soft tick, and a mite
2) Name and differentiate the two genera of ticks found most commonly on dogs in Ohio
3) Describe the development of a hard tick from egg to egg
4) Describe the concepts of 1-, 2-, and 3-host ticks and the mechanisms of disease transmission by ticks in each case
5) List and give examples of the morphological structures that are important for the identification of the genus of a tick.
6) List 5 ways that ticks can harm their hosts
7) Differentiate between Mesostigmata, Sarcoptiformes, and Trombidiformes mites (use *Demodex* as an example of Trombidiformes).
8) Describe and contrast the biology of each of these three groups
9) Describe and contrast the pathology caused by each of these groups
10) Describe the pathophysiology of the sarcoptic or psoroptic mange

**C. Example of a test question applicable to this lecture**:

*Boophilus* ticks can acquire the protozoan *Babesia* or the rickettsia *Anaplasma* from a bovine and transmit them to another animal although the tick only leaves its original host to oviposit and die. This is made possible because:

a) These pathogens are transmitted in the eggs between tick generations
b) Susceptible cattle get infected by eating ticks when they lick other bovine
b) Susceptible cattle get infected by eating fallen, infected ticks with the grass
c) Ticks crushed by casual contact release infective blood that infects new animals
d) Infections are transmitted by ticks carried accidentally to other animals

**LECTURE 6**. General concepts regarding nematodes (pages 110 to 125)

**A. Contents**:

1) Morphology and classification of the nematodes
2) Reproduction and development
3) Infection, medical importance, and survival in the external environment

**B. At the end of this lecture you should be able to**:

1) Identify a nematode and assign it to one of the seven orders
2) List the external structures of a nematode that are useful for classification
3) Describe three environments where an infective larva can develop
4) Describe five ways that a nematode can infect a definitive host
5) Define exsheathment, molting, and arrest, and explain their importance for the host or the parasite.
6) List the advantages and disadvantages that a parasite has living in a host
7) Describe the effect of temperature and humidity on the preparasitic stages of nematodes.

**C. Example of a test question applicable to this lecture**:

Which of the following conditions is the least suitable for the survival of a free-living, infective larvae in the external environment?

a) 25C and 95% humidity
b) 12C and 90% humidity
c) 32C and 90% humidity
d) 12C and 60% humidity
e) 32C and 60% humidity

**LECTURE 7.** The Nematodes: The *Trichuris*, Rhabditida and Horse Strongyles (pages 203 to 207 and 126 to 142)

**A. Contents**:

1) Morphology, life cycle, and medical importance of *Trichuris* spp.
2) Morphology, life cycle, and medical importance of *Strongyloides* spp.
3) Morphology and classification of the Strongylida
4) Morphology, life cycle, and medical importance of the large strongyles of horses
5) Morphology, life cycle, and medical importance of the small strongyles of horses

**B. At the end of this lecture you should be able to**:

1) Identify *Trichuris* spp. in the gut or feces of a host.
2) Describe their life cycle inside and outside the host
3) Describe their pathogenesis
4) Identify *Strongyloides* spp. in the gut or feces of a host.
5) Describe their life cycle inside and outside the host
6) List the ways that a host can be infected with *Strongyloides*
7) Describe their pathogenesis
8) Identify and differentiate between large and small strongyles of horses
9) Describe the preparasitic development of the strongyles of horses
10) Describe the development of each species of large strongyles from host invasion to oviposition.
11) Describe the development of the small strongyles from host invasion to oviposition.
12) Describe and contrast the damage caused by large or small strongyles to the host.

**C. Example of a test question applicable to this lecture**:

Which of the following lesions is uncommon in strongylosis *vulgaris* of horses?

a) Thrombo-endarteritis of the small intestinal arteries
b) Arteritis and fibrosis of the cranial mesenteric artery
c) Verminous aneurysm of the cranial mesenteric artery
d) Nodules containing juveniles in the intestinal wall
e) Small ulcers in the intestinal mucosa due to the bites of the adults

**LECTURE 8.** The Nematodes: The Nodular worms, Bowel worm, and Hookworms (pages 143 to 153)

**A. Contents:**

1) Morphology, life cycle, and medical importance of *Oesophagostomum* spp.
2) Morphology, life cycle, and medical importance of *Chabertia* sp.
3) Morphology, life cycle, and medical importance of the hookworms

**B. At the end of this lecture you should be able to:**

1) Identify and differentiate between *Oesophagostomum, Chabertia,* and hookworms.
2) List the structures that allow one to classify hookworms into genera or species
3) Describe the life cycle of *Oesophagostomum, Chabertia,* and hookworms outside the host
4) List the ways how *Oesophagostomum, Chabertia,* and hookworms infect their hosts
5) Describe the life cycles of *Oesophagostomum, Chabertia,* and hookworms inside the host
6) Describe the pathogenic mechanisms of *Oesophagostomum, Chabertia,* and hookworms
7) Explain what cutaneous larva migrans is and how the host gets infected.

**C. Example of a test question applicable to this lecture:**

Which of the following mechanisms of infection does NOT occur in the dog hookworms?

a) Ingestion of an infective larva in an egg-shell
b) Ingestion of an infective free living larva
c) Penetration of an infective larva through the skin
d) Ingestion of larvae with the mother's milk
e) Passage of larvae through the uterus

**LECTURE 9.** The Nematodes: The Trichostrongyloidea (pages 154 to 164)

**A. Contents:**

Morphology, classification, life cycle, and medical importance of the Trichostrongyloidea

**B. At the end of this lecture you should be able to:**

1) Identify the Trichostrongyloidea and differentiate them from other nematodes.
2) Differentiate between *Haemonchus, Ostertagia, Trichostrongylus, Cooperia,* and *Nematodirus*.
3) Describe their life cycles outside the host
4) Describe how they infects their hosts
5) Describe their life cycles inside the host
6) Describe the pathogenic mechanisms of each
7) Describe the influence of the climate on their transmission
8) Describe the influence of hypobiosis on their transmission

**C. Example of a test question applicable to this lecture:**

Which of the following signs is UNCHARACTERISTIC of ostertagiasis?

a) diarrhea
b) anorexia
c) anemia
d) poor growth
e) edemas

**LECTURE 10**. The Nematodes: The Metastrongyloidea and Filaroidea (pages 165 to 171 and 187 to 196)

**A. Contents**:

1) Morphology, classification, life cycle, and medical importance of the Metastrongyloidea
2) Morphology, classification, life cycle, and medical importance of the Filaroidea

**B. At the end of this lecture you should be able to**:

1) Identify a Metastrongyloidea and differentiate it from other nematodes
2) Differentiate between the larvae of sheep Metastrongyloidea
3) Describe and contrast the three types of life cycles that exist among the Metastrongyloidea
4) Describe the advantages and disadvantages of each type for the host or the parasite
5) Describe how the Metastrongyloidea infect their hosts
6) Describe how the Metastrongyloidea may cause pathology
7) Describe the influence of the climate on their transmission
8) Identify a Filaroidea and differentiate it from other nematodes
9) Describe how the Filaroidea infect their host
10) Describe how climate affects the transmission of the Filaroidea
11) Describe the pathophysiology of *Dirofilaria immitis*

**C. Example of a test question applicable to this lecture**:

Which of the following changes is the PRIMARY cause of pathogenesis in canine heartworm disease?

a) Impairment of the pulmonary arterial circulation
b) Obstruction of the venae cavae by the parasites
c) Obstacle to heart contraction by the parasites
d) Impediment of ventricular valves function by the parasites
e) Anemia due to blood whirlpools around the parasites

**LECTURE 11**. The Nematodes: The Ascaridida and Oxyurida (pages 172 to 186)

**A. Contents:**

1) Morphology, classification, life cycle, and medical importance of the Ascaridida
2) Morphology, classification, life cycle, and medical importance of the Oxyurida

**B. At the end of this lecture you should be able to:**

1) Identify an Ascaridida or an Oxyurida
2) Differentiate between an Ascaridida and nematodes of other orders
3) Differentiate between *Toxocara* and *Toxascaris* of dogs
3) Describe and contrast the three types of life cycles that exist among the Ascaridida
4) Describe the advantages and disadvantages of each type for the host or the parasite
5) Describe how the Ascaridida infect their hosts
6) Describe how the Ascaridida may cause pathology
7) Describe the influence of the climate on their transmission
8). Identify and differentiate Oxyurida from other intestinal nematodes
9). Describe their generalized life cycle
10). Define the pathology that they may cause

**C. Example of a test question applicable to this lecture**:

A woman brings her 3-month-old dog to your clinic with the story that he had vomited a "worm" the day before. She has the worm in a flask with water. You pour the content of the flask in a Petri dish and observe a white-yellowish thing that looks like a 3-inch-long spaghetti twisted in a C-shape. Your first decision is that the "worm" is effectively a nematode. Since you vaguely remember something about buccal capsules and copulatory bursas, you examine both ends with a 8X magnifying glass. One end looks pointed and the other somewhat blunt. Making a supreme effort you are able to come up with five nematodes of the dog gut that can be found in Ohio. They are listed below. Which of them you are more likely dealing with?

a) *Strongyloides stercoralis*
b) *Ancylostoma caninum*
c) *Toxocara canis*
d) *Toxascaris leonina*
e) *Trichuris vulpis*

**LECTURE 12**. The Platyhelminths: Cestoda (pages 226 to 243)

**A. Contents**:

Morphology, classification, life cycle, and medical importance of representative Cestoda that affect domestic animals and humans

**B. At the end of this lecture you should be able to:**

1) Identify a Cestoda and distinguish it from a Nematoda or Trematoda
2) Label the structures of a Cestoda that are important to their classification.
3) Name examples of adult Cestoda that infect dogs, cats, ruminants, horses, or humans
4) Name examples of larval Cestoda that infect ruminants, or humans
5) Describe the generalized life cycle of a Cestoda
6) Describe the pathology caused by an adult Cestoda and give examples
7) Describe the pathology caused by a larval Cestoda and give examples
8) Name five cestoda of public health importance

C. Example of a test question applicable to this lecture:

Which of the following tapeworms is NOT a zoonoses?

a) *Taenia saginata*
b) *Dipylidium caninum*
c) *Taenia pisiformis*
d) *Echinococcus granulosus*
e) *Hymenolepis nana*

**LECTURE 13**. The Platyhelminths: The Trematoda (pages 209 to 225). The Protozoa: generalities, the ciliates, the amoebae, and the flagellates (pages 244 to 256).

**A. Contents**:

1) Morphology, classification, life cycle, and medical importance of representative Trematoda affecting the liver, intestine, lungs, and blood vessels
2) Morphology, classification, and medical importance of the ciliates, the amoebae, and the flagellates

**B. At the end of this lecture you should be able to**:

1) Identify a Trematoda and distinguish it from a Nematoda or Cestoda
2) Label the structures of a Trematoda that are important to their classification.
3) Name examples of Trematoda that infect the liver, intestine, lungs, or blood vessels
4) Describe the life cycle of a Trematoda that infect the liver
5) Describe the life cycle of a Trematoda that infect the lungs
6) Describe the pathology caused by a liver Trematoda
7) Describe the pathology caused by a lung Trematoda
7) Describe the influence of the climate on the transmission of Trematoda
8) Name the most common Trematode of veterinary importance in Ohio and its hosts.
9) Identify and distinguish between ciliates, amoebae, and flagellates
10) Name examples of each group
11) Explain the pathogenicity of members of each group for domestic animals

**C. Example of a test question applicable to this lecture**:

Which of the following pathology is UNCOMMON in liver fascioliasis?

a) Traumatic hepatitis
b) Anemia
c) Liver fibrosis
d) Peritonitis
e) Fibrosis of the bile ducts

**LECTURE 14.** The Protozoa: Apicomplexa, Eucoccidiida (pages 257 to and 272)

**A. Contents:**

Morphology, classification, life cycle, and medical importance of representatives of the Eucoccidiida.

**B. At the end of this lecture you should be able to:**

1) Identify specimens of Apicomplexa based on their morphology
2) Distinguish between *Eimeria, Isospora, Criptosporidium, Toxoplasma, Neospora*, and *Sarcocystis* based on their morphology and/or biology.
2) Name one parasite representative of each genera and its host
3) Describe the importance of each genus for veterinary medicine
5) Describe the generalized life cycle of a coccidia
6) Describe the pathology caused by *Eimeria* or *Isospora*
7) Describe the pathology caused by *Cryptosporidium*
8) Describe the pathology caused by *Toxoplasma*
9) Describe the pathology caused by *Neospora*
10) Describe the pathology caused by *Sarcocystis*
11) Name the Eucoccidiida of public health importance

**C. Example of a test question applicable to this lecture:**

Which of the following mechanisms of infection is the LEAST probable in human toxoplasmosis?

a) Ingestion of dirt contaminated with cat's feces.
b) Congenitally from a mother with the acute infection
c) Congenitally from a mother with the chronic infection
d) By ingesting poorly cooked infected pork
e) By ingesting poorly cooked infected lamb

**LECTURE 15.** Immunity to parasitic infections and Parasite resistance to anti-parasitic drugs (pages 280 to 293)

**A. Contents:**

1) Differences between anti-prokaryote and anti-parasite immunology
2) Relevance of immunology to veterinary parasitology
3) Uses of immune diagnosis in parasitology
4) Immune-mediated pathology in parasitology
5) Mechanisms of immune protection against parasites
6) Evasion of host's immune responses by parasites
7) Epidemiological consequences of anti-parasite immunology
8) Generation of resistance to anti-parasitic drugs
9) Current status of the problem
10) Mechanisms of resistance to anti-parasitic drugs
11) Recommendations to delay the appearance of drug resistance

**B. At the end of this lecture you should be able to:**

1) List seven reasons that account for the differences between anti-prokaryote and anti-parasite immunology.
2) List five areas in which immunology is relevant to parasitology
3) List seven circumstances in which immune diagnosis is indicated in parasitology
4) List and give examples of four immune mechanisms of pathogenesis in parasitology
5) List two mechanisms of natural resistance characteristic of parasites
6) List three major mechanisms of immune protection against parasitic infections
7) List eight manners how parasites evade the host's immune responses
8) Describe how host's immunity affects the epidemiology of gastrointestinal nematodes of ruminants
9) Describe how antiparasitic treatment generates resistance against the drugs used
10) List 3 protozoa, 3 nematodes, and 3 arthropods that have developed resistance to anti-parasitic drugs.
11) Describe three mechanisms how parasites evade the effect of anti-parasitic drugs
12) List six actions that the a veterinarian can perform to delay the development of drug resistance

**C. Example of a test question applicable to this lecture:**

In a region of temperate climate (like Ohio), which of the followings is the best strategy to treat sheep against gastrointestinal parasites with the purposes of diminishing pasture contamination AND delaying development of anti-drug resistance?

a) To treat immediately before lactational rise and rest the pasture during winter
b) To treat immediately after lactation rise and leave the animals in the same pasture
c) To treat immediately after lactation rise and take the animals to a clean pasture
d) To treat at the end of the summer to dilute the resistant eggs in the pasture
e) To treat the animals as soon at symptoms of parasitism appear (start of fall)

## TABLE OF CONTENTS

# CHAPTER 1

# INTRODUCTION TO VETERINARY PARASITOLOGY

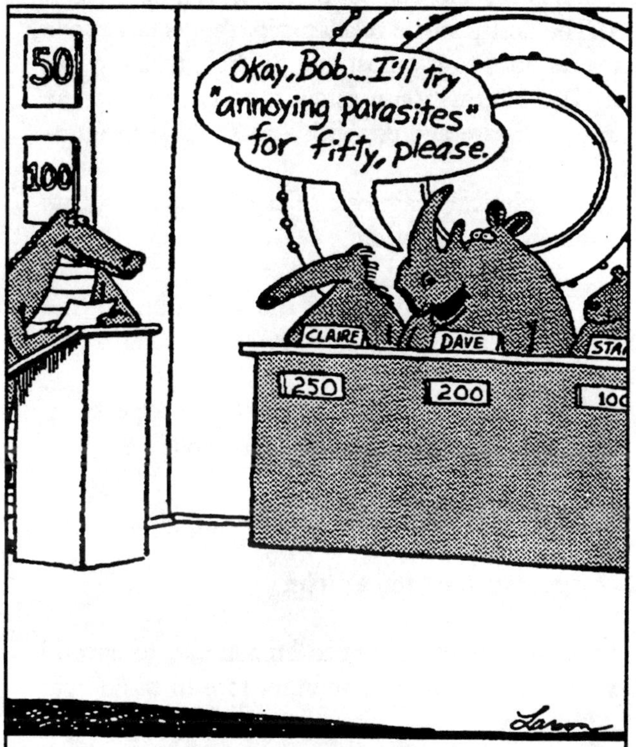
Okay, Bob... I'll try "annoying parasites" for fifty, please.
50
100
CLAIRE
DAVE
250
200

Animal game shows

**Preview.** In this chapter we will identify the aspects of parasitology that are of interest to a practicing veterinarian. We will also illustrate the importance of parasites as agents of human disease, deterrents to animal production, and tools in biologic investigation.

We will review and characterize the major types of associations between different biological species, types of parasites, types of hosts, and nomenclature of some common host-parasite associations. Finally, we will discuss the fundamentals of zoological systematics and its importance for a veterinarian practicing parasitology.

**Objectives**

Veterinary Parasitology is the study of the animal parasites of importance to veterinarians. It does not only include parasites pathogenic to domestic animals but also parasites that are of little danger for animals but may be transmitted to humans in which they cause disease (e.g., *Trichinella spiralis*).

A veterinarian is commonly interested in six aspects of parasitic infections:

1) The identification of the parasite and its place among other parasites. This information is often essential for treatment and control of parasitism.

2) The biology of the parasite to the extent that it helps explain the pathogenicity, diagnosis, transmission, and control of the infection,

3) The host-parasite relationship, this is, what the parasite does to the host and the host to the parasite. This information is essential to understand the parasitic disease and establish a reasonable prognosis.

4) The clinical diagnosis of the infection and its laboratory confirmation,

5) The treatment of the infection, and

6) The epidemiology of the infection to the extent that it explains how to prevent its transmission.

In this text we will discuss these aspects in regard to the principal parasites of veterinary importance.

## 2. Importance of parasitism

Parasites are important to human and to animal health and may be an important tool in biological studies.

In regard to human health, in 1947 Stoll[1] calculated the number of people probably affected with parasitic infections in the world. The improvements achieved in the developed countries in the following decades have been more than compensated by the worsening situation in the Third World. His estimates, then, are probably as valid today as they were originally. Table 1-I shows some interesting figures.

With the exception of pets, animal health is often regarded as an economic concept. Its deterioration is measured, therefore, as losses of money. Few world estimates have been made, and these only for a few parasites. The US Department of Agriculture calculated in 1965[2] the probable losses due to parasites of livestock in the United States. Since the situation has not changed drastically since then, these estimates are still considered to be valid. Table 1-II shows an update of the figures of the US Department of Agriculture based on the Producer Price Indexes for Meats and Dairy Products for 1988.

Biology often uses parasites as convenient tools for particular studies. For example, because nematodes do not replicate most of their somatic cells once they have reached the adult stage, they have been considered as an advantageous model to study aging at the cell level. Also, because parasites are subjected to a more constant environment than their hosts, they suffer less evolutionary pressures and are believed to change more slowly than their hosts. The presence of a same parasite in different hosts, therefore, constitutes one criterium to estimate the degree of relationship between the hosts. The phylogenetic relationship between the North African dromedary and the South American llama, for instance, is substantiated by the presence of the Anoplura louse, *Microthoracius*, on both ruminants. Finally, because parasites were present at the inception of immunity, they had a chance to detect flaws in the evolving immune function and take advantage of them to survive in immune competent hosts. Study of parasite-mediated immunomodulation, then, may reveal unsuspected weaknesses of the immune system.

## 3. Association between species

Biological individuals often have a better chance at survival as a species in nature when they live in association. These associations may be of individuals of a same species (e. g., pine forests, wolf packs) or of different species. The association in which two species live in close physical contact is called a **symbiosis** (from Gr *sum* = together, and *bios* = life).

Depending on the degree of metabolic dependency that develops between the associates, four major types of symbioses are recognized.

1) **Phoresis** (from Gr *phorein* = to carry): in this case one of the associates (phoron) is simply carried by the other (carrier) without establishing any metabolic relationship. An interesting example is the relationship of the parasitic fly, *Dermatobia*, with blood-sucking arthropods. The female *Dermatobia* glues her eggs on the ventral aspect of the

abdomen of mosquitoes or other hematophagous flies. The larvae develop in 4 or 5 days but they wait inside the eggshells until the carrier starts feeding on a mammal. At that time, they leave the eggshells and penetrate the skin of the host. Another example of interest to parasitologists is the relationship between mechanical vectors and the transmitted pathogen, to be discussed later.

2) **Commensalism**: in this association the larger species (host) provides some benefit (often food and/or shelter) to the smaller species (commensal). The metabolic dependance of the commensal on the host is minimal, however, and the commensal is perfectly capable of surviving as a species in the absence of the host. There are numerous examples of commensalism but the most interesting to the parasitologist may be the amebas, *Naegleria* and *Acanthamoeba*, and the nematode, *Pelodera*. These three organisms are free-living but occasionally they invade and establish themselves in mammalian tissues.

3) **Parasitism**: parasitism can be defined as that association in which one species (the host) is the ecosystem of another species (the parasite). This definition has several advantages. For example, it clearly separates parasitism, in which the parasite eats its host little by little without harming it, and predation, in which the predator kills the prey and often eats it all at once. The most important trait, however, is that it emphasizes that the parasite is affected by changes in the host but, in turn, it can use functions of its host (its environment) for its own benefit. For example, parasites can use the host's immune system to regulate the size of their own population[3] or fight other organisms that compete for the same niche.[4]

The identifying characteristic of parasites is that they depend metabolically on their hosts and cannot survive as a species without the host. This dependency is not restricted to nutrients but also includes biochemical signals that drive the development of the parasite while in the host. Actually, parasites can also be defined as organisms with biochemical deficiencies that must be supplied by the host. We will see examples in later chapters.

It is important to emphasize that the capacity to produce damage to the host is a medical and not a biological concept. As such, it is not an exclusive characteristic of any symbiosis in particular, and certainly not of parasitism. Actually, it is to the advantage of the parasite that the host flourish, since this will secure its home and food. Most of the modern parasites are comparatively little pathogenic which is probably the result of millennia of evolution that eliminated those that caused serious disease. Severe parasitism today is almost always attributable to man altering the balance of nature (by crowding the host and facilitating parasite transmission, for example). The evidence rather suggests that disease production is a feature of imperfect host-parasite adaptations.

4) **Mutualism**: in this case both partners have developed such a mutual metabolic dependence that neither can survive as a species without the other. The classic example of mutualism is the lichens, association of fungi and algae that lives in environments that would be insufficient to either of them alone. Another frequently mentioned example is the relationship between ruminants and the cellulose-degrading protozoa of the rumen. This may be mutualism in the making, however, because cattle can live rather well without these protozoa.

It is often speculated that symbioses begin as phoresis, then progress to commensalism, later evolve to parasitism, and finally become mutualism. This concept is based on the assumption that the parasite invades the host first (phoresis), starts eating from it later (commensalism), becomes more and more dependant on the food and shelter provided by the host (parasitism), until both associates adapt so much to each other that intermingle their metabolisms and forget how to live separately (mutualism). This may be true for free-living organisms that gradually became parasitic (although I cannot see the need for becoming mutualistic) but it does not apply to organisms that never developed, or suddenly lost (by mutation, for example), their capacity to manufacture their own food. Only three alternatives were open to these organisms: heterotrophy (from Gr *heteros* =

other, *trophe* = food), in which they adsorb organic molecules made by photosynthesizing organisms (e.g., the fungi); holotrophy (from Gr *holos* = entire), in which they ingest and digest whole organisms (e.g., the free-living animals); or parasitism.

## 4. **Types of parasites**

To facilitate the rapid transmission of accurate information, parasites are often identified with adjectives that inform about some of their characteristics. The followings are widely used:

1) **Endoparasites** (from Gr *endon* = inside) are parasites that live inside their host, like the gastrointestinal nematodes. **Ectoparasites** (from Gr *ektos* = outside) are parasites that live on the surface of their host, like the lice.

2) **Permanent** parasites are those that live all or a considerable part of their lives in or on the host, like the gastrointestinal nematodes and the lice. **Temporary** or **periodic** parasites are those that visit the host only occasionally, like the mosquitoes and fleas.

3) **Obligatory** parasites are those that require the presence of the host to survive as a specie. Those than can live as free-living organisms if necessary are often called **facultative** parasites. Actually, by definition, all parasites need the host to survive as a species. Those that do not, are commensals. This peculiar classification tries to accommodate organisms (like *Naegleria*, *Acanthoameba*, and *Pelodera*) that appear to be in transition between the commensal and the parasitic modes of life.

4) **Erratic** or **aberrant** parasites are those found in an unusual location in their normal host (e.g., an ascarid in the peritoneal cavity). **Incidental** parasites are those found in an unusual host (e.g., *Haemonchus* of ruminants in humans).

5) **Hyperparasites** (from Gr *huper* = above, beyond) are parasites of a parasite. For example, the microsporidian, *Nosema helminthorum*, that parasitizes the tapeworm, *Moniezia*. Attempts at using hyperparasites for the control of parasites of medical or veterinary importance have not succeded so far.

6) **Pseudoparasites** (from Gr *pseudos* = false) are structures that are confused with parasites. Beginners often confuse hairs with larvae and grains of pollen with nematode eggs in fecal exams.

## 5. **Types of hosts**

As with the parasites, the hosts are often given adjectives that inform about some of their characteristics. The most common ones are:

1) **Definitive** or **final** host is the host that supports the life of the adult, reproductive parasite (e.g., sheep for *Fasciola hepatica*, dogs for *Dirofilaria immitis*). **Intermediate** host is that one that supports the development of the preadult (larval) stages of the parasite (e.g., snails for *F. hepatica*, mosquitoes for *D. immitis*).

2) **Paratenic** (Gr *para* = beside, Lat *tenere* = to maintain) or **transport** host is that one that supports the life but not the further development of a larval parasite. For example, the larvae of the dog ascarid, Toxocara *canis*, can infect and survive in mice for months but do not develop in them. Differently from the intermediate host, the paratenic host is an option and not a requirement in the life of the parasite. This host often acts as a "waiting" reservoir in nature until the parasite is able to reach the definitive host and begins reproduction again.

3) **Vectors** are arthropods that actively transport a pathogen from an infected individual to a susceptible one. There are two major types of vectors: **Biological vectors** that are required for the development of the parasite (e.g., *Anopheles* mosquitoes for malaria, *Boophilus* ticks for babesiosis), and **Mechanical vectors** that only act as carriers of the parasite (e.g., housefly for cysts of protozoa, horsefly for trypanosomas).

In the first case the vector is really an intermediate (and sometimes a definitive) host for the parasite so the elimination of the vector would also eliminate the parasite from nature. In the second, the vector acts only as a convenience for the parasite to reach a new host so the elimination of the vector rarely has drastic consequences for the life of the parasitic species.

6. **Types of host-parasite associations**

Here we will mention only some common expressions that are necessary to the understanding of the relationship among host and parasite.

1) **Infection** is the presence of a parasite *in* a host, **infestation** is the presence of a parasite *on* a host. Infestation also includes the presence of arthropods or rodents in a dwelling. A dog, for example, may be infected with intestinal worms and infested with lice. Its house may be infested with fleas.

Several decades ago the term infection was reserved for vegetable parasites (fungi, bacteria) and viruses and the term infestation for animal parasites. That was a misleading separation because it implied that the infections by animal parasites were inherently different from those by the other organisms, which is not true.

2) **Disease** is a manifestation of physiological disfunction. It reveals a failure of the host's homeostatic mechanisms to compensate for the damage caused by the agent of disease. In the case of parasitism, disease is an infection or infestation in which the damage caused by the parasite is severe enough to result in symptoms and/or signs.

It is important to keep in mind that parasites often cause moderate damage that is not enough to produce overt symptoms and signs but is sufficient to diminish production. It is also interesting to notice that, from the epidemiological point of view, a diseased host is less important than a solely infected host. In the first case, it is evident that the host is infesting the environment. In the second case, a long time may pass before the owner or the veterinarian realize that the asymptomatic animal is infecting the rest of the herd.

3) **Contamination** is the presence of a pathogen on a surface, including the skin. In the case of the skin, however, the parasite does not establish any metabolic relationship with the individual and, for all practical purposes, it regards the individual as inert matter. A pasture seeded with eggs of a parasite is said to be contaminated.

7. **Principles of systematics**

Systematics is the arrangement of the living organisms according to their evolutionary relationships. Since the paleontologic register of parasites is virtually nonexistent, these relationships are mostly assumed from morphological, ecological, and, recently, biochemical and genetic similarities.

The basis for the organization is the **species**, which is defined as a group of similar individuals that can interbreed and produce fertile descendence. This is a mostly genetic criterium that is difficult to apply to protozoa and hermaphroditic metazoa. In these cases, it is often replaced by morphological and biochemical observations. Groups smaller than species are often referred to as **strains** or **demes** (Gr *demos* = common people). Samples of *Toxoplasma gondii* with different pathogenicity for their host, for example, are called *nosodemes* (Gr *nosos* = disease).

Depending on selected similarities, the **species** are grouped in **genera**, the genera in **families**, the families in **orders**, the orders in **classes**, and the classes in **phyla**. When necessary, groups of intermediate hierarchy are created (e.g., superfamilies, suborders, etc.). Since Linnaeus (1758), each species is identified by two latin words, in italics or underlined, and with the initial of the first word capitalized. The first word indicates the genus and the second, the species.

In the original language, Latin, each systematic category has a typical ending but many of these names have been translated into English. Table 1-III gives an example of the classification of a common nematode of ruminants.

Because this hierarchic organization of parasites is based on morphologic and biologic similarities, it stands to reason that all parasites in a same group must share certain characteristics. This may help the study of parasites a great deal because the simple identification of a parasite as belonging to a given group often provides abundant information about its biology. For example, the presence of a copulatory bursa and a large mouth with teeth or cutting plates on a nematode recovered from the small intestine identifies it as a hookworm (Family Ancylostomatidae). By extension of what we know of the hookworms, we may assume that this parasite is hematophagous, that the females lay oval eggs with a thin shell and a few blastomeres when passed in the feces, that the eggs develop outside the host under appropriate conditions (conditions that we can also guess), that the infective element for the host is a free-living third stage larvae, that young hosts are more susceptible than older animals, that the larvae may penetrate the host by mouth or through the skin, that in the later case they will migrate through the lungs, that under repeated infections they may cause dermatitis and/or pneumonia, etc., etc.

## 8. Classification of animal parasites

Parasites are found in every phylum of the animal kingdom. Those of medical or veterinary importance, however, belong to the groups Arthropoda, Nematoda, Acanthocephala, Trematoda, Cestoda, and Protozoa. The nematodes, acanthocephalans, trematodes, and cestodes are commonly referred to as **helminths** or **worms**. We will mention the identifying characteristics and the classification of each group in the discussion of the respective group.

## 9. Additional readings

Further information about the subjects discussed in this text can be found in the followings books:

1) Barriga OO. 1981. *The immunology of parasitic infections*, University Park Press, Baltimore, 354 pp. An introductory textbook on the immunological aspects of parasitic infections of humans and domestic animals.

2) Sloss MW, Kemp RL and Zajac, AM. 1994. *Veterinary Clinical Parasitology*. 6th ed. Iowa State Press, Ames, Iowa, 198 pp. An excellent collection of photographs of diagnostic elements in veterinary parasitology. Essential to the clinician.

3) Georgi JR and Georgi ME. 1990. *Parasitology for veterinarians*, 5th ed., Saunders, Philadelphia, 412 pp. Excellent illustrations, weak in ecology.

4) Kreier JP and Baker JR (eds). 1991-1994. *Parasitic Protozoa*. 2nd ed. 8+ vol. Academic Press, New York. A comprehensive, multi-authored review of the protozoa parasitic of humans and domestic animals.

5) Lancaster JL and Meisch MV, 1986. *Arthropods in livestock and poultry production*, Horwood, Chichester, 402 pp.

6) Levine ND, 1980. *Nematode parasites of domestic animals and man*, 2nd ed., Burger, Minneapolis, 477 pp. Possibly the most comprehensive textbook on parasitic nematodes.

7) Soulsby EJL, 1982. *Helminths, arthropods and protozoa of domesticated animals*. 7th edition. Lea and Febiger, Philadelphia, 809 pp. The most comprehensive text of veterinary parasitology that still remains within the area of interest of practicing veterinarians.

8) Urquhart GM et al., 1987. *Veterinary Parasitology*. Longman, Essex, 286 pp. Brief discussions of the parasites of veterinary importance in the United Kingdom.

9) Williams RE (ed), 1985. *Livestock entomology*, Wiley and Sons, New York, 335 pp. With interesting discussions of epizootiological and clinical aspects.

**Table 1-I. People infected with parasites in the world**

| Infection | % of people, 1947 | # of people, 1987 |
|---|---|---|
| Ascariasis | 30% | 1,500 millions |
| Hookworm | 21% | 1,050 millions |
| Trichuriasis | 16% | 800 millions |
| Filariasis | 12% | 600 millions |
| Schistosomiasis | 5% | 200 millions |
| Amebiasis | - | 300 millions |
| Malaria | - | 500 million |
| Chagas' disease | - | 18 millions |

**Table 1-II. Annual losses due to parasitism in US livestock**
(USDA, adjusted to millions of 1988 dollars)

| Livestock | Mortality | Morbidity | Total |
|---|---|---|---|
| Cattle | | | |
| Internal parasites | 109.0 | 340.5 | 449.5 |
| External parasites | | 2097.8 | 2097.8 |
| Total | 109.0 | 2538.3 | 2547.3 |
| Sheep and goats | | | |
| Internal parasites | 21.1 | 47.7 | 68.8 |
| External parasites | | 82.1 | 82.1 |
| Total | 21.1 | 129.8 | 150.9 |
| Swine | | | |
| Internal parasites | 9.4 | 172.9 | 182.3 |
| External parasites | | 8.3 | 8.3 |
| Total | 9.4 | 181.2 | 190.6 |
| Horses | | | |
| Internal parasites | 0.4 | 2.6 | 3.0 |
| Poultry | | | |
| Internal parasites | 84.4 | 130.4 | 214.8 |
| External parasites | | 247.5 | 247.5 |
| Total | 84.4 | 377.9 | 462.3 |
| Total | | | |
| Internal parasites | 224.3 | 693.6 | 917.9 |
| External parasites | | 2435.7 | 2435.7 |
| GRAND TOTAL | 224.3 | 3129.3 | 3354.1 |

**Table 1-III. Systematics of *Haemonchus contortus***

| Category | Latin name | English name |
|---|---|---|
| Phylum: | Nemathelmint*a* | Nemathelminthes |
| Class: | Nematod*a* | Nematodes |
| Order: | Strongyl*ida* | Strongylid |
| Superfamily: | Trichostrongyl*oidea* | Trichostrongyloid |
| Family: | Trichostrongyl*idae* | Trichostrongylid |
| Genus: | *Haemonchus* | None |
| Species: | *contortus* | None |
| Name: | *Haemonchus contortus* | Barber's pole worm |

**Summary:**

1. The purpose of this book is to discuss the identification, biology, host-parasite relationship, diagnosis, treatment, and control of parasites of significant veterinary importance.

2. Parasites cause harm to human health and animal production but are useful as tools in some biological studies.

3. The physical association of individuals of different species is called **symbiosis**. Depending on the metabolic dependence between the associates, symbioses can be described as **phoresis,commensalism**, **parasitism**, or **mutualism**.

4. Parasites can be described as ecto- or endo-parasites, permanent or temporary, obligatory or facultative, erratic or incidental.

5. Hosts can be described as definitive or intermediate, paratenic, or vectors. In this last case, they can be biological or mechanical vectors.

6. **Infection**, **infestation**, and **contamination** describe different host-parasite associations.

7. Parasites are classified into systematic catregories (phylum, class, order, family, genus, and species). The characteristics of the category to which a parasite belongs often provide valuable information about the parasite.

## REFERENCES

1. Stoll NR, 1947. This wormy world. J. Parasit. 33:1-18.

2. US Department of Agriculture, 1965. *Losses in Agriculture*, USDA ARS Agr. Handbook # 291, 120 pp.

3. Dineen JK, 1963. Immunological aspects of parasitism. Nature 197:268-269.

4. Schad GA, 1966. Immunity, competition, and natural regulation of helminth populations. Amer. Naturalist 100:359-364.

# CHAPTER 2

# THE ARTHROPODS

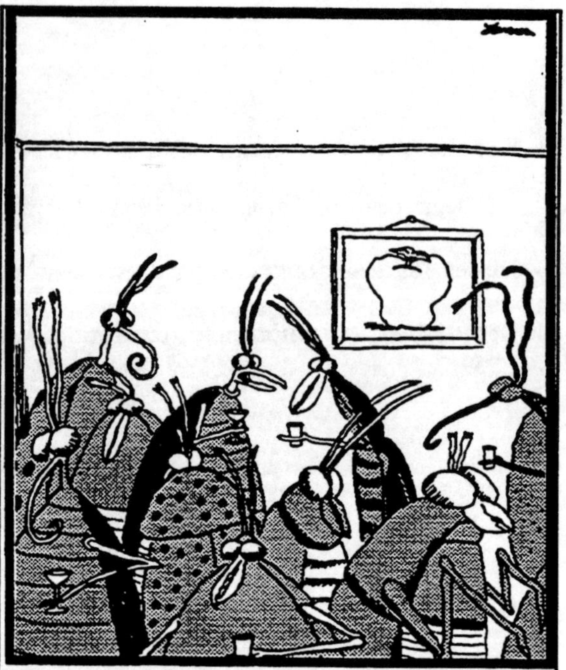

"Think about it, Ed.... The class Insecta contains 26 orders, almost 1,000 families, and over 750,000 described species—but I can't shake the feeling we're all just a bunch of bugs."

**Preview**. In this chapter we will discuss the external and internal morphology of arthropods with emphasis on those structures useful for classification or that help explain peculiarities of the biology of these organisms. We will mention the way to recognize an arthropod and the subdivisions of veterinary importance within the phylum.

We will examine in some detail the development of the arthropods and will allude to some of its control mechanisms. We will also mention the means by which parasitic arthropods locate their host and the response of the host to arthropod bites. Finally, we will discuss the general mechanisms by which arthropods harm their host and the general procedures of arthropod control.

## 1. Morphology

### 1.1. External morphology

**A. Exoskeleton**. In the arthropods, the body rigidity necessary for movement is given by a hard covering called **exoskeleton** (from Gr *exo* = outside). It is made of a monolayer of epidermal cells that secrete a cuticle of a nitrogenous polysaccharide **(chitin)** combined with tanned proteins that encloses the arthropod like a suit of armor. In some arthropods, the exoskeleton has thickened areas called **plates** that are useful in their classification. This rigid structure is replaced by flexible membranes in the parts that must bend, such as the joints. The exoskeleton supplies the arthropod with the same functions that the skeleton and skin afford in the vertebrates: support, avoidance of mechanical injury, protection against invasion by pathogens and chemicals, and retention of body water.

**B. Segmentation**. The embryo of the arthropods is made of a number of traversal segments that can be still seen in some larvae like the caterpillars. Originally, all the segments are identical but, as the arthropod develops, some segments fuse together and lose their original structure. In the Insects, a group of anterior segments forms a fairly spherical capsule that becomes the head. The three following segments form the thorax, and the remaining segments constitute the abdomen (Figure 2.1). The final division is somewhat different in the Arachnids (see the respective chapter).

**a. The head**. The head of an insect bears the mouthparts, the eyes, and the antennae.

The **mouthparts**, from the front to the back, are formed by a movable upper lip (**labrum**), two lateral **mandibles** that move horizontally, two lateral **maxillae** which are similar to the mandibles but that bear some joined appendices called **palpi**, and a lower lip (**labium**) that also bears palpi (Figure 2.1). A tongue-like structure (**hypopharynx**) arises from the oral aspect of the labium, The original mouthparts were adapted to chewing but they have been strongly affected by evolution and have become adapted to absorbing fluids, piercing or cutting skin, etc. in different species. These adaptations will be described with the corresponding arthropod groups.

The **eyes** of the arthropods are simple structures sensitive to light (**ocelli**). Most insects have three single eyes and two compound eyes made out of many ocelli.

The **antennae** exist only in the Insects and Crustacea. They are formed by a variable number of segments the number and shape of which are often used for identification purposes. The antennae are involved with the senses of tact and smell, and partially with those of hearing, and tasting.

**b. The thorax**

The thorax is formed by three rings that originate from three primitive segments of the embryo. From the front to the back, they are called **prothorax** (Gr *pro* = in front of), **mesothorax** (Gr *meso* = middle), and **metathorax** (Lat *meta* = end). The lateral walls of each ring are the **pleura** (sing. **pleurum**), the roof is the **tergum** or **notum**, and the floor is the **sternum**.The complete structure of the insect thorax is rather complex (with a number of grooves, sutures, and hairs) and its knowledge is of little use to the practicing veterinarian. We will give some further details when discussing the flies. The thorax is specialized for locomotion. In the Insects, each segment bears a pair of legs, and the meso- and metathorax often bear a pair of wings each. For the characteristics of the thorax of the Arachnids, see the respective chapter.

Each **leg** is composed of 5 segments. From the body to the distal end, they are: coxa, trochanter, femur, tibia, and tarsus (Figure 2.1). At its end the tarsus has a sculptured and often sticky surface that allows the arthropod to walk on vertical walls or on the ceilings.

The **wings** are thin expansions of the external cuticle of the body supported by sclerotized braces that enclose smaller portions of the cuticle. The braces are called **veins** (although they are really tracheae) and the spaces between them are called **cells**. The veins and cells have standard names that are useful in the identification of certain groups. We will give further details in the chapter about flies.

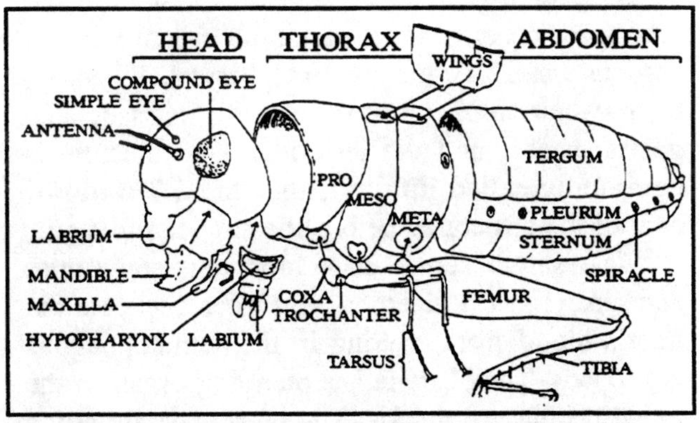


**Figure 2.1**. External morphology of a typical insect (modified from Hardwood and James, 1979)

**c. The abdomen**. Except in the Crustaceans, the abdomen is almost devoid of appendages. The last segments are modified into a copulatory organ in the male, and into an organ to lay eggs and place them in the appropriate microhabitat (ovipositor) in the female. In a few insects (bees and wasps, for example) the ovipositor has been further modified into a sting.

1.2. **Internal morphology** (Figure 2.2)

A. **Respiratory system**. The air penetrates the body of the arthropods through openings at the body surface **(spiracles)** that lead to a system of tubes (tracheae) that are reinforced with a spiral of chitin. These tubes ramify into the tissues reaching to the vicinity of the mitochondria where they constitute an air-tissue fluid interface for the interchange of gases. The spiracles have valves that keep the opening closed unless muscle activity forces air in or out.

B. **Circulatory system**. The circulatory system is constituted by a dorsal vessel that sucks the fluid (hemolymph) from the general body cavity (hemocele) and impels it forward towards the body cavity again.It is in charge of the circulation of nutrients, hormones, cells, and heat (produced mainly by the flying muscles) but is not related to respiration. The hemolymph has cells that are involved in clotting, phagocytosis, and encapsulation of parasites.

C. **Digestive system**. The digestive system of the arthropods consists of six parts: the mouth with its associate salivary glands, the pharynx, the crop, the proventriculus, the stomach with its associated gastric caeca, and the intestine. The intestine is commonly called **hindgut**, the stomach **midgut**, and all the structures before the stomach **foregut**.

The saliva serves as a lubricant, sometimes participates in the digestion, and often prevents the host's blood from clotting in the hematophagous arthropods. The pharynx is a pumping organ in the bloodsucking arthropods. The crop is essentially a storage organ. The proventriculus is a valve that

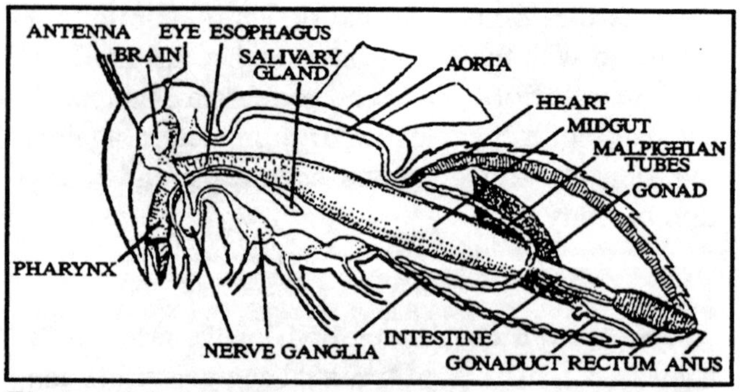


**Figure 2.2**. Internal morphology of a typical insect (modified from Belding, 1965)

avoids reflux and is often provided with teeth for trituration of the food. The stomach digests the food with the enzymes provided by the gastric caeca, and participates in the absorption. The intestine is mainly an organ of absorption.

The stomach of many arthropods contains bacteria and protozoa that provide the vitamins absent in the diet and (in the case of termites and roaches, for example) enzymes to digest some foodstuffs.

D. **Excretory system**. The excretory function is produced in the arthropods by the **Malpighian tubes**, blind tubules that arise from the anterior part of the intestine, and by the final portion of the intestine, the rectum. They take the excretions from the body fluid by an active mechanism (since there is not blood pressure to push them through) and secrete them into the digestive tract. They not only excrete catabolites but also regulate the osmotic pressure of the arthropod.

E. **Nervous system**. The nervous system is constituted by three pairs of supraesophageal ganglia fused into a brain, three more fused into a subesophageal ganglion, and a pair of single ganglia per each thoracic and abdominal segment. They have nerves connecting all the ganglia, and other nerves going into the organs. The arthropods have a variety of **neurotransmitters**. Some of them are identical to the neurotransmitters in the vertebrates but other are exclusive to the arthropods. These latter should allow to devise insecticides that would be atoxic for vertebrates.

F. **Reproductive system**. In the males, there are two testes, two sperm ducts, and two seminal vesicles where the sperm is stored. During copulation, the sperm passes through a common ejaculatory duct where it receives some fluid from a pair of accessory glands, and through the copulatory organ into the female body. In the female, there are two ovaries, two oviducts (that often store the eggs in the species that lay a large number of eggs at a time), and a vagina. Two other organs open in the vagina: a **spermatheca** (Lat *sperm*, and *theca* = case, sheath) that may store viable sperm for long periods, and two accessory glands that may cover the eggs with a sticky fluid during oviposition.

## 2. Identification and classification

The arthropods are easily identified by the presence of an exoskeleton and of jointed appendices. They are the only invertebrates with striated muscles which is of diagnostic value when one tries to identify a parasite in a section of host's tissue. The arthropods are divided into several sub-phyla and classes but the only ones of interest to us here are the classes Insects, Arachnids, Pentastomids, and Crustaceans. Key 2.1 will help identify the arthropods of veterinary importance.

The **Insects** are arthropods with three pairs of legs and a pair of antennae at the adult stage. Their body is generally divided into three distinct parts. The orders important to medicine are the Hemiptera or True Bugs, the Mallophaga or Chewing Lice, the Anoplura or Sucking Lice, the Siphonaptera or Fleas, and the Diptera or Flies. We will discuss their identification and classification in the respective chapters.

The **Arachnids** are arthropods with four pairs of legs and devoid of antennae at the adult stage. Their body is generally formed by a single sack in the species of veterinary importance. The orders important to medicine are the Acarina that contains the ticks and mites, and to a much lesser extent the Araneida or Spiders, and the Scorpionida or Scorpions. The larvae of many arachnids have only three pairs of legs and the morphology of this class differs substantially from that of the insects. We will discuss this and their identification and classification in the chapter on Acarina.

The **Pentastomids** are arthropods highly modified by parasitism. They have a worm-like body and are believed to be distantly related to the Acarina and Crustacea. Only a few species are important to veterinary medicine.

The **Crustaceans** are arthropods with five or more pairs of legs and two pairs of antennae at the adult stage. Their importance to medicine is only as intermediate host of parasites.

## 3. Biology

### 3.1. Reproduction

All arthropods are **dioecious** (Gr *di* = two, *oikos* = house), this is, there are male and female individuals (as opposed to **monoecious** [G *monos* = single] or hermaphrodites). The females receive the sperm and save it in the spermatheca for weeks (bed bugs) or for years (queen ants). Fertilization of the ova occurs only shortly before oviposition. In some species, particularly in the absence of males, the eggs can develop without fertilization (**parthenogenesis**, Gr *parthenos* = virgin). This may be an emergency solution of nature, however, because the parthenogenetic offspring lacks the genetic variety that facilitates adaptation.

Most arthropods are **oviparous** (Lat *ovum* = egg, *parere* = give birth to), this is, they lay eggs that develop outside the body of the female. A few species are **ovoviviparous**, this is, the female retains the eggs inside her body until they hatch (e.g., the sarcophagids or flesh flies). The embryo still feeds on the egg yolk, however. Although ovoviviparity usually means that fewer eggs are produced, the protection afforded to the eggs and the laying of active stages may be advantageous for the survival of the species. Stil other species are **viviparous** (Lat *vivus* = alive), this is, the female not only retains the eggs in her body but also contributes to the feeding of the larvae (e.g. the African flies, tsetses).

### 3.2. Development

The eggs are usually deposited by the female in microenvironments that assure their further development. Under these conditions, embryonic development proceeds until an immature stage of the arthropod hatches from the egg. The changes that this juvenile arthropod must undergo to become a fully functional adult or **imago** (Lat *imago* = image) are called **metamorphosis** (Gr *meta* = change, *morphe* = form).

In some species, the newly hatched arthropods are small, wingless, sexually immature, and have body proportions different from those in the adult. Still, their general morphology, behavior, and habitat are very similar to those of the adult. These stages are called **nymphs**. The moderate transformations that the nymphs require to become adults are referred to as **incomplete metamorphosis** (Figure 2.3).

In other species, the hatched arthropod looks like a little worm (the maggots, for example). This stage is called a **larva** and must go through an intermediate stage of **pupa** before becoming an imago or adult arthropod. Whereas larvae are normally quite active and voracious eaters, many pupae are quiet transformation stages. The imago, in turn, is specialized in reproduction and dispersal. This development, that comprises drastic changes involving extensive histolysis and histogenesis, is referred to as **complete metamorphosis** (Figure 2.4).

As opposed to the nymphs of the incomplete metamorphosis, the morphology, behavior, and habitat of the larval and pupal stages are vastly different from those of the corresponding adult. Because of these differences, and contrarily to what happens with the incomplete metamorphosis, the control measures applied against adult arthropods with complete metamorphosis rarely are effective against its larval and pupal stages.

### 3.3. Growth

One of the most serious problems faced by developing arthropods is growth. Because their hard exoskeleton does not stretch, they must cast

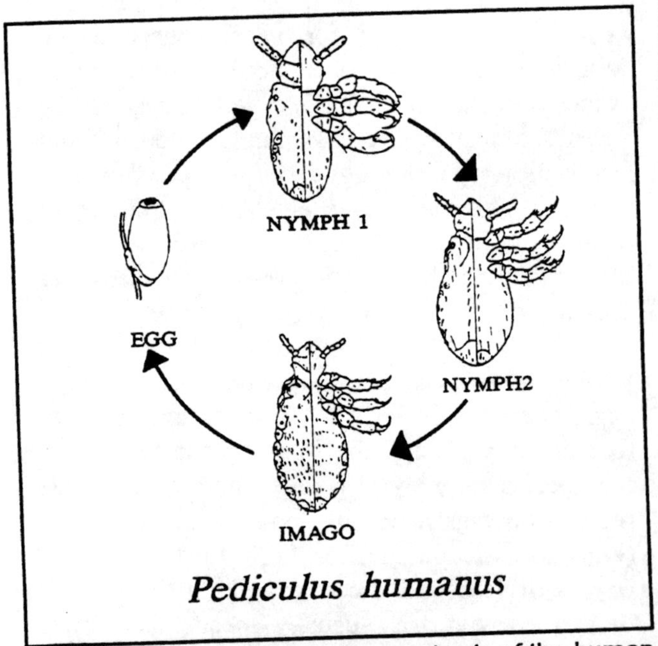


**Figure 2.3.** Incomplete metamorphosis of the human louse, *Pediculus humanus* (modified from Kim et al., 1986).

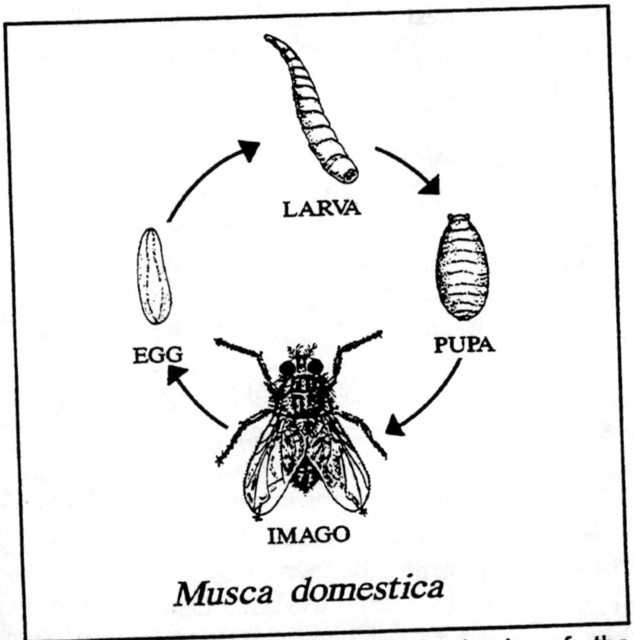


**Figure 2.4.** Complete metamorphosis of the common house fly, *Musca domestica* (Modified from Belding, 1961).

it off to increase in size. These changes of exoskeleton (molts or **ecdyses**) take place several times during metamorphosis. Each stage between molts is called an **instar**. Usually, there are 5 nymphal, 4 larval, and 1 pupal instars, but their number may vary with the species. To molt, the arthropod loosens the old covering, produces a soft one underneath, and then it draws in air and contracts its muscles to increase the volume of its body. This ruptures the old exoskeleton which is cast off and distends the new one. When tanning hardens the new covering, the arthropod relaxes and a space for growth is created under the new exoskeleton.

### 3.4. Diapause

Most arthropods have the ability to go through periods of arrested development with a severe metabolic reduction (**diapause**, **dormancy**, or **hypobiosis**). This phenomenon can affect any stage in the life cycle of the arthropod and is usually triggered by stimuli that anticipate unfavorable ecologic conditions (e.g., decreasing hours of light, falling temperature, desiccation, scarcity of food, crowding). The stimuli that terminate diapause are less well known but the reverse of the initiating stimulus works with some species.[1] In *Aedes* mosquitoes, for example, egg development enters in diapause when the hours of daylight shorten in the Fall, and comes out of it when they lengthen again in the Spring. The larva inside the egg also enters in dormancy automatically upon formation, and only hatches when it is immersed in water and the oxygen pressure is lowered.

Diapause is a valuable mechanism to avoid potentially dangerous situations that may affect seriously the survival of the arthropod species. Because of the reduced metabolism, dormant arthropods are also quite resistant to the action of pesticides.

### 3.5 Arthropod hormones

Many physiological functions of the arthropods are directed by a number of hormones. The best known of these hormones are the **prothoracicotropic hormone** that is produced by the brain and regulates the secretion of ecdysones; the **ecdysones** that control molting and induce differentiation to the adult stage; and the **juvenile hormones** that inhibit differentiation to adult and force the arthropod to remain a larva despite molts and growth. These and other hormones have also a critical influence on the phenomena of diapause and reproduction.

Although arthropod endocrinology is a highly specialized area of study, its fundamentals are of interest to the veterinarian because synthetic arthropod hormones may replace the conventional insecticides in the near future.

Close relatives to the hormones are some substances secreted externally that influence the behavior of other members of the same species (**pheromones**). The pheromones are highly diffusible substances that operate in extremely small quantities. Some of the best known are the **sex pheromones** that are produced by females and attract males; the **alarm pheromones** that induce enhanced activity of the arthropods; and the **social pheromones** that keep the colonies together. The imaginative use of these substances may help control the parasitic arthropods some day.

### 3.6. Locating the host

Differently from the helminths and protozoa, the arthropods have the possibility to move freely in search of their hosts. For the flying insects, visual stimuli, particularly movement and color of the host, are the principal attractants. Once the arthropods are close to the host, its odor and the increasing temperature and $CO_2$ gradient near the host drive them to enter in actual contact with it.

Most biting arthropods explore the host's skin before the bite. They are guided in this activity by the temperature of, and the contact with, the skin. The location and subsequent suction of blood depends on the osmotic and chemical composition of the host's fluids, especially on the presence of nucleotides which are abundant in erythrocytes and platelets. A host who does not provide the right stimuli will not be attacked.[2] Actually, feeding on an inappropriate host may be lethal to an arthropod; if the hemoglobin crystals are too large, they may destroy the arthropod's gut.

### 3.7. **Host immunity**

The host generally responds to the inoculation of arthropod's saliva or body components with production of allergic reactions. Protective immunity has been found in virtually all the few cases in which it has been studied seriously.[3] In nature, however, immune resistance is believed to play only a minor role to prevent further attacks but there is evidence that artificial immunization with selected antigens may induce significant protection.[4]

## 4. Medical importance

Not all arthropods are harmful. Honey bees and silkworms have been highly regarded by man since ancient times. Many arthropods are essential for polinization, others are food for birds and animals, still others (like spiders) help in the control of pests, and *Drosophila* flies have done much for our knowledge of genetics. Still, 14% of all known insects are parasitic at some time of their lives, and about 6,000 species are ectoparasites of homothermous. Of these, 60% affect mammals and 40% birds; 51% are lice, 34% fleas, 11% flies, and 2% true bugs.[5]

Arthropods can affect directly the well being of their host in several ways. The simplest is the **annoyance** of an insect flying constantly around its host (e.g., the face fly, *Musca autumnalis*). This activity often interferes with grazing and with the desirable rest of the animals.

Other arthropods can also inject **allergens** (e.g., fleas, mosquitoes, bees, wasps) or **venoms** (e.g., spiders, scorpions) with their **bites** or **stings**.

The hematophagous arthropods cause annoyance, **remove blood,** and even **damage the hides** (e.g., tabanid flies, ticks).

Finally, others actually **invade the body of the host**, either with its larval stages (e.g., the myiasis-producing flies) or by themselves (e.g., the *Sarcoptes* and *Demodex* mites).

In addition to the direct damage, arthropods can act as **biological or mechanical vectors** for other organisms. For example, *Anopheles* mosquitoes are the biological vectors of human malaria and many species of mosquitoes are biological vectors of equine encephalitides. *Boophilus* ticks are the biological vectors of babesiosis of bovines and *Dermacentor* ticks the biological vectors of the Rocky Mountain spotted fever of humans. The tabanid flies are biological or mechanical vectors of trypanosomiases and the common house fly can carry over 100 different pathogens on its body or in its digestive tract.[6]

An estimation in 1976, put the annual losses due to arthropods in the United States at 2,495 million dollars for the cattle industry (8.1% of the total annual production), 43 million (8.5% of the production) for the sheep industry, 100 million (1.3% of the production) for the swine industry, and 100 million (1.4% of the production) for the poultry industry.[7] Steelman[8] made detailed estimations of losses due to parasitism in domestic animals. We will quote updated figures in the proper places.

It is important to keep in mind that regardless how staggering these figures are, the U.S. livestock is little affected by parasitism in comparison to less developed countries. The losses per head of livestock must be considerably higher in those nations then.

## 5. Control

Because of the important losses that they may cause, control of arthropods is an important concern of veterinarians. There are five major approaches to the control of arthropods: **physical means**, that pretend to establish an actual physical barrier between the pests and the host; **chemical means**, particularly repellents and insecticides (acaricides in the case of the acarina); **environmental manipulation**, that pretends to make the environment inappropriate for the proliferation of the arthropod; **biological means**, that try to interfere with the biology of the pests; and **immunological means**, that try to increase the resistance of the host to the arthropod attack. Currently, chemical control is by far the most developed and popular method of control. However, arthropods are developing resistance to the action of insecticides very rapidly. It is widely predicted that chemical control will have to be complemented or replaced by other methods in the near future if efficient control of arthropods is to continue

**Summary:**

1. The arthropods are invertebrates characterized by having an exoskeleton and joined appendages.

2. The major groups of veterinary importance are the **Insects** (with three pairs of legs, one pair of antennae, and their body divided into three parts), and the **Arachnids** (with four pairs of legs, no antennae, and their body generally forming a single sac-like portion).

3. The main parts of the insect body are: the **head** that bears the mouth parts, eyes, and antennae; the **thorax** that bears the legs and wings; and the **abdomen**. The morphology of all these parts is useful for the identification of diverse groups.

4. Most arthropods are oviparous, a few are ovoviviparous, and even fewer are viviparous. Development to adult involves a number of changes called **metamorphosis**.

5. The developing stages of the arthropods may have morphology, habitat, and behavior very similar to, or very different from, those of their parents. These two modalities are called **incomplete** and **complete metamorphosis**, respectively.

6. The type of metamorphosis that an arthropod possesses is important to understand its pathogenesis and its control.

7. Development and behavior of arthropods are largely dependant on specific hormones and neurotransmitters. Interference with these substances may produce effective insecticides.

8. Many arthropods are able to go through periods of metabolic reduction (diapause) to avoid external factors that may endanger their existence.

9. Arthropods produce losses of animal production by interfering with the feeding and rest of livestock, injecting allergens or venoms, biting, sucking blood, invading their tissues, and transmitting pathogens.

10. The losses caused by arthropods in the United States have been estimated in 8% of the cattle or sheep industries, and 1.3% of the swine or poultry industries.

**KEY 2.1. Key for the identification of the major groups of ectoparasites of domestic animals**

| | | |
|---|---|---|
| 1. | Elongated body without legs | go to 10 |
| | Body with legs, sometimes with antennae | go to 2 |
| 2. (1) | With three pairs of leg | go to 3 |
| | With four pairs of legs | go to 9 |
| 3. (2) | Body dorso-ventrally compressed (nearly ovoid when fed), 2nd and 3rd pair of legs comparable in size | go to 4 |
| | Body laterally compressed, 3rd pair of legs much larger than 1st or 2nd pair | **SIPHONAPTERA** |
| 4. (3) | Thorax fused to the abdomen forming a single sac | go to 9 |
| | Thorax distinct from the abdomen | go to 5 |
| 5. (4) | Non retractable beak running backward under head and thorax | go to 6 |
| | Other kind of buccal parts | go to 7 |
| 6. (5) | Winged, head much longer than broader, transverse groove between the eyes | **HEMIPTERA, Reduviidae** |
| | Wingless, head broader than longer, prothorax with lateral expansions | **HEMIPTERA, Cimidae** |
| 7. (5) | Piercing buccal parts retracted when not in use | go to 8 |
| | Chewing buccal parts on a head broader than the thorax | **MALLOPHAGA** |
| 8. (7) | Wingless, head narrower than, and separated from the thorax, massive grasping claws | **ANOPLURA** |
| | Winged or wingless, head in a depression of prothorax, small paired claws | **DIPTERA, Hippoboscidae** |
| 9. (2, 4) | Buccal parts with a toothed hypostoma, usually longer than 1 mm | **ACARINA, ticks** |
| | Buccal parts without a toothed hypostoma, usually shorter than 1 mm | **ACARINA, mites** |
| 10. (1) | Body with transverse divisions, longer than 1.5 mm and stout, clearly visible | **DIPTERA, Cyclorrhapha (larva)** |
| | Body without transverse divisions, smaller than 1.5 mm and very thin, microscopic | **NEMATODA, Rhabditida** |

## REFERENCES

1. Tauber MJ and Tauber CA, 1976. Insect seasonality: diapause maintenance, termination, and postdiapause development. Ann. Rev. Entomol. 21:81-107.

2. Friend WG and Smith JJ. 1977. Factors affecting feeding by blood sucking arthropods. Ann. Rev. Entomol. 22:309-331.

3. Wikel SK. 1982. Immune responses to arthropods and their products. Ann. Rev. Entomol. 27:21-48.

4. Barriga OO. 1994. A review on vaccination against protozoa or arthropods of veterinary importance. Vet. Parasit. (in press).

5. Marshall AG, 1981. *The ecology of ectoparasitic insects*, Academic Press, New York, 459 pp.

6. Greenberg B, 1971-73. *Flies and disease.* 2 vols. Princeton Univ. Press, Princeton, 856 and 447 pp.

7. Burridge MJ. 1982. Effects of disease on animal productivity. In Rechcigl M Jr (ed.), *CRC handbook of agricultural productivity*, vol. II. CRC Press, Boca Raton, Florida, 319-343.

8. Steelman CD, 1976. Effects of external and internal arthropod parasites on domestic livestock production. Ann. Rev. Entomol. 21:155-178.

# CHAPTER 3

# THE ORDER HEMIPTERA OR TRUE BUGS

**Preview.** The Hemiptera or True bugs are hematophagous insects that hide in cracks near the host dwelling during the day and go out to feed at night. The bed bugs and assassin bugs belong to this group. The former infest especially humans, laboratory rodents, and chickens. They can cause cutaneous allergies and draw significant amounts of blood. The latter affect humans and animals in the peridomestic environment. They can produce cutaneous allergies, draw large amounts of blood, and transmit the trypanosome of Chagas' disease.

The Hemiptera constitute only an occasional problem in veterinary medicine but the assassin bugs are a major concern of human public health in many rural areas of Latin America.

## 1. Morphology

The medically important **Hemiptera** (Lat *hemi*= half, Gr *pteron* = wing) or **True Bugs** are insects 4 to 30 mm long. Their first pair of wings are leathery at the base and membranous at the tip. The second pair is entirely membranous and covered by the first pair. In some species, both pairs are absent. The mouth parts are modified to form a jointed tube, the **beak** or **proboscis**, with four stylets inside (Figure 3.1). Characteristically, this beak arises from the front of the ventral aspect of the head and runs backward underneath the head and part of the thorax when at rest. Since the Hemiptera have an incomplete metamorphosis, the nymphs look like the adults but are smaller, and have much reduced or no wings.

## 2. Identification and Classification

The typical structure of the wings and mouthparts is enough to identify an insect as an Hemiptera. Only the order Homoptera (Gr *homo* = equal) may lead to some confusion but the Homoptera feed only on plants, their first pair of wings is uniformly leathery or membranous, and their beak

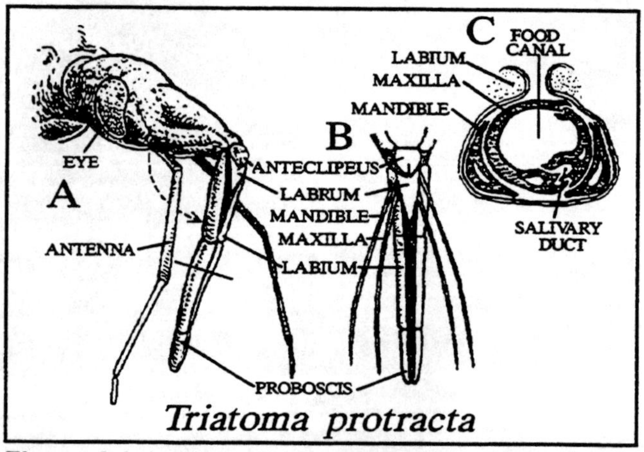


**Figure 3.1**. Lateral (A), frontal (B) and cross section (C) view of the mouth parts of a assassin bug (modified from Furman, 1961)

runs forward rather than backward. Among more than 60,000 species of Hemiptera known, only two families and a few species are important to medicine.

The family **Cimidae**[1] contains the **bed bugs** and related insects. These are wingless, reddish-brown arthropods, with a oval and flat body about 4-7 mm long (Figure 3.2). They are always found in the proximity of their hosts.

The Cimidae are parasites of bats and secondarily of birds (for example, *Haematosiphon* and *Ornithocoris* on chickens). The best known species, however, *Cimex lectularius* and *C. hemipterus*, are parasites of man. These species are of cosmopolitan distribution but while *C. lectularius* prefers temperate climates, *C. hemipterus* is particularly prevalent in tropical ones.

The family **Reduviidae** contains the **assassin bugs**, also known as **conenoses** or **kissing bugs**. The species important to medicine are about 20 to 30 mm long. The Reduviidae are distinguished from other Hemiptera because they have elongated heads with a transverse groove between the eyes, their curved beaks have their tip resting in a depression on the thorax, and their flat abdomen (when unfed) is broad with the lateral borders extending beyond the wings (Figure 3.3).

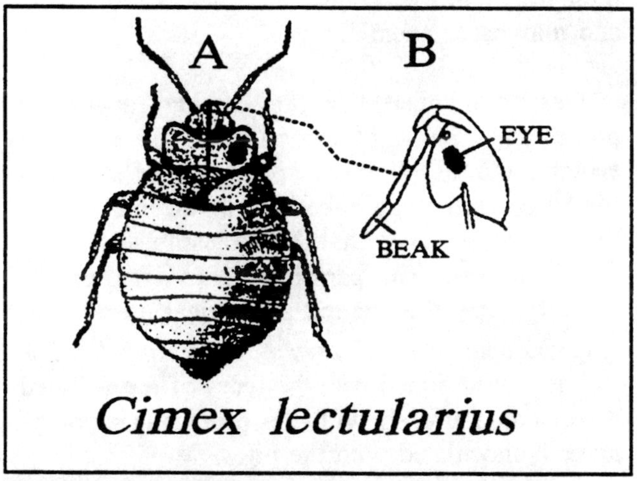


**Figure 3.2**. Specimen of *Cimex* (A) with a lateral view (B) of its buccal parts (modified from CDC, 1969).

The Reduviidae are distributed almost exclusively in the Americas, from central Chile to southern and western United States. Because of their importance as vectors of *Trypanosoma cruzi*, the best known genera are: *Triatoma*, mainly in North and Central America and the southern half of South America; *Panstrongylus* in Brazil and northern South America, and *Rhodnius* in Central America and the northern portion of South America. Plate I will help in the identification of some common Hemiptera of medical importance.

### 3. Biology

All the Cimidae and about 110 species of Reduviidae that belong to the subfamily Triatominae are temporary ectoparasites of vertebrates. The remaining Reduviidae are predators on other insects or feed on plant juices. The males and females of the parasitic species require a blood meal before each moult and before attaining fertility. Although they have clear preferences in regard to hosts, the parasitic Hemiptera are only moderately host specific and will feed, at least

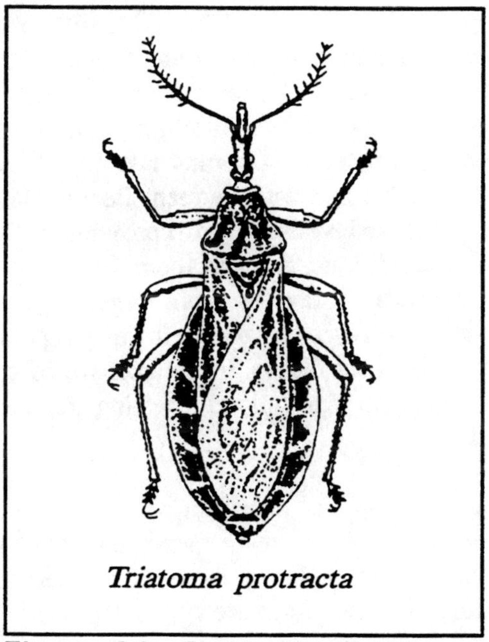


**Figure 3.3.** Specimen of *Triatoma protracta* (CDC, 1969)

temporarily, on a variety of host species if necessary.

During their meal, the Hemiptera introduce only the stylets in the skin of the host and tap a blood vessel to suck 2 to 10 times their own weight in host's blood. Commonly, they take one or two meals per week that last 3 to 10 minutes for the bed bugs, and 10 to 20 minutes for the kissing bugs. Some species defecate during or immediately after a meal and soil the host's skin with their feces. In the vectors infected with *Trypanosoma cruzi*, these feces are loaded with protozoa.

The females lay 10 to 15 eggs after each meal. The eggs are operculated (= capped), whitish, 1 to 2 mm long, and are often glued to materials in the hiding places of the female. The total number of eggs laid by a female in her lifetime varies with the species and alimentation but often reaches a few hundreds. The eggs hatch in 4 to 20 days depending on the prevalent temperature, and five nymphal stages ensue before the appearance of the adults. The Hemiptera usually produce only 1 or 2 generations per year.

The Cimidae are rather tolerant to variations of relative humidity but become inactive below 14C and begin to die over 37C. The life cycle of *Cimex lectularius* from egg to adult takes 120 days at 18C, 30 days at 28C, and 34 days at 33C. The adults live about 2 months under conditions that keep them well active but may last for 18 months in cold weather and with frequent fasting. The life cycle of the Reduviidae is more prolonged.[2] Under optimal conditions, it takes them from 3 to 5 or more months to develop from egg to egg but it may take well over a year at lower temperatures and with frequent fasting. In the absence of a host, the Hemiptera can tolerate fasting for several months.

The Hemiptera parasitic on vertebrates are nocturnal creatures that spend the day hours hidden in cracks and crevices near their host's dwelling. The bed bugs are typically found in the unions of wooden bedsteads, seams of mattresses and box springs, under loose wall paper, and behind pictures close to the wall. The domestic kissing bugs are found in the cracks of adobe or mud walls and in the breaks of thatched roofs. At night they crawl out of their hiding places in search of an appropriate source of blood.

**4. Medical importance**

The parasitic Hemiptera are important on account of their bites, their blood letting activities, and their role as vectors.

With most domestic species, the bite is painless and usually goes unnoticed by the host. The saliva injected during the suction of blood, however, often induces a delayed type, and less often an immediate type, hypersensitivity in the host that may result in more severe reactions to subsequent bites.[3,4] A skin swelling of the eyelids with enlargement of the satellite lymph node that is often found in patients of acute Chagas' disease may be a manifestation of this allergy.[5] It is called "Romañas's sign" and is regarded as a clinical manifestation of the infection.

The importance of the blood letting activity becomes evident when one learns that 100 *Cimex* can remove 1 ml of blood, and that close to 2000 specimens have been recovered from a single owl. A single kissing bug may take up to 1 ml of blood during a meal. Intense attacks by hemipterans, then, can remove a significant amount of blood and may cause anemia.

Despite the fact that the Cimidae appear to possess all the right attributes to be effective vectors, and that they have proven to be susceptible to a number of infections in the laboratory, there is no evidence that they transmit any infection in nature.[6] The parasitic Reduviidae, on the contrary, are the natural biological vectors of *Trypanosoma cruzi* and *Trypanosoma rangeli*.[7] The former is transmitted with the feces of the infected insect contaminated with the protozoan, and the latter is inoculated with the bites.

Every Reduviidae that has been tried has demonstrated to be able to support the infection with *T.*

*cruzi*. Only a score of species, however, feed regularly on man or his animals in the peridomestic environment and defecate before leaving the host. These are the species that have a practical importance as vectors for humans. The species that are not found in the vicinity of humans, or do not bite man, or defecate after leaving the host have little opportunity to transmit the infections to other than wild life (which may eat the infected bugs). For example, more than a third of 2000 specimens of *Triatoma protracta* (mostly a wild species) examined in California has been found infected with *Triatoma cruzi* but the human infection is exceptional in that locality.

The parasitic Hemiptera are commonly regarded as a concern of human rather than of veterinary medicine.[8] The Cimidae, however, may become an important problem in chicken houses and in laboratory animal quarters, particularly with rats and rabbits. Studies with domestic Reduviidae, on the other hand, showed that almost all the species studied fed on humans, dogs, cats, and chickens.

Cases of severe or lethal Chagas' disease in dogs and cats are reported occasionally in the literature.

## 5. Diagnosis and control

Other than the Romaña's sign, the bites by Hemiptera appear as a nonspecific arthropod bite with or without an allergic component. There is no reliable clinical ground to distinguish them from other arthropod bites. The diagnosis of the infestation of the premises is done by observation of the insects crawling about, or of eggs and/or molts in their places of hiding.

Control of hemiptera is established by proper construction and upkeeping of living quarters that avoid the cracks and crevices where they proliferate. This is often impossible to achieve in poor rural communities, or in the surrounding animal quarters that are often the reservoir of human infestations. Spraying the habitat of the insects and, the inner walls of the infested buildings with residual insecticides has produce satisfactory results to eliminate the infestation. However, resistance of bedbugs to DDT, malathion, dieldrin, and BHC, and of assassin bugs to dieldrin and BHC has already been reported. Toxicity for humans or domestic animals and regulations on pesticides residues in animal products must be regarded.

**Summary:**

1. The Hemiptera or True bugs include the bedbugs (Cimidae) and the kissing or assassin bugs (Reduviidae).

2. They reproduce by incomplete metamorphosis in cracks and crevices in the host dwellings where they hide during the day.

3. They go out by night to look for an appropriate source of blood.

4. In veterinary medicine, they are found most often as parasites of laboratory rodents or chickens.

5. They are important because they may extract large amounts of blood and cause cutaneous allergies. The Reduviidae are also the biological vectors of Chagas' disease in the Americas.

6. Control is achieved by elimination of the habitats that favor their proliferation and/or spaying of residual insecticides.

## REFERENCES

1. Usinger RL, 1966. *Monograph of Cimidae (Hemiptera-Heteroptera)*, Entomol. Soc. Amer., vol. 7, 585 pp.

2. Zeledon R and Rabinovich JE, 1981. Chagas' disease: an ecological approach with special emphasis on its insect vector. Ann. Rev. Entomol. 26:101-133.

3. Ryckman RE, 1979. Host reactions to bug bites (Hemiptera, Homoptera): a literature review and annotated bibliography. Part I. Cal. Vector Views 26:1-24.

4. Ryckman RE and Bentley DG, 1979. Host reactions to bug bites (Hemiptera, Homoptera): a literature review and annotated bibliography. Part II. Calif. Vector Views 26:25-50.

5. Lumbreras H, Flores W and Escallon A, 1959. Allergishe Reactionen auf Stiche von Reduviiden und ihre Bedeutung ber der Chagas Krankheit. Z. Tropenmed. Parasitol. 10:6-9

6. Burton GJ, 1963. Bedbugs in relation to transmission of human disease. Publ. Health Rep. 78:513-524.

7. Zeledon R, 1974. Epidemiology, modes of transmission and reservoir hosts of Chagas' disease. In Ciba Foundation Symposium 20 (new series), Elsevier, Amsterdam, 51-71.

8. Brenner RR and Stoka AM (eds), 1987. *Chagas' Disease Vectors*. 3 vols. CRC Press, Boca Raton, Florida, 155 + 136 + 156 pp.

## PLATE I. PICTORIAL KEY TO SOME SPECIES OF HEMIPTERA

(Harry D. Pratt and Chester J. Stojanovich)

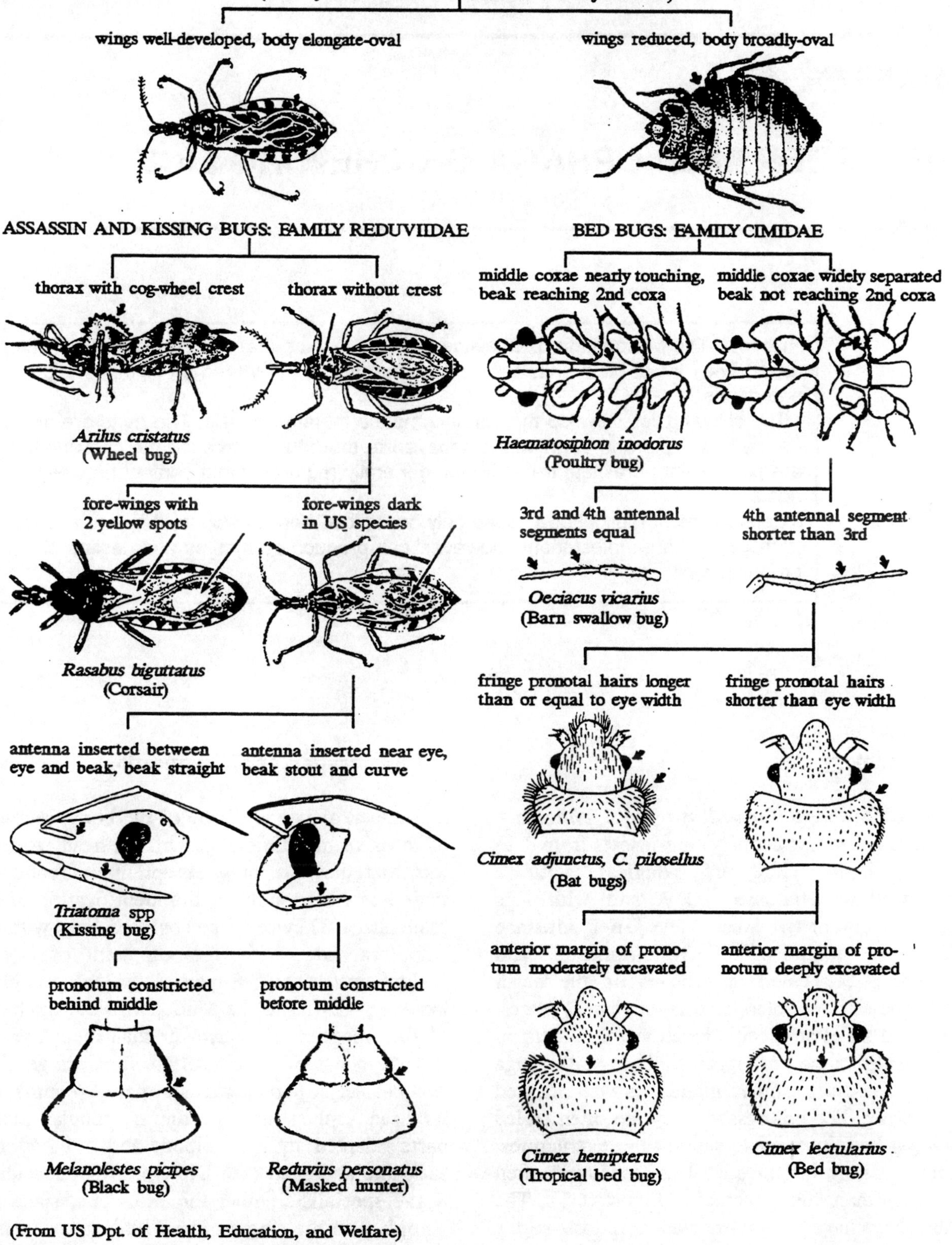


(From US Dpt. of Health, Education, and Welfare)

# CHAPTER 4

# THE ORDER MALLOPHAGA OR CHEWING LICE

**Preview**. The Mallophaga or Chewing Lice are insects that live permanently on their hosts. They infest birds and, secondarily, mammals. They feed on skin secretions and debris.

The chewing lice develop through incomplete metamorphosis. The eggs are glued on the host hairs and the nymphs behave like the adults. Because the chewing lice are permanent parasites, transmission generally requires direct contact between hosts.

Because most Mallophaga cause only superficial skin abrasions, they are not very pathogenic. Large infestations, however, can produce dermatites and decline of production.

## 1. Morphology

The **Mallophaga** (Gr *mallos* = wool, *phagein* = to eat. A misnomer actually) are insects from 1 to 5 mm long. They are wingless, with a dorso-ventrally flattened body, and with legs ending in one or two weak claws. Their antennae are short, composed of 3-5 segments, and sometimes concealed in grooves on the head. Their bodies have sclerotized (= hardened) plates, hairs, and scales at specific locations, that assist in the identification of species. The Mallophaga possess massive, toothed mandibles well adapted to chewing. For this reason, they are often called **chewing lice**. In order to support these structures, their heads are large, as least as broad, and often broader, than their thoraces (Figure 4.1). The Mallophaga have incomplete metamorphosis so the nymphs look like a reduced version of the adults.

## 2. Identification and classification

The lack of wings, shape of the body, presence of massive mandibles, size of the head, and the fact that they are only exceptionally found off their hosts is enough for the identification of the Mallophaga. They could be confused only with the Anoplura and with the dipteran of sheep, *Melophagus ovinus*. Superficially, the Anoplura look very similar to the Mallophaga but the heads of the Anoplura are narrower than their thoraces and the claws on their legs are much larger (see next chapter). *Melophagus* is larger (4-7 mm), has its head sunken into the thorax, tubular mouth parts adapted to suck blood, and a broad and sack-like abdomen (see Diptera, Hippoboscidae). Some specialists gather the Mallophaga and the Anoplura in the single order Phthiraptera or lice. Here we will consider them separately.

The almost 3,000 species of Mallophaga identified at present are distributed in 3 suborders and several families. The description of them is of no particular benefit to the practicing veterinarian. The most important species of chewing lice on domestic animals are:

2.1. **On mammals**:

*Bovicola bovis*, about 1.5 mm long, the reddish biting louse of cattle (Figure 4.1),

*Bovicola ovis*, about 2 mm long, on sheep,

*Bovicola caprae*, about 1.6 mm long, on goats,

*Bovicola limbatus*, about 2 mm long, on Angora goats,

*Bovicola equi*, about 2 mm long, on horses and other equids,

*Heterodoxus spiniger*, about 2.5 mm long and with a pointed head, on dogs and other canids,

*Trichodectes canis*, about 1.5 mm long and with an anteriorly rounded head, on dogs and dingos,

*Felicola subrostratus*, about 1.2 mm long, on cats,

*Gliricola porcelli*, the slender louse of guinea pigs, and *Gyropus ovalis*, the oval louse of guinea pigs. Both are yellowish and about 1.2 mm long.

2.2. **On birds**:

*Menacanthus stramineus*, about 3 mm long, the yellow body louse of chicken and many other domestic and game fowl. It is found in areas with relatively few feathers (breast, thighs, around the anus) and is probably the most dangerous louse of chickens,

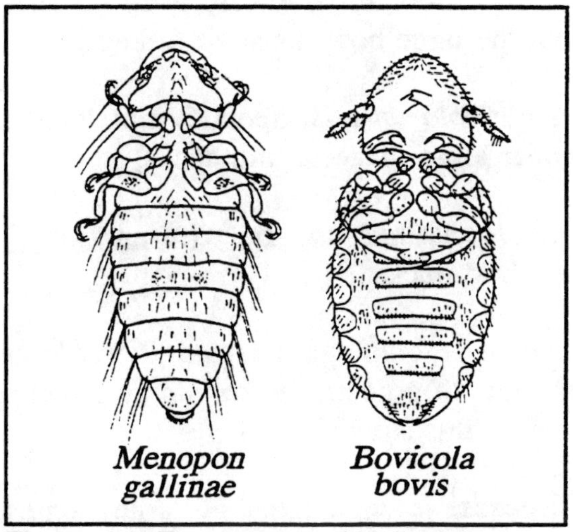


**Figure 4.1**. Two species of Mallophaga. Compare the shape of the head with that of the Anoplura (from Borror et al., 1976).

*Cuclotogaster heterographus*, about 2 mm long, the gray head louse of chicken and pheasants. It may become a serious pest,

*Goniocotes gallinae*, about 1.4 mm long, the yellow fluff louse of chicken and other fowls,

*Goniodes dissimilis*, about 3 mm long, the brown body louse of chicken,

*Menopon gallinae*, about 2 mm long, the yellow shaft louse of chicken and other fowl (Figure 4.1),

*Lipeurus caponis*, about 2.5 mm long, the gray wing louse of chicken,

*Oxylepeurus polytrapezius*, about 3.3 mm long, the slender body louse of turkeys,

*Chelopistes meleagridis*, about 3.3 mm long, the large body louse of turkeys,

*Anaticola anseris*, about 3 mm long, the slender louse of geese and ducks,

*Anatoecus dentatus*, about 1.8 mm long, on geese and ducks.

Some entomologists regard *Bovicola* as a subgenus of a genus *Damalinia*. We will not consider this subdivision here.

Because each species of large domestic mammals commonly harbors only one species of Mallophaga, for practical purposes the preliminary identification of the species of *Bovicola* can be done on the basis of the host from where the parasite was collected. The same criterium may be used for the preliminary identification of *Felicola* since this is the only common Mallophaga of cats.

The two common chewing lice of dogs can be distinguished by their sizes and the shape of their heads. The species of Mallophaga of guinea pigs can be distinguished by several well evident body characteristics.[1] The identification of Mallophaga of birds requires careful study of the characteristics of the antennae, plates, hairs and scales, which is best left to the specialist.[2] Plate II will assist in the identification of some of the most common species on chickens.

## 3. Biology

The chewing lice are essentially ectoparasites of birds that spend their entire lives on their hosts. Only 15% of the species known today affects mammals. Most of the Mallophaga are very host specific and do not live on animals other than their natural host. The specificity even extends to particular areas of the body. For example, *B. bovis* is found preferentially around the base of the tail, shoulders, and back of cattle, and *C. heterographus* lives only on the head and neck of fowl. This specificity is attributed to differences in temperature, relative humidity, and density of the body coverings of the various regions of the body. A few Mallophaga have a broader specificity, however. For example, *H. spiniger* is found on a number of canids, and *M. stramineus* on a number of galliformes birds.

Most chewing lice feed on skin secretions and debris. Some also eat feathers but they are not known to feed on hair (or wool, for that matter). A few species, such as *M. stramineus*, *M. gallinae*, *H. spiniger* and, possibly *T. canis*, regularly gnaw the skin and draw blood. Lice have rickettsia-like symbiotes in their intestine that synthesize the vitamins and other nutrients that are absent in the regular insect's diet. Elimination of these microorganisms would presumably be lethal to the louse.

The females of Mallophaga lay whitish, operculated, and about 0.7 mm long eggs, one at a time, which are immediately glued at the base of the hairs or feathers (see Figure 5.3). The eggs of lice are commonly called **nits**. The chewing lice are little prolific, a female typically lays 15 to 20 eggs in her lifetime and *M. stramineus* does not produce more than 4. *B. bovis* (and possibly other species of the same genus) is facultatively parthenogenetic, this is, their eggs may develop without fecundation if males are not available. Hatching takes place in 4 to 7 days for the species on birds, and in 7 to 12 days for the species on mammals. This difference may be due to the higher body temperature of the avian hosts that accelerates the development of the embryo. Three nymphal stages take place, and the adults appear about a month after oviposition. *M. stramineus* seems to be the only marked exception to these periods; its life cycle from egg to adult takes only 9 to 13 days.

The life span of the adult chewing lice on the host is only 2 to 6 weeks. They are sensitive to starvation and variations of temperature and relative humidity, and do not survive off the host for more than 3 to 7 days under optimal conditions (about 33 to 40C and 70 to 90% relative humidity). In cold, dry weather, they live less than a day off the host. Incubation may proceed on detached hairs or feathers off the host for up to 3 or 4 weeks in warm weather (22 to 45C and less than 92% relative humidity for *B. ovis*, for example) but the resulting nymph will die in 2 or 3 days unless it finds an appropriate host.[3]

## 4. Medical importance

The Mallophaga are very active parasites that gnaw the skin on a place and move rapidly to other places. Although they rarely produce visible wounds, the constant chewing irritates the skin of the host which provokes rubbing, scratching, and biting of the affected areas. This self-inflicted damage may be as important to the pathology by chewing lice as the activity of the arthropods themselves. The secretions of the inflamed skin and the excretions of the parasite may give the hair a matted aspect. Although Mallophaga infestations may produce intense pruritus which is often interpreted as a manifestation of allergy, there is no evidence that the host develops protective immunity: chickens infested with three lice had more than 12,000 four months later.[4] Grooming by the animals themselves, however, is quite efficient in reducing the number of lice.

Mallophaga are of limited concern in mammals unless they are present in large numbers. They may be significant, nevertheless, in cases in which production of high quality wool (mohair, for example) is the goal.

The pathogenicity of chewing lice for birds has been a matter of dispute. Some authors deny them any effect but others consider them serious pests. Possibly the degree of damage produced is directly related to the intensity of the infection. It is difficult to accept that infestations with more than 35,000 chewing lice per hen, as has been reported in the literature, are harmless. Estimations of 7% losses in weight and 10% in egg production,[5] and reports of losses of 450 g in body weight in 12 weeks and 46% in egg production[6] have been published. It is believed that *M. stramineus* and *C. heterographus* can kill young chicks. The highest prevalence of lice typically occurs in confined animals and during the winter in temperate regions, or at the end of the late dry season in tropical areas. Young, malnourished, or ungroomed animals seem to be more susceptible to the infestation and its pathology.

Since most Mallophaga eat only superficially on the skin, they have little chance to act as vectors of infections. Nevertheless, *T. canis* can be the biological vector of the cestode *Dipylidium caninum* when it gets to eat its eggs, and *H. spiniger* supports the development of the filarial worm, *Dipetalonema reconditum*.[7]

## 5. Diagnosis and control

Here we will deal with the lice of poultry. The lice of mammals will be discussed in the next chapter.

Because fowl lice as not very pathogenic, the presence of louse infestation on birds is commonly established by examination of the birds and observation of the arthropods or their eggs on the animals. It is important to exclude other causes of low production before attributing this effect to lice. Overt infestations are controlled by spraying caged birds, o dusting the litter of birds raised on the floor.

Carbaryl, coumaphos, malathion, or stirofos are insecticides in common use. New infestations are generally introduced through infested equipment or new birds. When the risk and the possibilities make it practical, control of these sources can be intended.

**Summary:**

1. The Mallophaga or Chewing Lice are permanent ectoparasites of birds and, secondarily, mammals.

2. They are distinguished from the Anoplura or Sucking Lice because the Mallophaga are skin-feeders with a broad and blunt head whereas the Anoplura are hematophagous with a narrow and pointed head.

3. Each species of Mallophaga is very specific about the host species it infests.

4. The females glue their eggs (or nits) to the hairs or feathers of the host. The development proceeds through an incomplete metamorphosis.

5. Because most Mallophaga feed on skin secretions and debris, they are not very pathogenic or important vectors of diseases.

6. Because they remain constantly on their host, transmission commonly occurs by direct contact between infested animals.

7. Because the Mallophaga are not very pathogenic, it is important to exclude other causes of disease before attempting their control.

## REFERENCES

1. Emerson KC and Flynn RJ, 1973. Lice. In Flynn RJ (ed.), *Parasites of Laboratory Animals*, Iowa St. Univ. Press, Ames, Iowa, 376-393.

2. Emerson KC, 1956. Mallophaga (chewing lice) occurring in the domestic chicken. J. Kansas Entomol. Soc. 29:63-79.

3. Saxena AK and Agarwal GP, 1983. Review article: In vitro rearing of Mallophaga. Angew. Parasitol. 24:178-186.

4. Stockdale HJ and Ruan ES, 1960. Economic importance of the chicken body louse, *Menacanthus stramineus*. J. Econom. Entomol. 53:421-423.

5. Drummond Ro, Lambert G, Smalley HE Jr and Terrill CE, 1981. Estimated losses of livestock to pests. In *Handbook of pest management*, CRC Press, Boca Raton, Florida, 111-127.

6. De Vaney JA, 1976. Effect of the chicken body louse, *Menacanthus stramineus*, on caged layers. Poult. Sci. 55:430-435.

7. Pennington NE and Phelps CA, 1969. Canine filariasis in Okinawa, Ryukyu Islands. J. Med. Entomol. 6:59-67.

# PLATE II. PICTORIAL KEY TO SOME MALLOPHAGA OF CHICKENS

(Chester J. Stojanovich and Harry D. Pratt)

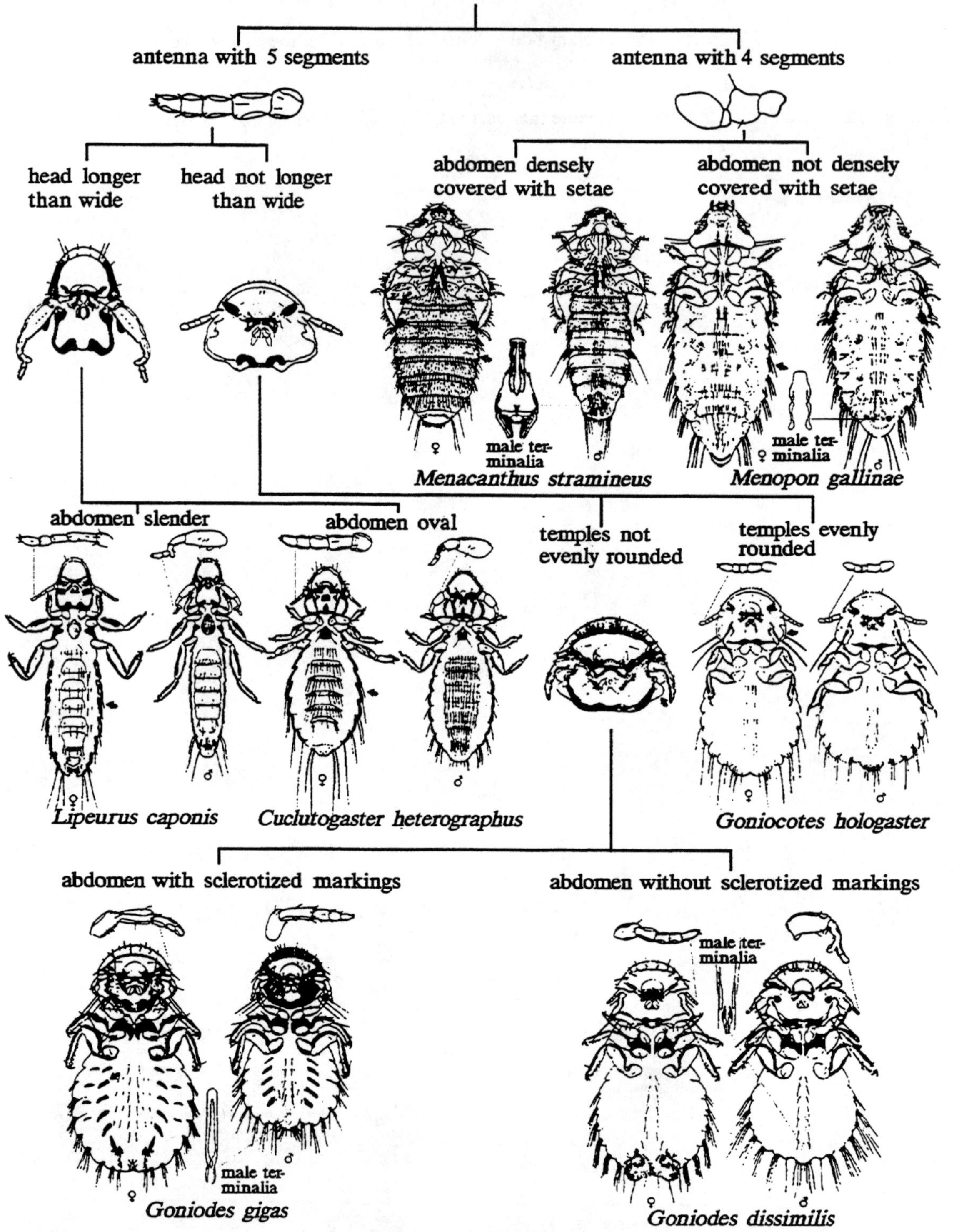


(From the US Dpt. of Health, Education, and Welfare)

# CHAPTER 5

# THE ORDER ANOPLURA OR SUCKING LICE

**Preview.** The Anoplura or Sucking Lice are insects that live permanently on their hosts. They affect mammals exclusively, and feed on blood.

The females glue their eggs to the hairs of the host. Because the Anoplura have an incomplete metamorphosis, their preadult stages also live and feed on their hosts. Because they are permanent parasites, transmission usually occurs by direct contact among infested animals.

The punctures to suck blood, the allergy caused by the insects' saliva, the loss of blood, and the scratching by the host may produce important damage to health and/or production. The habit of sucking blood also favors the transmission of infections.

## 1. Morphology

The **Anoplura** (Gr *an* = without, pleura= la teral walls of the insect's thorax, because their pleura are very small) are arthropods about 0.5 to 7 mm long. They are wingless, with a dorso-ventrally flattened body, and with legs ending in a large claw that forms a grasping organ in association with a lobe of the leg tibia (Figure 5.1). Their antennae are short, with 2 to 5 segments. Only a few species have eyes but others have prominent knobs (ocular points) at the place where the eyes are usually located. Others species have neither eyes nor ocular points. Their maxillae and hypopharynx are transformed into stylets that remain in a sac inside the head when at rest (Figure 5.2). The sac has internal hooklets that become in contact with the host's skin when the sac is everted to feed, and anchor the louse during feeding. Because the Anoplura are obligatory hematophagous, they are often called **sucking lice**.

The head of the Anoplura is rather pointed, and narrower than their thorax. Their bodies have sclerotized (= hardened) plaques, hairs, spines, and scales at specific locations which assists in the identification of the species. Since the Anoplura have an incomplete metamorphosis, their nymphs look like tiny adults.

## 2. Identification and classification

The lack of wings, shape of the body and legs, presence of concealed piercing mouth parts, size of the head, and the fact that they are only exceptionally found off their hosts is enough for the identification of the Anoplura. They are distinguished from the Mallophaga because these latter have heads as broad or broader than their thoraces and smaller claws (Figure 4.1). *Melophagus* of sheep is more massive, has the head sunken into the thorax, a broad and sac-like abdomen, and small paired claws (see Diptera, Hippoboscidae).

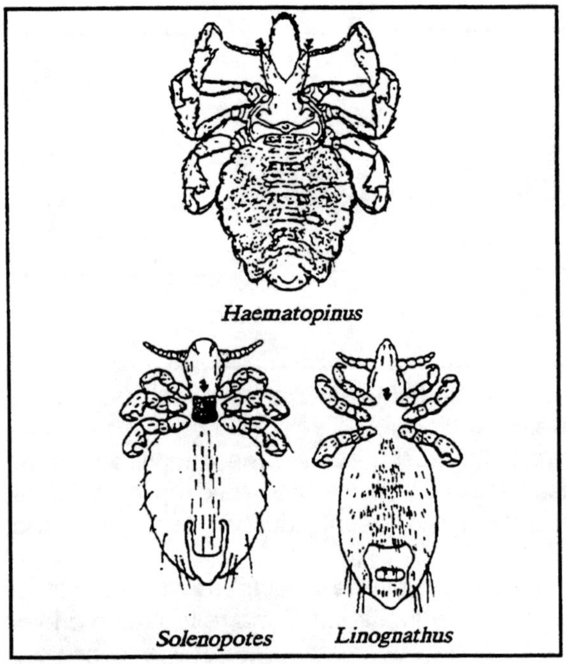


**Figure 5.1**. Representatives of the Anoplura (modified from CDC, 1969)

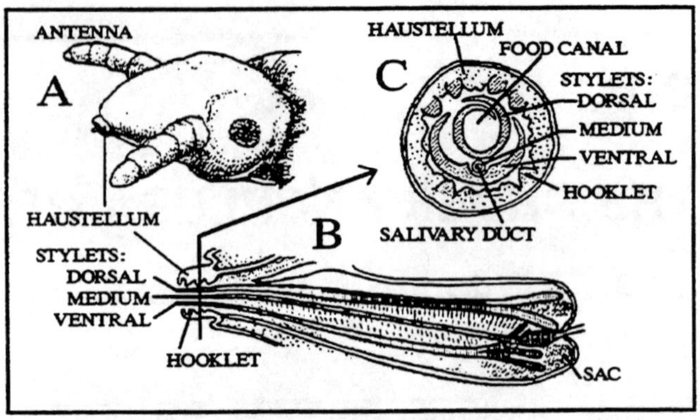


**Figure 5.2**. External (A), longitudinal section (B), and cross section (C) of the mouth parts of a sucking louse (modified from Furman, 1961)

Almost 500 species of Anoplura, distributed in15 families, are known at present.[1] Six of these families contain species of medical importance but their individual description is of no particular benefit to the practicing veterinarian. The most important species of sucking lice are:

*Haematopinus eurysternus*, about 4 mm long, the shortnosed louse of cattle, found mostly in the neck and ears of cattle, particularly prevalent in temperate climates,

*Haematopinus quadripertusus*, about 5 mm long, the brown tail louse of cattle, prevalent in tropical climates, specially in the summer,

*Haematopinus tuberculatus*, about 5.2 mm long, the louse of buffalos, on water buffalos and cattle,

*Linognathus vituli*, about 2.3 mm long, the blue longnosed louse of cattle, particularly on the dewlap and shoulders of cattle,

*Solenopotes capillatus*, about 1.4 mm long, the little blue louse of cattle,

*Linognathus pedalis*, about 1.7 mm long, the foot and leg louse of sheep,

*Linognathus ovillus*, about 2.8 mm long, the blue face louse of sheep,

*Linognathus stenopsis*, about 2.6 mm long, the body louse of goats,

*Linognathus africanus*, about 2.1 mm long, the African blue louse of small ruminants, on the body of goat, sheep, and deer,

*Microthoracius* spp., 1.5 to 4 mm long, species on camels, dromedaries, and llamas,

*Haematopinus suis*, about 5.5 mm long, the louse of hogs,

*Haematopinus asini*, about 3.2 mm long, the louse of horses, on equids,

*Linognathus setosus*, about 2.1 mm long, the blue louse of dogs, on canids and, occasionally, rabbits,

*Haemodipsus ventricosus*, about 2 mm long, the body louse of rabbits,

*Polyplax spinulosa* and *Hopopleura pacifica*, about 1.2 mm long, the lice of rats,

*Polyplax serrata* and *Hopopleura captiosa*, about 1.2 mm long, the lice of mice,

*Pediculus humanus*, about 2.5 mm long, the head and body lice of man, with a variety that lives on the head (*capitis*) and another on the body coverings (*vestimenti*),

*Phthirus pubis*, about 1.7 mm long, the pubic louse of man.

The common genera of Anoplura can be differentiated by the characteristics shown in Plate III. Identification of species of *Haematopinus* of cattle is discussed by Meleney and Kim.[2] Preliminary identification of *Linognathus* of sheep can be done on the basis of their size, distribution on the host, and observation of the head: *L. africanus* is the only of the common sucking lice of small ruminants that has a marked lateral expansion of the head behind the antennae. The books by Ferris[3] (dated by now) and by Kim et al.[4] are excellent sources for the identification of Anoplura.

## 3. Biology

The sucking lice are parasites exclusive to mammals but its biology is very similar to that of the chewing lice. All the stages remain on the host for their entire lives. They exhibit such a strict host specificity that the adaptation of a strain of *Pediculus humanus* to feed on rabbits was considered a major accomplishment. Many species show well defined preferences for certain regions of the host's body but may invade other areas in heavy infestations.

The Anoplura are avid hematophagous that must take blood before attaining fertility. Each meal last 5 to 30 minutes and is repeated every 3 to 5 hours. They tap a vessel with their stylets and take a third to a fourth of their body weight at each meal (1 mg in the case of *Pediculus humanus*). Like with the Mallophaga, rickettsia-like organisms in their guts supplement nutrients that are not present in their regular diet.

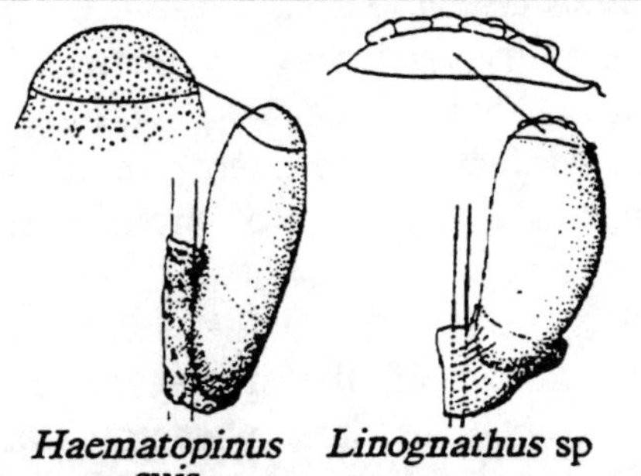


**Figure 5.3**. Examples of Anoplura eggs (nits) (modified from Ferris, 1951)

The females are little prolific. They usually lay 1 to 3 eggs per day for a total of 20 to 80 in their lifespan. The eggs, commonly called **nits**, are operculated, about 0.8 mm long, and often brownish or bluish. They are glued on the hairs, near the base, at the moment of oviposition (Figure 5.3). Hatching occurs in 7 to 20 days for most species. In the case of *Haematopinus asini*, *L. setosus* and *Polyplax* spp., incubation may be as short as 5 days. Three nymphal stages take place and the adults appear about 9 to 18 days after hatching. The life cycle from egg to egg takes usually from 3 to 5 weeks. In the case of *H. suis*, 6 or more generations can occur in one year. On the host, the adults live for 2 to 4 weeks. Off the host, most of them die in less than 4 days at low temperatures (10 to 12C), and sooner in warmer weather. As an exception, *L. pedalis* has been reported to survive up to 18 days away from the host. Lice are more common in winter than in the warmer months of the year.

## 4. Medical importance

The sucking lice are important as direct agents of disease and as vectors.

Although they are less active than the Mallophaga, the Anoplura produce small wounds in the skin when they feed and inoculate a saliva that causes immediate and delayed types hypersensitivity. The subsequent inflammation of the skin is very pruriginous and is aggravated by the rubbing, scratching and biting by the host that tries to relieve its discomfort. As a result, the hair looks rough and dry, and may be matted. In severe cases, it may be loss of hair, scarifications, and secondary infections. In overt clinical cases, loss of weight and reduction of production may be important.

Replacement of the blood taken by the Anoplura occupies host's energy that could otherwise be used for production. The blood loss may also produce anemia in massive infestations. The presence of sucking lice may help maintain fungal infections of the skin of cattle.[5] Studies have estimated that heavy infestations may cause losses of 250 g of daily weight gain in calves,[4] and of 2% of weight in pigs.[6] In sheep, only the production of clean wool appears to be affected but this may be reduced by 2.6%.[7]

Studies with laboratory animals indicate that the host begins to develop immune resistance to the arthropods after several weeks of infestation. This immunity prevents the feeding of the lice but does not kill them. They usually abandon the immune host, however. Grooming by the host itself is still an important mechanism of control of lice infestations.

Because of their blood-sucking habit, the Anoplura are particularly suited to act as vectors. They do not tolerate variations of temperature of more than a few degrees and soon leave the hosts when this becomes febrile or dies. This peculiarity makes them extremely effective as vectors. The most common infections transmitted by sucking lice are:

1. **Epidemic typhus**: a human infection caused by *Rickettsia prowazekii* and transmitted by *Pediculus humanus vestimenti*. The rickettsiae penetrate the louse with the host's blood, multiply in their intestinal epithelium, and are discharged with the feces. Most of the infected lice die within two weeks but a few survive and remain infective for life. The human infection is acquired by inhalation of the dried louse's feces, self-inoculation with them during scratching, or infection of conjunctives or mucosas with contaminated fingers. Crushing infected lice with the fingers can also lead to contamination and infection.

2. **Trench fever** is another rickettsial infection of humans (by *Rochalimaea quintana*) transmitted by the body louse. In this case the rickettsia multiplies in the lumen of the louse's intestine so the arthropod lives as long as a non-infected one but carries the infection for life.

3. **Epidemic relapsing fever** is the infection of humans by the spirocheta, *Borrelia recurrentis*, that is also transmitted by the body louse. In this case, the spirochete leaves rapidly the louse's intestine after ingestion and multiplies in its hemocele without invading other organs. The only way for humans to get the infection, then, is by crushing the louse, releasing the pathogens, and contaminating their skin. *Borrelia* does not affect the lifespan of the louse which carries the infection for life.

4. **Dipetalonemiasis**. This is the infection of dogs with the filarial worm, *Dipetalonema reconditum*. This blood nematode may be also transmitted by the chewing louse, *Heterodoxus spiniger*, the sucking louse, *Linognathus setosus*, or several species of fleas.[8] Because, differently from the fleas, *H. spiniger* does not suck blood regularly and *L. setosus* does not change hosts frequently, fleas are probably more important vectors than lice.

## 5. Diagnosis and control

The diagnosis of louse infestation is based on the observation of the actual insects, or of viable eggs on the host. Empty eggshells, particularly when they are located high on the hairs and away from the skin, may not represent current infestations. Spontaneous cure of louse infestations is infrequent, however, so the presence of empty eggs still should be regarded with suspicion. The marked reduction of the infestation and clinical improvement that commonly occur in the summer must not be confused with definitive cure.

Because lice complete their entire life cycle on the host but their embryos are protected for one to three weeks inside the eggshells, control of louse infestations normally requires the application of insecticides with residual power, or the repeated application of nonresidual insecticides. The choice of chemicals is restricted not only by their toxicity for the host, but also by government regulations on pesticide contamination of food of animal origin.

Because of their persistance in the animal tissues the organochlorine insecticides (but lindane, methoxychlor, and toxaphene are still in use) have been largely replaced by the organophosphates (e.g.; chlorpyrifos, coumaphos, dichlorvos, diazinon, fenthion, malathion, ronnel, etc.) and carbamates (e.g.; carbaryl). Synthetic pyrethroids (e.g.; fenvalerate, permethrin), formamidines (e.g.; amitraz) and injectable ivermectin have proved to be also effective (see chapter on Parasiticides). Ivermectin is much less effective against chewing lice which do not ingest host's blood.

**Summary:**

1. The Anoplura or Sucking Lice are permanent ectoparasites of mammals that affect all domestic animals and humans.

2. They are distinguished from the Mallophaga or Chewing Lice Because the Anoplura are hematophagous with a narrow and pointed head whereas the Mallophaga are skin-feeders with a broad and blunt head.

3. Like the Mallophaga, the different species of Anoplura are very specific in respect to the species of hosts they infest.

4. The females glue their eggs (or nits) to the hairs of the host and the further development is through an incomplete metamorphosis.

5. Damage results from the bites, allergy to the insect's saliva, loss of blood, and scratching by the host itself. They are also vectors of the human epidemic typhus and other infections.

6. Because they are permanent ectoparasites, transmission commonly occurs through direct contact between hosts.

7. Because they are permanent ectoparasites, control consists of insecticide treatment of the infested host.

8. Because the embryos are protected from insecticides inside the eggshells for 1-3 weeks, treatment must span this period.

## REFERENCES

1. Kim KC and Ludwig HW, 1978. The family classification of the Anoplura. System. Entomol. 3:249-284.

2. Meleney WP and Kim KC, 1974. A comparative study of cattle-infesting *Haematopinus* with redescription of *H. quadripertusus* Fahernholz, 1919 (Anoplura: Haematopinidae). J. Parasit. 60:507-522.

3. Ferris GF, 1951. *The sucking lice*, Pacific Coast Entomol. Soc., San Francisco, 320 pp.

4. Kim KC, Pratt HD and Stojanovitch CJ, 1986. *The sucking lice of North America*, Penn. St. U. Press, University Park, Pennsylvania, 241 pp.

5. Kamyszek F and Tratwal Z, 1977. Ectoparasites in pigs and cattle. IV. Influence of diseases caused by skin parasites on gain in weight in cattle. Wiad. Parazyt. 23:425-430.

6. Drummond RO, Lambert G, Smalley HE Jr and Terrill CE, 1981. Estimated losses of livestock to pests. In *Handbook of pest management*, CRC Press, Boca Raton, Florida, 111-127.

7. Kettle PR and Watson AJ, 1982. Long-term effect of sheep body lice (*Damalinia ovis*) on body weight and wool production. N. Z. J. Agric. Res. 25:531-534.

8. Pennington NE and Phelps CA, 1969. Canine filariasis in Okinawa, Ryukyu Islands. J. Med. Entomol. 6:59-67.

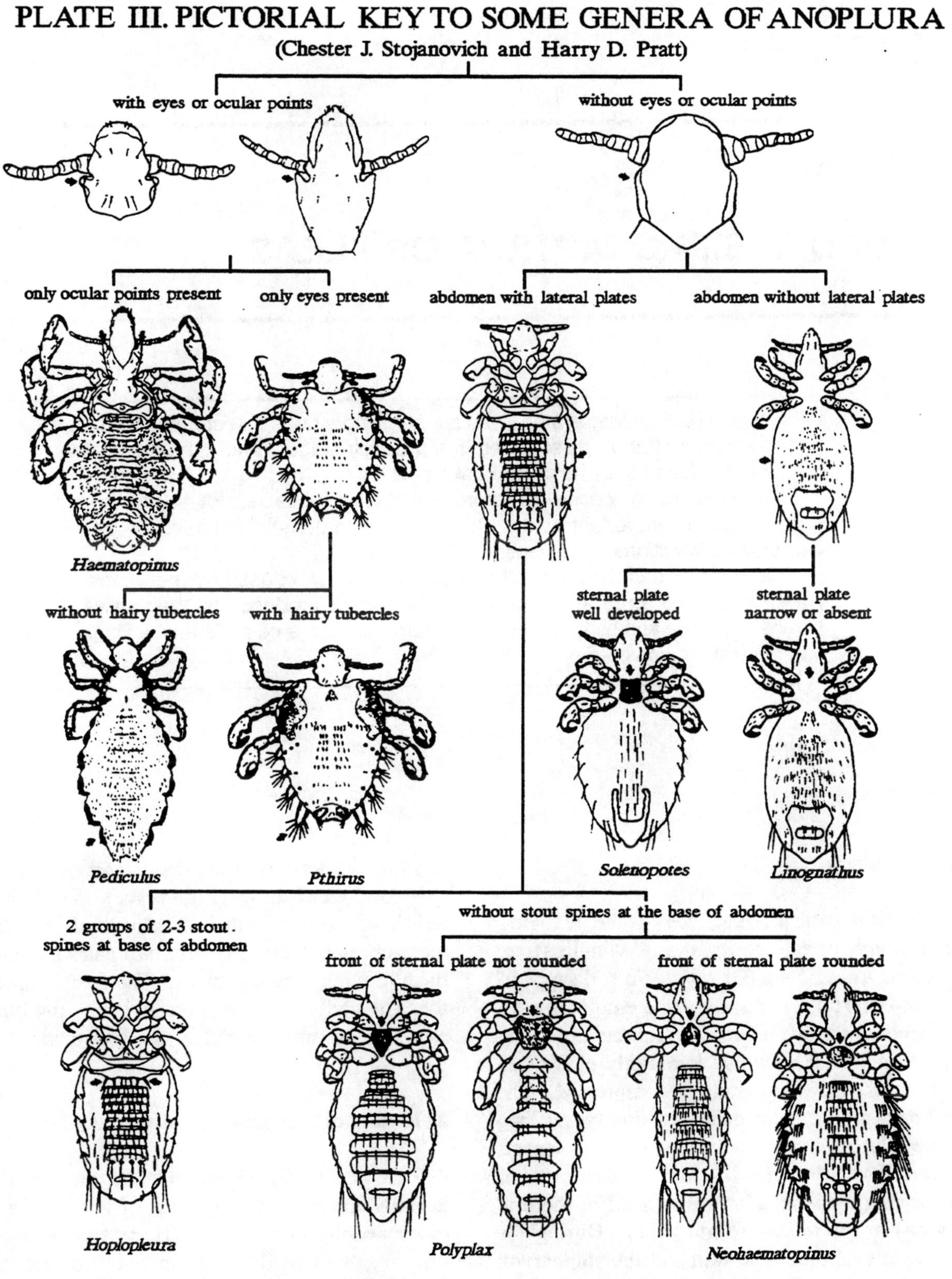

(From the US Dpt. of Health, Education, and Welfare)

# CHAPTER 6

# THE ORDER SIPHONAPTERA OR FLEAS

**Preview.** The Siphonaptera or Fleas are hematophagous insects that feed on their host but reproduce off it. In most cases, the preadult stages, and the adults between blood meals, are found in or near the host's nest.

Fleas infest many species of mammals and birds, especially during the summer. They are particularly important as agents of disease in domestic carnivores, and as vectors of serious infections in humans.

Fleas affect their host's health by the annoyance caused by their constant activity, their bites, the removal of blood, and the allergy produced by their saliva. They also transmit plague and endemic typhus to humans, and a cestode and a filarial nematode to domestic carnivores.

## 1. Morphology

The **Siphonaptera** (Gr *siphon* = tube, referring to the mouth parts, and *apteros* = wingless) are also called Aphaniptera (Gr *aphaneia* = disappearance, and *pteron* = wing) by some entomologists. They are small brownish-reddish insects from 1 to 6 mm long with a body that is roughly oval when seen from the side, and laterally compressed. The mouthparts are of the piercing-sucking type. Two grooved labial palps enclose two long lancets derived from the maxillas and a thin tubular epipharynx (a prolongation of the roof of the oral opening) in the middle (Figure 6.1). During the bite, the lancets break the skin and the epipharynx is inserted into a vessel to pump blood out.

Some species have a row of spine-like structures called **ctenidia** (sing. ctenidium, Gr *kteis* = comb, *ideium* = diminutive) or **combs** along the ventral border of the head (**genal ctenidium**) or the caudal border of the first thoracic segment (**pronotal ctenidium**) (Figure 6.2). Very characteristic of the fleas is their third pair of legs that is more developed that the first two pairs and allows them to jump long distances. The female spermatheca is visible by transparency from the outside as a sack toward the end of the abdomen.

## 2. Identification and classification

Fleas are easily identifiable by their oval and laterally compressed body, lack of wings, and well developed third pair of legs. There are about 2,000 known species of fleas distributed into four major families. The unequivocal identification of families and of individual species is best left to the specialist[1],[2] but a preliminary identification of some important fleas can be done by some easily observable characteristics (Plate IV). The followings are some important species:

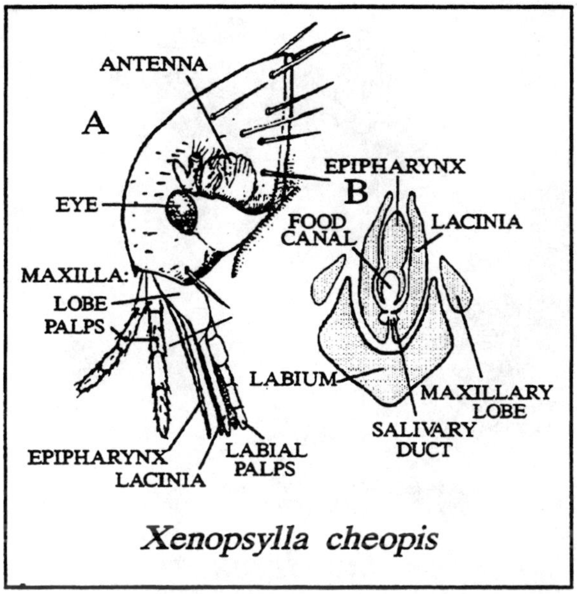


**Figure 6.1**. Lateral (A) and cross section (B) view of the mouthparts of a flea (modified from Furman, 1961).

*Pulex irritans*, of cosmopolitan distribution, is considered the **human flea** but occurs on a wide range of animals, particularly on pigs. It lacks genal and pronotal ctenidia.

*Tunga penetrans*, the "**chigoe**" or sand-flea, is a small flea of the tropical and subtropical regions of America, Africa, and Asia that attacks humans and, occasionally, pigs.

*Ctencephalides canis* and *C. felis* are considered to be the **dog** and **cat fleas**, respectively, but they attack either species as well as humans and other animals. Both have genal and pronotal ctenidia but the first tooth of the genal ctenidium of *C. canis* is about half as long as the second tooth. The first and second teeth are about the same size in *C. felis*. *C. felis* is the most common flea of dogs and cats and also infests raccons, opposums, and other wild animals.

*Xenopsylla cheopis*, called the **Oriental rat flea**, is of almost cosmopolitan distribution. This andother *Xenopsylla* species of more restricted geographic distribution are primarily fleas of rats but feed on man freely if necessary. They do not have ctenidia.

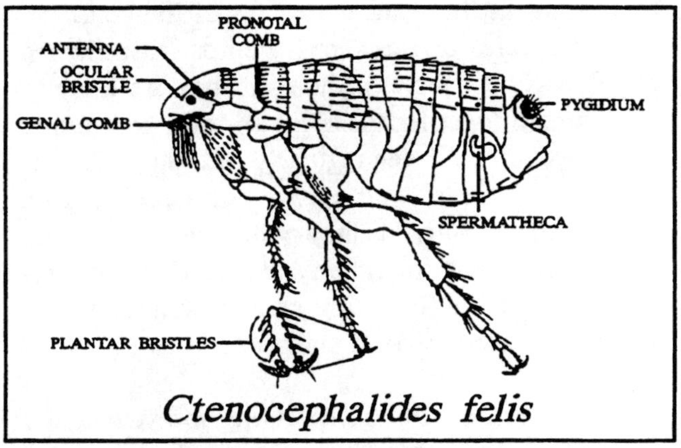


**Figure 6.2**. External morphology of a typical flea (modified from CDC, 1969).

*Nosopsyllus fasciatus* is the **Northern rat flea**, common in North America and Europe. It has only pronotal ctenidium and occurs on rats, mice, humans, and many other mammals.

*Leptopsylla segnis*, the **European mouse flea**, is cosmopolitan and occurs on mice and rats. It attacks humans only rarely. It has genal and pronotal ctenidia but the former one has only four teeth.

*Ceratophyllus* spp. are fleas of chicken that also infest cats, dogs, humans and other mammals.

*Echidnophaga gallinacea*, the **sticktight flea** of poultry, particularly prevalent in tropical areas. It is easily recognized because its head is sharply angular rather than smoothly rounded. Besides birds, it attacks cats, dogs, horses, rabbits, and humans.

## 3. Biology

Adult fleas are temporary, hematophagous ectoparasites. Most species spend from a few minutes to a few hours on their host every day and the rest of their time in or near the host's nest (but see exceptions below). They must feed on blood to lay fertile eggs and the females need mate only once since they store the sperm in the sperma-theca. Unlike the lice, fleas are more common on their hosts in the warmer months of the year.

Most species of fleas are little host-specific and attack diverse species of hosts if they are hungry. They tend to wait for the approach of a host rather than seek for it. When regularly fed, they can live for three months to well over a year depending on the species. Starved, they will live one to four months in a cool, humid environment. High temperature and low humidity shorten their life considerably, particularly if starved.

Fleas breed continuously during the year under tropical and temperate conditions but suspend breeding when exposed to cold winters. The female flea lays a few white, 0.5 mm long, oval eggs every day that may amount to several hundreds during her life. The eggs are usually laid in the host's nest and develop in four to six days under ideal conditions (18 to 27C and 75% or higher relative humidity). Under conditions other than ideal, hatching may take from two to 21 days. Eggs do not develop above 38C or below 5-12C, or with relative humidity less than 70%. The flea larvae are yellow-white and look like a mosquito larva. They moult twice and reach a maximum size of 5-10 mm. Flea larvae are very active and feed on any organic material available, particularly on the droppings left by the adult fleas. At 25C and 85% relative humidity, they complete their development in one or two weeks. Low temperature or lack of food can prolong their development for up to seven months. Humidity below 60% kills them rapidly. At the end of its development, the larva spins a whitish, loose, ovoid cocoon of 1x1x3 mm, and becomes a pupa. Debris adheres easily to the outside of the cocoon that soon looks like a speck of dirt (Figure 6.3).

The length of pupation is highly influenced by temperature. The shortest time is about four days at 35C, but it takes eight days at 18C. At lower temperature, pupation can last nearly a year. The entire life cycle, from egg to adult, may take from 18 days to 20 or more months. Pupae are a little more resistant to desiccation than eggs and larvae, they still develop at 50% relative humidity. In the absence of a host, the pupa can remain in the cocoon for long periods.

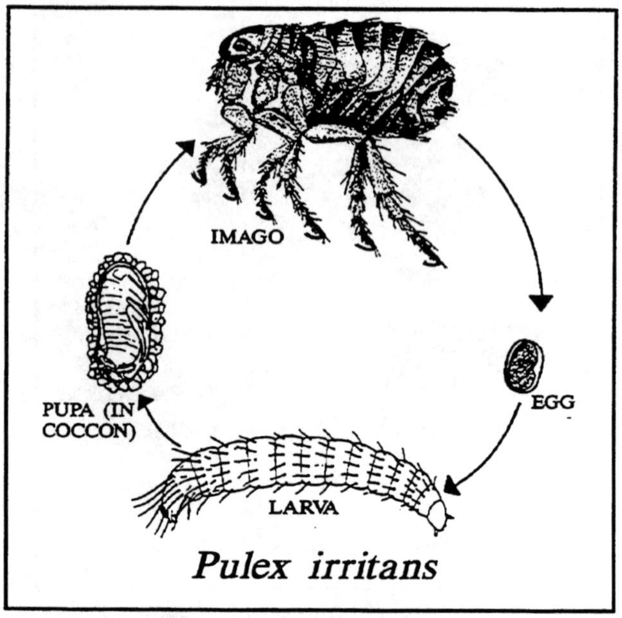


**Figure 6.3**. Life cycle of a typical flea.

The adults emerge when increase in temperature, physical pressure, or air vibrations indicate that a host is approaching. This is the reason why people that return to summer cottages that are empty most of the year are attacked by an army of new, hungry fleas.

*C. felis*, *E. gallinacea* and *T. penetrans* are partial exceptions to the condition of fleas of temporary parasites.

*C. felis* spends most of its adult life on its host. Once they have fed for a few days, they cannot live off the host for more than one to four days. The female takes long blood meals that may last more than an hour and defecates while feeding. Seventy two fleas may take 1 ml of blood per day. The eggs are usually laid on the host and roll off to accumulate in the places where the host usually rests.[3]

The female of *E. gallinacea* attaches firmly by its mouth parts to the skin of the host during its first blood feeding, mates, and start laying eggs. The females are often seen in clusters of many fleas on the comb, wattles, around the eyes and beak, and around the anus of the chicken.

The female of *T. penetrans* burrows into the skin and becomes soon surrounded by inflamed tissue that leaves only a small opening through which the eggs are discharged to the exterior.

The rabbit fleas, *Spilopsyllus cuniculi* and *Cediopsylla simplex*, control their own sexual cycles according to the level of sexual hormones in the blood of their host.[4] This dependence has not been found in other flea species.

## 4. Medical importance

Fleas are important to medicine as agents of disease, cause of allergies, and vectors of infections.

The constant activity of fleas is enough to cause annoyance and interfere with the tranquility of the host. Although individual fleas takes little blood, massive infestations in very young or malnourished hosts may result in anemia.[5] *E. gallinacea* causes ulcerations, swelling, and wartlike lesions that interfere with production and may result in blindness and even death of the affected chicken. *T. penetrans* undergoes hypertrophy after establishment under the skin and causes extreme irritation and, quite often, facilitates secondary bacterial infections.

Like most hematophagous insects, fleas inoculate saliva during blood feeding. Many components of the saliva behave as allergens and trigger the corresponding allergies in the host. Studies with laboratory animals subjected to continuous attack by fleas have demonstrated that cell-mediated hypersensitivity develops first, and immediate type hypersensitivity may appear later.[6] These two allergies can evolve concurrently and become very severe in dogs and cats. The lesions occur preferentially on the lumbosacral and tail areas in the dog and on the back, neck, and face in cats. The pruritus causes the infested animal to rub and bite the area which makes the inflammation more severe and often favors secondary infections. Self-inflicted trauma is not rare. In the acute disease, the skin shows alopecia, erythema, papules, crusts, and, often, self-trauma and pyogenic infection.. In chronic cases, seborrhea, hyperkeratosis and hyperpigmentation are also present.

If the infestation continues, it is possible that the host reaches a refractory stage and the allergies disappear spontaneously, first the delayed hypersensitivity and then the reaginic hypersensitivity. In nature, however, spontaneous resolution of flea allergy is seen only in massive and continuous infestations that are unlikely to occur in owned animals.

The hematophagia, frequent changes of host, and long life of fleas favor the transmission of a number of pathogens. The most common are:

1. **Myxomatosis.** The rabbit flea, *Spilopsyllus cuniculi*, can transmit the myxomatosis virus mechanically among rabbits with its bites. Although multiplication of the virus in the flea has not been demonstrated, it remains in starved fleas for 105 days.

2. **Plague.** Fleas that feed on rats infested with *Yersinia pestis* acquire the infection themselves. The bacterium multiplies in the stomach of the flea and blocks its digestive tract. When the infected flea feeds on another animal, the host's blood cannot pass the blockage and is regurgitated back into the bite wound carrying bacteria washed from the flea's stomach. Because rats die from plague, epizootics of the disease in rats commonly result in large populations of fleas searching for new hosts. Since the infected fleas cannot feed properly, they go hungry and become very aggressive in this search. These two events may explain why human epidemics of plague commonly appear very rapidly after rat epizootics. The most important vector of plague to man is *Xenopsylla cheopis*.

3. **Endemic typhus.** Typhus caused by *Rickettsia typhi* (syn. *R. moosery*) is called flea-borne typhus or murine typhus to differentiate it from the epidemic or louse-borne typhus by *R. prowazekii*. *R. typhi* infects rats and humans. When acquired by a flea, the rickettsia multiplies in its intestinal epithelium without killing it, and numerous bacteria are discharged with the fleas' feces.

Humans become infected with these feces by self-inoculation when they scratch their contaminated skin, or by contamination of their conjunctive or mucous membranes, or by inhalation of dried feces. Probably the major mechanism of infection for the rat is the ingestion of infected fleas during grooming. The most important vector is *Xenopsylla cheopis* but the sucking louse, *Polyplax spinulosa*, can also transmit the rickettsia among rats.

4. **Dipylidiasis.** Fleas are also the intermediate host of the cestode of dogs and cats, *Dipylidium caninum*. The eggs passed by infected hosts are eaten by the flea larva and develop to a larval stage called cysticercoid in the resulting adult flea. When dogs or cats (or an infant!) ingest the infected flea during grooming, the cysticercoid develops into the adult cestode in their intestine.

5. **Dipetalonemiasis.** *Ctenocephalides* spp. are the intermediate hosts of the filarial worm of the dog, *Dipetalonema reconditum*. Microfilariae are taken with the blood of an infected dog and develop to a third stage, infective larvae in the hemocele of the flea in about a week. During a next feeding, these larvae leave the flea by the mouth during the blood meal and contaminate the host's skin. These larvae are believed to invade the host by the puncture wound left by the flea bite.

### 5. Diagnosis and control

The diagnosis of flea infestation commonly relies on the declarations of the owner of the animal. The veterinarian may confirm the condition by observing fleas or flea's feces on the patient's skin. Flea feces look like tiny black pellets that dissolve slowly in water giving a reddish color due to the undigested hemoglobin.

Flea allergy dermatitis is suspected in flea infested animals by the intense pruritus, typical characteristics and location of the lesions, its occurrence in animals over a year of age and, commonly, in the late summer which corresponds to the peak of flea infestations. Intradermal skin testing is little reliable with the commercially available whole flea extracts. Because the antigens responsible for flea allergy are just being investigated, preparations with specific antigens are unlike to be available soon. Treatment of flea allergy dermatitis consists of the elimination of the fleas. The use of glucocorticoides or antihistaminics is only a palliative to relieve the animal's discomfort while the problem is solved. Similar to skin testing, hyposensitizing preparations with whole flea extracts (rather than the specific antigen) are unreliable.

Elimination of fleas from a household is a rather complex proposition.[7] First, the places most likely to contain preadult stages of fleas (sites where the dog or cat usually rests) must be identified and cleaned from flea stages. Outdoor sites such as places with dense vegetation and damp soil must be defoliated and soil debris removed to permit penetration of sunlight and drying of the ground. Indoor sites such as pet nests, carpets, chairs, beneath tables or beds, etc., must be vacumed to remove eggs, larvae, and pupae. This vacuuming also brings the pupae from the depth of the carpets and stimulate the emergence of the new adults which makes them more susceptible to the action of the insecticides.

Once mechanical control has been achieved, insecticides with or without insect growth regulators should be applied to the places where fleas accumulate (doghouses, beneath Spot's favority shrub, carpets, grooves in hardwood floors, behind baseboards, beneath tables, beds, and sofas, in closets, etc.) and on the pet itself. Application to the environment can be done with hand-held spayers or, more conveniently indoors, with total-release aerosols or foggers. Chlorpyrifos at 0.25% kills 97% of the fleas and its activity on a carpet lasts for 6 weeks. Permethrin at 0.5% kills 100% of the fleas and lasts for 3 weeks. Methoprene and Fenoxycarb are juvenile hormone analogues that acts on the eggs and larvae. Used indoors, both are active for more than 6 months but methoprene is unstable to ultraviolet light outdoors.

Treatment of pets is normally done with non-residual insecticide flea shampoos, dips, sprays, or foams at the same time that the environment is treated. The directions of the manufacturer must be followed strictly because many shampoos require up to 10 minutes of soaking time to be effective If environmental control is deficient, preparations with residual insecticides may be necessary. Lufenuron (not available in the USA yet) is a chitin synthesis inhibitor that is administered orally to pets and produces effective blood levels for up to one month. Female fleas that ingest the chemical with their blood meal fail to produce viable larvae. Dichlorvos-impregnated collars (that kill the adults) or methoprene-impregnated collars (that render the flea eggs sterile) are effective in association with an adequate environmental control. Ultrasonic flea collars do not appear to affect the fleas but bother considerably some pets.

## Summary

1. The Siphonaptera or Fleas are temporary, hematophagous parasites of domestic animals and humans.

2. They are particularly important as agents of disease in domestic carnivores and as vectors of infections in humans and carnivores.

3. They are little specific for the species of host they infest.

4. They are easily recognized by their laterally compressed body and well developed third pair of legs.

5. The eggs, larvae, and pupae are found in or near the host's nest. With theexception of *C. felis, E. gallinacea*, and *T. penetrans*, the adults are found in or near the nest, or on the host.

6. Fleas are particularly prevalent in the summer.

7. They annoy their host with their activity and bites, draw blood, cause cutaneous allergies, and transmit *Dipylidium* and *Dipetalonema* infections to domestic carnivores, and plague and endemic typhus to humans.

8. Control of fleas is based on insecticide application and must include the habitat of the preadult stages.

## REFERENCES

1. Hopkins GHE and Rothschild M, 1953-1971. *An illustrated catalogue of the Rothschild collection of fleas (Siphonaptera) in the British Museum (Natural History)*. Br. Mus. Nat. Hist., London, 5 vols., 2,385 pp.

2. Holland GP, 1964. Evolution, classification, and host relationships of Siphonaptera. Ann. Rev. Entomol. 9:123-146.

3. Dryden MW. 1993. Biology of fleas of dogs and cats. Compendium, Sm An. Sect., 15:569-78.

4. Rothschild M, 1965. The rabbit flea and hormones. Endeavour 24:162-168.

5. Yeruham I, Rosen S and Hadani A. 1989. Mortality in calves, lambs, and kids caused by severe infestation with the cat flea *Ctenocephalides felis felis* (Bouche, 1835) in Israel. Vet. Parasit. 30:351-356.

6. Feingold BF, Benjamini E and Michaeli D, 1968. The allergic responses to insects bites. Ann. Rev. Entomol. 13:137-158.

7. Dryden MW and Prestwood AK. 1993. Successful flea control. Compendium, Sm. An. Sect. 15:821-831.

# PLATE IV. PICTORIAL KEY TO SOME SPECIES OF SIPHONAPTERA

(Harry D. Pratt)

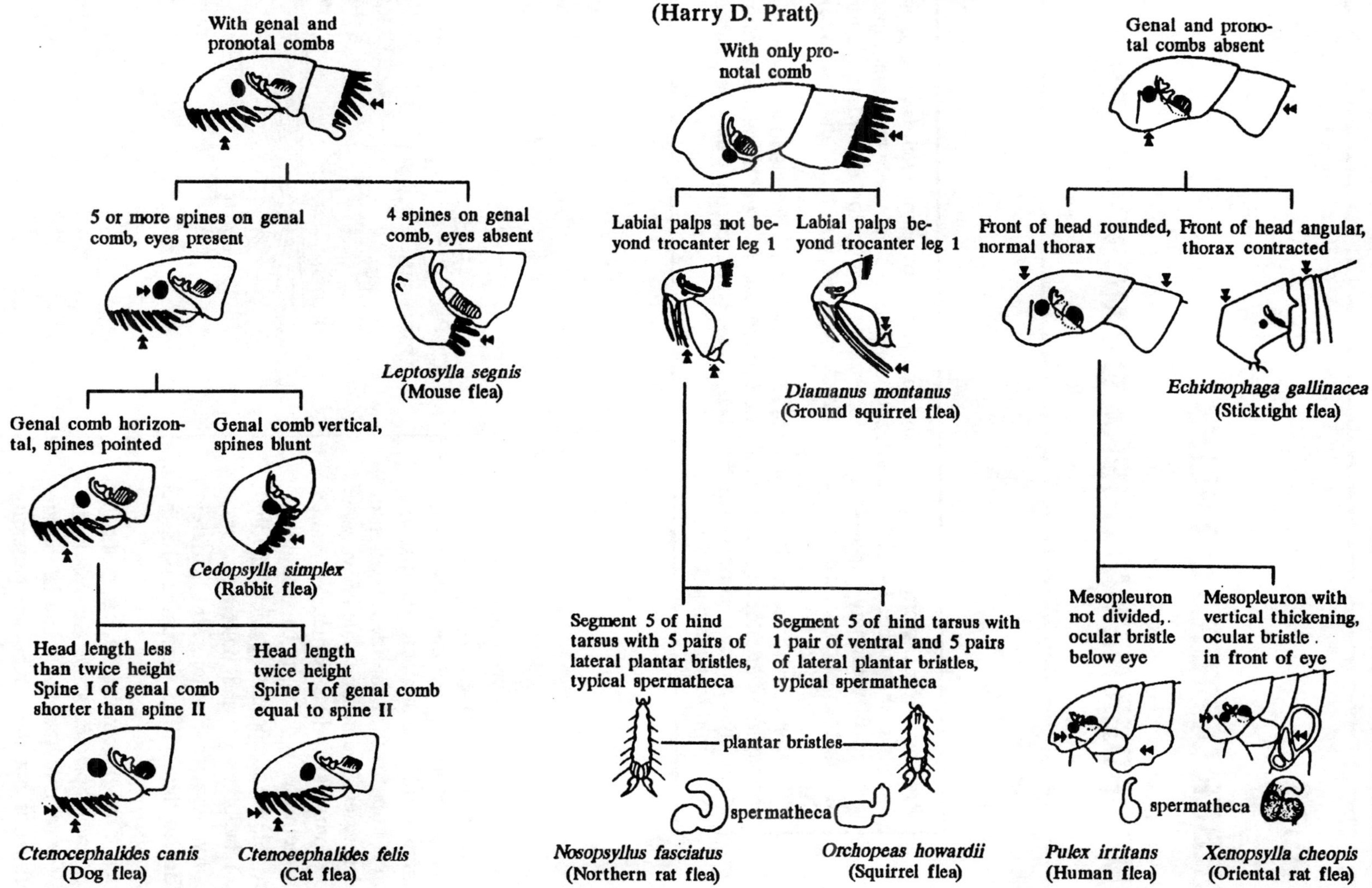


(From the US Dpt. of Health, Education, and Welfare)

# CHAPTER 7

# THE ORDER DIPTERA OR FLIES.

# THE SUBORDER NEMATOCERA OR MOSQUITOES

**Preview**. The Diptera are insects with the first pair of wings well developed and the second pair replaced by knob-like structures. All have a complete metamorphosis. The species of veterinary importance are distributed among the suborders Nematocera (mosquitoes, gnats, and relatives), Brachycera (horse flies and relatives), and Cyclorrhapha (house fly and relatives).

The Nematocera are small and delicate Diptera with long and slender antennae. Many species are hematophagous and all need an aquatic or semi-aquatic environment to breed. They annoy their hosts with their bites, draw blood, produce allergies, some inject toxins, and many transmit diseases.

The **Diptera** (from Gr *di* = two, and *pteron* = wing) are arthropods that have only the first pair of wings well developed. These are membranous and have a number of veins and cells the distribution of which is important for the identification of families and species. The second pair of wings is reduced to some knob-like structures called **halteres** that help the fly keep its balance during flight (Figure 7.1). An important species (*Melophagus ovinus*) lacks wings and halteres. Other structures vary somewhat among the different groups of flies so they will be discussed with the respective group.

All Diptera have incomplete metamorphosis. Most species are oviparous, some are ovoviviparous, and a few are viviparous. The larvae are active in all cases but the pupae are generally inactive.

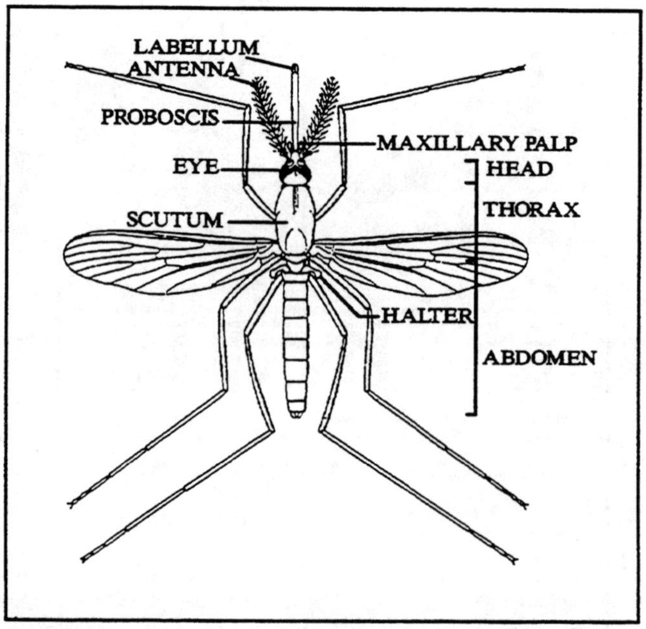


**Figure 7.1**. External morphology of a mosquito.

The Diptera is a very large group that contains perhaps 100,000 species. Once an arthropod has been identified as a dipteran by the presence of only one pair of developed wings and one pair of halteres, consideration of its size and of characteristics of its wings and its antennae (Figures 7.2 and 7.3) should permit to assign it to one of the three suborders of veterinary importance: Nematocera, Brachycera, or Cyclorrhapha.

The **Nematocera** (mosquitoes and relatives) are small and delicate flies with their antennae composed of more than six segments and usually long.

The **Brachycera** (horse flies and relatives) are stout flies with very characteristic antennae.

The **Cyclorrhapha** (house fly and relatives) are medium to large size flies with short and also very characteristic antennae.

The structure of the mouth parts is also important for the classification of some groups. Because each of these suborders has very distinctive morphological and biological characteristics and contains representatives of importance to veterinary medicine, we will discuss them separately.

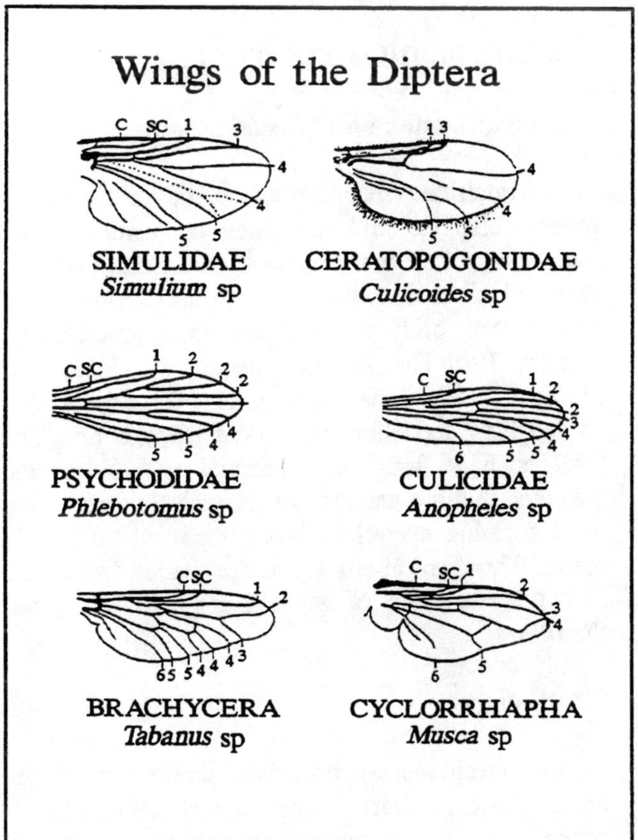


**Figure 7.1.** Typical wings of some dipteran groups. The veins are identified according to the old nomenclature (modified from Beldings, 1965)

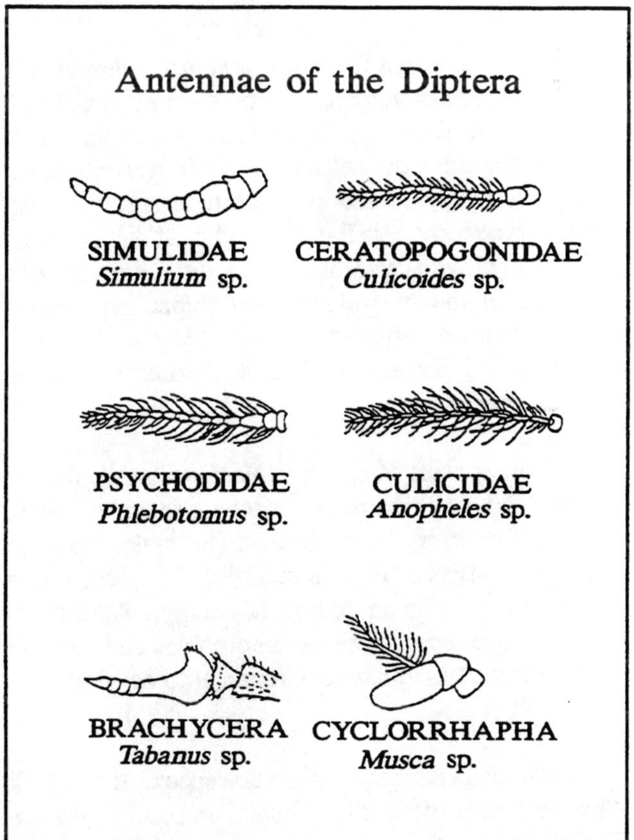


**Figure 7.3.** Typical antennae of some dipteran groups (modified from Belding, 1965).

# THE SUBORDER NEMATOCERA: MOSQUITOES, GNATS, AND RELATIVES

The **Nematocera** (from Gr *nematos* = thread, and *keron* = horn or antenna) are by the most part small and delicate Diptera with long and slender antennae. In some species the antennae are relatively short but they are always made by more than six segments. The larvae have a well-developed head distinct from the body, with mandibles that bite horizontally. Except in the mosquitoes, the pupae are resting stages that do not move around. They are free, this is, they are not enclosed in a capsule like in the Cyclorrhapha.

In most species of parasitic Nematocera the female must feed on blood before reaching sexual maturity and before every oviposition. The males, and the females between blood meals, feed on plant juices which is their main source of energy. All Nematocera have a complete metamorphosis and need an aquatic or semiaquatic environment to develop their preadult stages.

All Nematocera families include species that attack humans, their domestic animals, or both. They are important as a source of annoyance, blood suckers, agents of allergies or toxicosis, and vectors of infections.

The Nematocera of veterinary importance belong to four families: Simuliidae, Ceratopogonidae, Psychodidae, and Culicidae.[1] We will discuss them separately.

## 1. THE SIMULIIDAE OR BLACK FLIES

### 1.1. Identification and Classification

The Simuliidae (from *Simulium*, the most common genus), also called **black flies** or **buffalo gnats** (because of their humped back), are small (1-5 mm long), black to dark-grey or even dark-yellow flies, with a stout body and a prominent thoracic hump (Figure 7.4). The antennae usually have 11 short segments and, unlike the other Nematocera discussed here, look like little horns (Figure 7.3). The females have long and serrated mandibles and maxillae that are used to cut through the host's skin until forming a pool of blood from where the fly feeds. There are about 1,300 species of Simuliidae and three fourths of them belong to the genus *Simulium*.

### 1.2. Biology

The Simuliidae are particularly prevalent in the temperate and subartic zones of the northern hemisphere but many species exist also in the subtropical and tropical zones. They are strong fliers that are active in daylight and commonly fly in enormous swarms. Although they can disperse for many miles, particularly with the help of strong winds, they often remain close to the water courses where they breed. They are outdoor feeders and many have preferences for some host species (humans, livestock, birds).

The females live for 2-4 weeks and lay several hundreds eggs in that time. They oviposit in swiftly flowing streams with well-aerated water. The eggs (rather triangular and 0.1-0.4 mm long, Figure 7.4) are deposited on the water surface or on objects over or near the water where the relative humidity is over 95% and the larvae will fall into the water on hatching. The eggs develop in 4-30 days according to the temperature and species but in some simuliids they will still develop at 5C. The eggs can remain dormant for long periods under extremes of temperatures if the humidity is high.

The larvae, black to light brown, up to 15 mm long, and quite active, require rapidly flowing water, and fix themselves by a caudal sucker to submerged objects about one inch below the surface. They may be so abundant that look like moss. Under optimal conditions, the larvae develop in 7 to 12 days but low water temperature and poor availability of food may prolong development for months. When ready to pupate, the larvae produce a boat- or basket-shaped cocoon, up to 5 mm long, that is attached to the substrate where the larva lived. The pupae develop in 2 to 6 days under ideal conditions but, like with the eggs and larvae, adverse conditions can greatly retard development. The imagoes often emerge simultaneously creating enormous swarms.

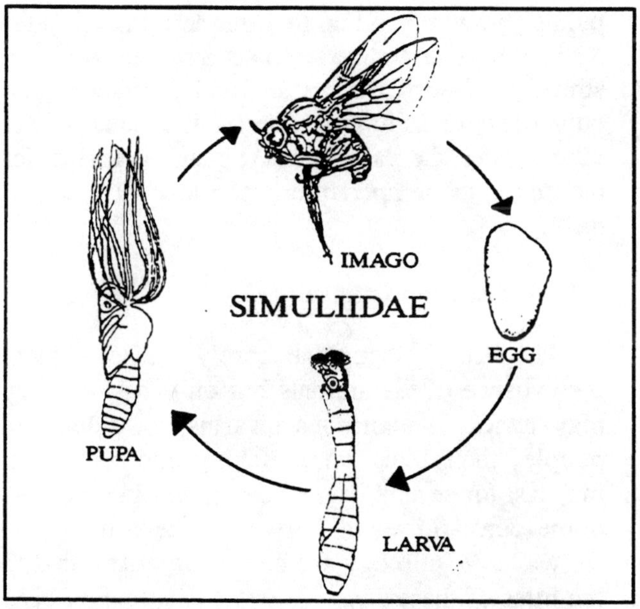


**Figure 7.4.** Stages in the life cycle of Simuliidae.

## 1.3. Medical importance

The Simuliidae are commonly temporary pests that are around for about a month in the spring or early summer. They inflict painful bites that frequently cause panic among the animals and greatly disturb grazing with the subsequent losses in production. Losses of 2-15% of milk production have been reported.[2] The bites cause large welts and itching which is generally interpreted as an allergic reaction (although it may be also caused by histaminic substances in the fly's saliva). Some experimental evidence suggests that bitten animals develop type III (immune complex) and IV (cell-mediated), but not type I (anaphylactic), hypersensitivities.[3] Further work in this area is necessary, however.

Although each fly takes little blood, their bites leave small oozing wounds which contributes to the blood loss. Because they may attack in large swarms and inflict as many as 25,000 bites per animal,[4] simuliids may kill cattle and smaller animals by exsanguination.

Animals that suffer severe attacks (or are injected with black fly extract) show depression, a stiff walk, a rough coat, and do not eat. Subcutaneous edemas develop in several areas of the body. Edema of the throat and inhalation of flies, particularly in agitated animals trying desperately to escape from these pests, may cause deaths by asphyxia.

Massive attacks have resulted in the death of hundreds or thousands of farm animals in the past.[5] Killed animals present extensive petechiae in the skin, subcutaneous edema, and occasional necrosis of the epidermis. Animals that have been previously exposed to simuliid bites are more resistant to the effect of the attacks. Inoculation of serum from exposed animals prevents the systemic, but not the cutaneous, signs caused by the injection of black fly extracts. Although at least part of the damage by simuliid bites may be attributed to histaminic substances in the saliva of the arthropod and allergic reactions of the host, the rapid death of livestock under massive attack, the general signs and pathology, its replication with fly extracts, and the protective effect of the serum suggest the action of a toxin, possibly with effect on the vessels.

Apart from causing direct damage, the simuliids act as biological vectors of **onchocercoses** of humans, cattle, and horses (see Filarial nematodes) and **leucocytozoonosis** of birds (see Haemosporina), and probably as mechanical vectors of some viroses. Although eastern equine encephalitis and vesicular stomatitis are commonly transmitted by mosquitoes and sandflies, respectively, simulids are suspected in the transmission of both viruses.

## 2. THE CERATOPOGONIDAE OR BITING MIDGETS

### 2.1. Identification and classification

The Ceratopogonidae, also called **biting midgets, pinkies**, or **no-see-ums**, are also small (1-3 mm long), dark flies. They can be distinguished from the Simuliidae because the Ceratopogonidae are smaller, have a slender abdomen, longer antenna, shorter front tarsi, and different wing venation (Figure 7.5). Their antennae bear bristles, more abundant in the males than in the females.

Like the black flies, the female biting midges cut the skin to obtain blood from the wound they inflict. Of the 4,000 species described, in only about a fourth the females are hematophagous and most of these belong to the genus *Culicoides* and *Leptoconops*.

### 2.2. Biology

The Ceratopogonidae are prevalent in tropical and temperate zones. They are fairly strong fliers but usually are found within a couple of miles of their breeding places. They are outdoor feeders and while many species of *Culicoides* prefer to feed in the early morning or late afternoon and many of *Leptoconops* during the day, a few important vectors feed at night. Many ceratopogonids show clear preference for a particular species of host.

The females deposit their eggs (up to 0.5 mm and cigar-shaped, Figure 7.6) in masses in slow-moving streams, polluted still waters, or in decaying, moist vegetation. Under optimal conditions they hatch in

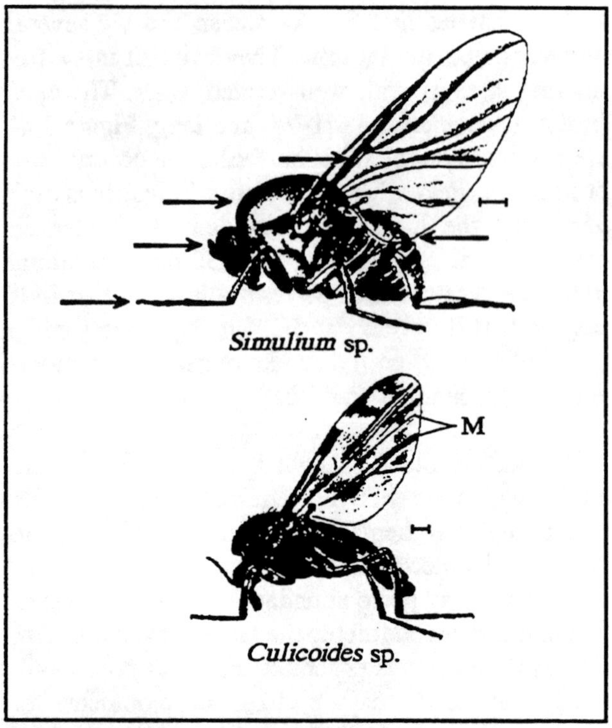


**Figure 7.5**. Morphological differences between Simuliidae and Ceratopogonidae (modified from Borror and White, 1970).

2 to 8 days and produce a whitish larva up to 6 mm long. The larvae of most species are found in moist environments (like the mud on the margins of streams) rather than under water, and develop in about 3 weeks under ideal conditions. The quiet pupae (brownish and up to 4 mm long) develop for 3 to 10 days in conical cocoons attached to a substrate. Although the entire development can last only a few weeks in some species, it is much slower others, and the larvae can remain dormant for months if the temperature is too low for development.

### 2.3. Medical importance

The Ceratopogonidae rarely cause evident disturbance of the animals but on occasions they may attack in enormous swarms.[6] At least in people, their bites cause itching and welts that may last for several days in sensitized individuals. Some dermatitides of horses or sheep of apparently allergic etiology are commonly attributed to the bites of these flies.

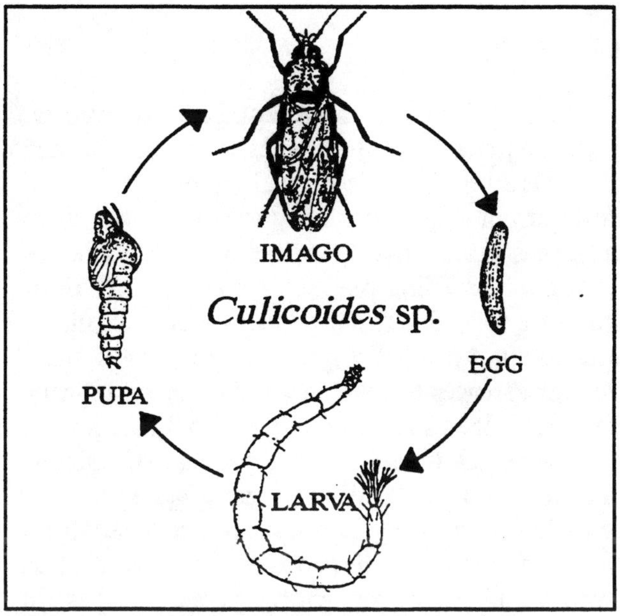


**Figure 7.6.** Life cycle of Ceratopogonidae.

Their major role as vectors is in the transmission of the blue tongue virus of cattle and sheep, and the African horse sickness virus. They may act as biological vectors of some filarial nematodes (see respective chapter) and are suspected as vectors of the Venezuelan equine encephalitis virus.[7]

## 3. THE PSYCHODIDAE OR SANDFLIES

### 3.1. Identification and classification

The Psychodidae important to medicine (Subfamily Phlebotominae), also called **sandflies**, are small (2-5 mm), brownish flies, with slender bodies, and quite long legs, antennae and palps. Their body and wings are covered with hairs what gives them the appearance of tiny, hairy mosquitoes (Figure 7.7). The females obtain blood by piercing the skin and tapping a capillary vessel. About 600 species of Psychodidae are hematophagous. About half of them belong to the genus *Lutzomyia* which is restricted to the American continent, and most of the remaining to the genera *Phlebotomus* and *Sergentomyia* which are found in the Old World. The Phlebotominae can be distinguished from other Psychodidae because they are less hairy and keep their wings erect rather than folded over the abdomen when at rest.

### 3.2. Biology

The Psychodidae of medical importance are distributed mainly in the tropical and subtropical zones. They are weak flyers that rarely venture too far away from their breeding places. They bite indoors or in deeply shaded places outdoors, and attack in the evening or at night, particularly when there is no wind. During the daylight, they hide in buildings, burrows, or thick vegetation. Many species feed on cold-blooded animals but others attack livestock or humans. They exhibit some host preference but it is not too strict.

The female lays batches of eggs in places that provide darkness, very high humidity, and organic matter to feed the larvae (stables, poultry houses, rodent burrows, dead leaves between stones in the woods, etc.). The eggs are ovoid, about 0.1 by 0.3-0.4 mm, and white when laid but become brown or black when they mature. They hatch in 6 to 17 days and produce whitish larvae that feed on decaying organic debris. The larva looks like a tiny caterpillar up to 6 mm long and pupate in 3 to 8 weeks. The inactive pupae give origin to the adults in about 10 days (Figure 7.7). The egg-to-egg cycle may require only 7 to 10 weeks but the larvae may enter in dormancy for up to several months when the temperature or humidity are too low.[8]

### 3.3. Medical importance

The Psychodidae are rarely considered as important hematophagous flies because they inflict a painless bite, remove only small amounts of blood, and are seldom seen since they usually attack by night. They are very important, however, as biological vectors of leishmaniases (see Trypanosomatidae). They are also vectors of the virus of the sandfly fever and of *Bartonella bacilliformis* of humans.

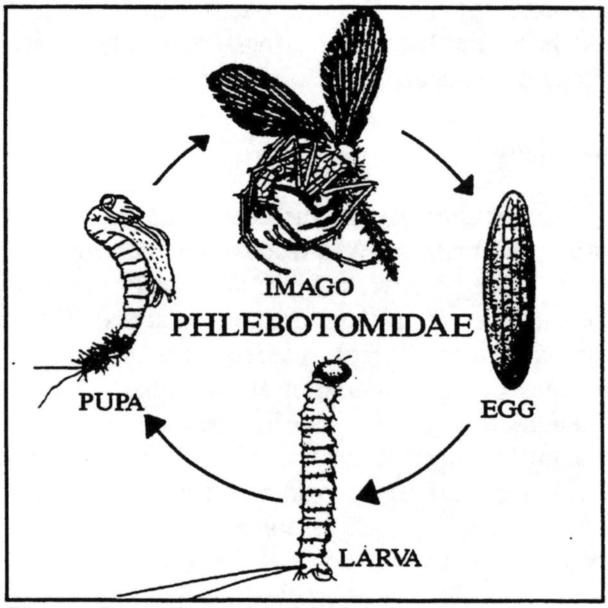


**Figure 7.7**. Life cycle of Phlebotomidae.

## 4. THE CULICIDAE OR MOSQUITOES

### 4.1. Identification and classification

The Culicidae, also called **mosquitoes**, are small to medium size (3-6 mm, few species larger) Nematocera with long legs and antennas, and mouth parts that form an elongated proboscis directed forward (Figure 7.8). The antenna are plumose (= feather-like) in the males and pilose (with tufts of hairs) in the females. The females obtain blood by piercing the skin and tapping a capillary vessel. Characteristically of the Culicidae, the veins and borders of their wings are covered with scales. The long proboscis and the scales on their wings are useful to distinguish the mosquitoes from other insects that may look alike. About 3,000 species of mosquitoes belonging to several genera have been described.[9] Because of their abundance and their role as vectors, the genera *Anopheles, Aedes,* and *Culex* are of particular importance. Plate V shows some characteristics of these three genera.

### 4.2. Biology

The Culicidae are truly cosmopolitan insects. They are found from the tropics to the Arctic, and from 1,160 m below sea level (in gold mines) to elevations of 4,300 m. They are not strong fliers but occasionally may be found at 40 or more km from their breeding places. Although most mosquitoes bite at dusk, many species do it at night, and others during daylight. Some species show clear preferences to feed on animals or on humans but others feed indiscriminately. All mosquitoes need water to develop but the range of habitats that are adequate to diverse mosquito species is remarkable, as long as they are protected from waves and wind. Collections of water as large as swamps, lakes, or sea shores or as small as tin cans, tree holes, or hoof prints are appropriate to some species. Clean, polluted, or black waters, fresh or salty water are suitable to others.

The females lay the eggs on water, either singly (e.g., *Anopheles* and *Aedes*), or glued together in a floating raft (e.g., *Culex* and *Culiseta*). Some

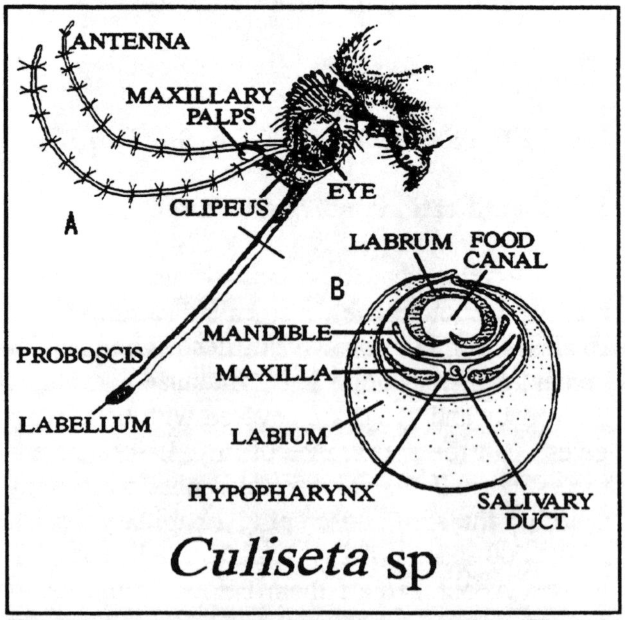


**Figure 7.8.** Lateral (A) and cross-section (B) view of the mouthparts of a mosquito (modified from Furman, 1961).

eggs have lateral floats (e.g., *Anopheles*). Although it varies depending on the species and the amount of blood ingested, each female lays about 50 to 150 eggs per oviposition, and repeats the oviposition at about two week intervals. Under ideal conditions the eggs hatch in 1 to 4 days but low temperatures may inhibit their development for a year or longer.

The larvae have a distinct head, thorax, and abdomen and, in many species, an air tube that arises from the caudal respiratory opening. They lie just under the surface of the water and move with a wiggling movement that has earned them the common name of **wigglers**. With optimal temperature and food supply, they develop in 1 to 3 weeks. The pupae consists of a capsular head and thorax with an air tube, and a coiled abdomen. They usually lie quietly underneath the surface but dart down with a tumbling motion when disturbed. They are commonly called **tumblers**. They develop in 2 or 3 days (Figure 7.9). The adult males live for about a week and need fecundate the females only once. The females live from about 2 weeks at maximum activity (summers or tropical zones) to up to 5 months at reduced activity or under hibernation. They rarely oviposit more than four times in their lives.

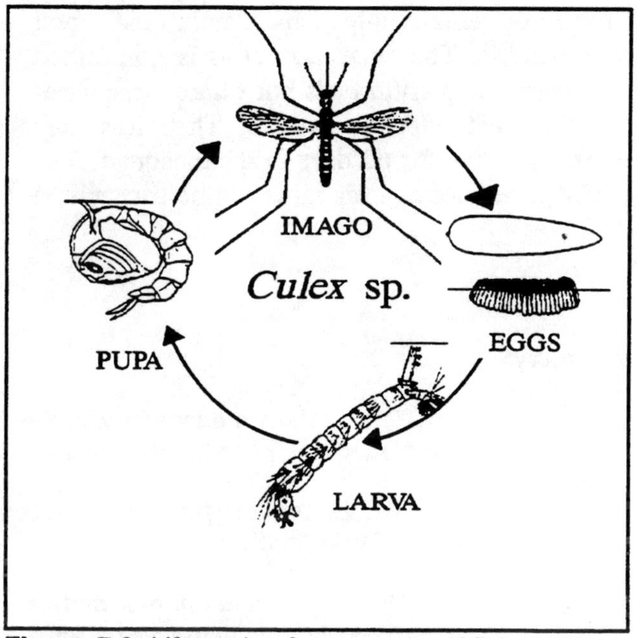


**Figure 7.9**. Life cycle of a mosquito (CDC, 1961).

### 4.3. Medical importance

The Culicidae are persistent pests that may greatly disturb the activities of humans or animals. Mosquitoes almost prevented the construction of the Panama canal and, in one study, reduced the weight of cattle by 21 kg (45.5 lb). Although each mosquito removes only a tiny amount of blood, there are reports of cattle killed by exsanguination due to mosquito attacks.

The bites of mosquitoes often produce cutaneous hypersensitivities in the same sequence described for fleas: delayed hypersensitivity first, and immediate hypersensitivity later. Spontaneous resolution of these allergies is rare.

Mosquitoes are particularly important as vectors of infections:

- *Anopheles* mosquitoes are the vectors of **mammalian malarias** (see Haemosporina),

- Several genera of mosquitoes are the biological vectors of **filarial nematodes** including *Dirofilaria immitis* of dogs (see Filarial Nematodes).

- About a hundred viruses that infect humans and/or domestic animals have been isolated from different species of mosquitoes. For example, *Aedes* mosquitoes transmit the viruses of the Eastern equine **encephalitis** and the **yellow fever**, *Aedes* and other genera transmit the viruses of the California group encephalitides, *Culex* mosquitoes transmit the viruses of the Japanese B and Saint Louis encephalitides, *Culex* an *Culiseta* transmit the virus of the Western equine encephalitis, *Culex* and other genera transmit the virus of the West Nile encephalitis, and many species transmit the virus of the Venezuelan equine encephalitis.

- Mosquitoes also transmit other viruses important to veterinary medicine such as those of the avian (fowl) pox, equine infectious anemia, and rabbit myxomatosis. The **avian pox** virus is transmitted by several biting arthropods but *Culex* mosquitoes are the most effective vectors. The virus may remain infective for 60 days in the mosquito. The **equine infectious anemia** virus can be transmitted mechanically by virtually any blood sucking arthropod. **Rabbit myxomatosis** can also be transmitted mechanically by almost any blood sucking arthropod but mosquitoes are the vectors most often implicated.

**Summary:**

1. The Diptera are insects with the first pair of wings well developed and the second pair replaced with knob-like structures (= halteres). All have a complete metamorphosis.

2. The Diptera of veterinary importance belong to the suborders Nematocera, Brachycera, and Cyclorrhapha.

3. The Nematocera are mall and delicate Diptera with antenna with more than six segments and usually long. In many species the females need a blood meal before sexual maturation and oviposition.

4. The Nematocera of veterinary importance belong to the families Simuliidae (black flies), Ceratopogonidae (biting midges), Psychodidae (sandflies), or Culicidae (mosquitoes).

5. All Nematocera need an aquatic or semiaquatic environment to breed: swiftly moving streams for the black flies, quiet waters for the biting midgets and mosquitoes, and wet soil for the sandflies.

6. The black flies attack in large swarms and mostly in daylight. They annoy the animals with their bites, may cause suffocation, draw blood, produce cutaneous allergies, inject a toxin, and transmit infections.

7. Most biting midgets attack at sunrise or sundown. Although their bites are painful and may produce cutaneous allergies, their major importance is as vectors of infections, particularly blue tongue.

8. The sandflies inflict painless bites and mostly by night. They are important because they transmit leishmaniases and other infections.

9. The mosquitoes are persistent pests that may attack in large swarms. They cause annoyance, draw blood, produce cutaneous allergies, and transmit important diseases (malaria, yellow fever, encephalitides, etc.).

## REFERENCES

1. Smith KGV (ed), 1973. Insects and other arthropods of medical significance. Br. Museum (Nat. Hist.), London, 561 pp.

2. Hunter DM and Moorhouse DE. 1976. The effect of *Austrosimulium pestilens* on the milk production of daily cattle. Austr. Vet. J. 52:97-99.

3. Beck BE. 1980. Clinical studies of the effect of the black fly *Simulium arcticum* on cattle. Tech. Rep. Pollut. Ctrl. Div., Alberta Environment, p. 233-237.

4. Noirtin C and Boiteux P. 1979. Death of 25 farm animals (including 24 cattle) attributed to the bites of Simuliidae (black flies) in the Vosges. Bull. Mens. Soc. Vet. Pract. France 63:41-54.

5. Steelman CD. 1976. Effect of external and internal arthropod parasites on domestic livestock production. Ann. Rev. Entomol. 21:155-178.

6. Nielsen BO and Christensen O. 1975. A mass attack by the biting midget *Culicoides nubeculosus* (Mg.) (Diptera, Ceratopogonidae) on grazing cattle in Denmark. Nord. Vet. Med. 27:365-372.

7. Jones RA, Porter HWJr and Rhodes HA. 1972. Ceratopogonidae attacking horses in south Texas during the 1971 VEE epidemic. Mosquito News 32:507-509.

8. Lewis DJ, 1974. The biology of Phlebotomidae in relation to leishmaniasis. Ann. Rev. Entomol. 19:363-384.

9. Knight KL and Stone A, 1977. A catalogue of the mosquitoes of the world (Diptera: Culicidae), 2nd ed., Entomol. Soc. America, 611 pp.

## PLATE V. CHARACTERISTICS OF THREE IMPORTANT GENERA OF MOSQUITOES

(K. S. Littig and J. Stojanovich)

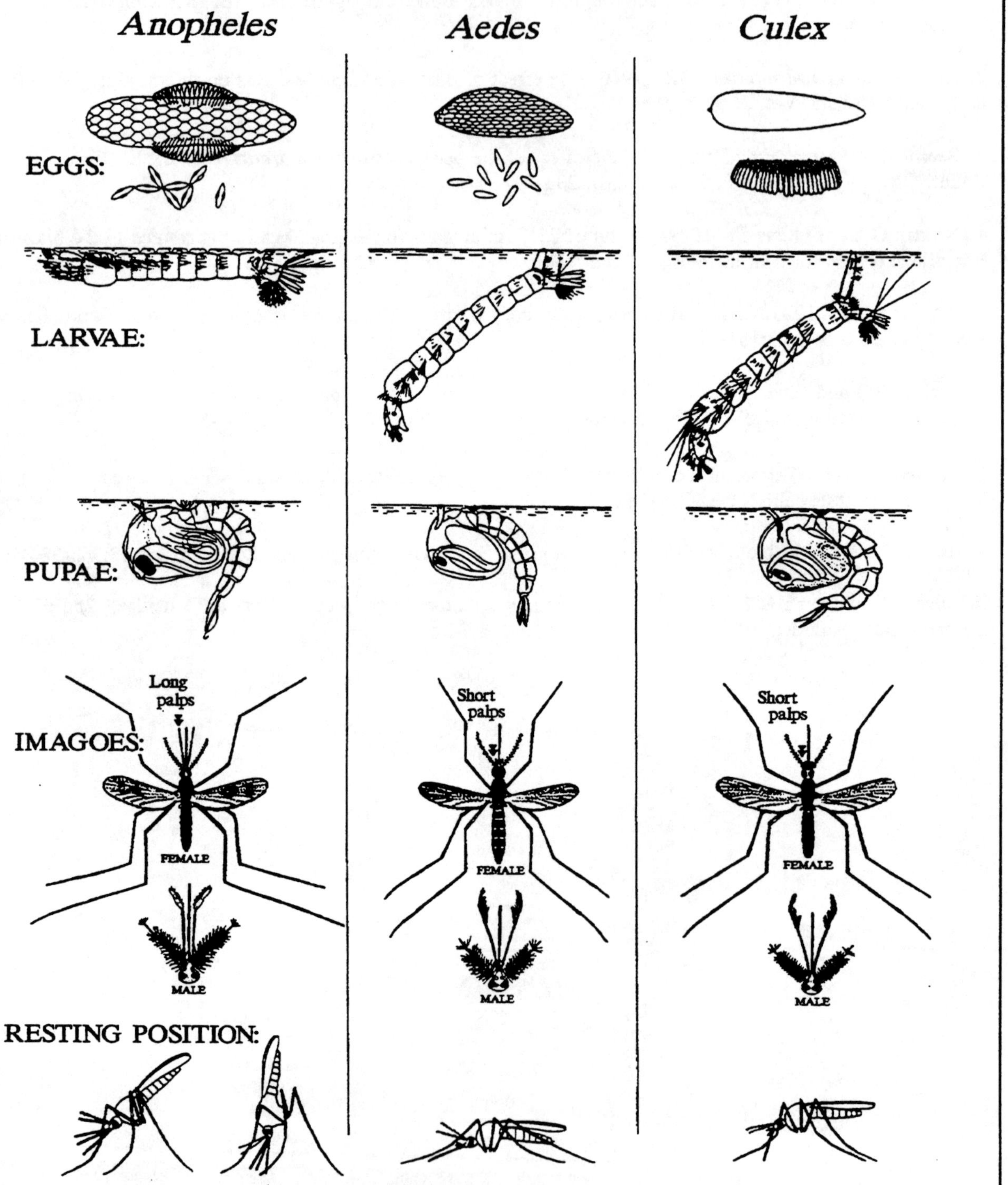


(Modified from the US Dpt. of Health, Education, and Welfare)

# CHAPTER 8

# THE SUBORDER BRACHYCERA: HORSE FLIES AND RELATIVES

**Preview.** The horse flies are robust, mostly dark flies the females of which cut the skin of mammalian hosts to adsorb blood. They develop slowly (about one generation per year) but the adults emerge synchronously so they may cause sudden outbreaks.

The horse flies are feared by the domestic animals, they inflict painful bites that draw abundant blood, and are mechanical vectors of a number of infections.

## 1. Identification and classification

The Brachycera (from G *brakhus* = short, *keron* = antenna) are stout, medium to large size flies. Only the family Tabanidae is important to medicine. Members of this family are commonly called **horse flies, deer flies, gad flies**, or **clegs**. They are robust flies, 8 to 25 mm long, and mostly dark. The tabanids are recognized because their antennae have three segments with the distal one bearing annulations (that make the antennae appear as having six to ten segments) but no arista (Figure 8.1) and because the R4 and R5 veins of their wings diverge and enclose the wing tip (Figure 8.2). The antennae are quite different from those of the nematocera or cyclorrhapha (Figure 7.3). The females have blade-like mandibles and maxillae that they thrust into the tissues with a scissorlike motion (Figure 8.3). A vast head that looks like a crescent when viewed from the dorsum, and large eyes (sometimes iridescent) that occupy most of the head are also very typical of the tabanids (Figure 8.4).

The tabanids comprise several dozens genera[1] with almost 4,200 species. The most common genera are:

a) *Tabanus* (**horse flies**): large to medium, black or gray, and stout flies. Their wings, uniformly clear or smoky, are held flat on the abdomen and separated in an inverted V when at rest. Their antennae are as shown in Figure 8.1. They are cosmopolitan.

b) *Chrysops* (**deer flies**): black or brown flies, about the size of the house fly. Their wings are held like in the *Tabanus* but bear a conspicuous dark transverse band. Their antennae are as shown in Figure 8.1. They are particularly common in the American continent.

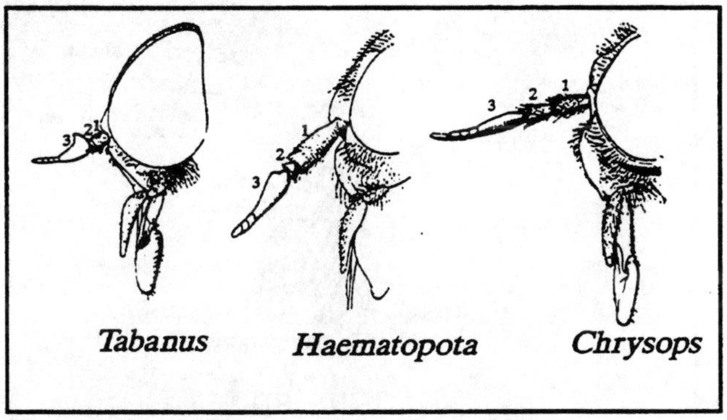


**Figure 8.1**. Antennae of the Tabanidae.

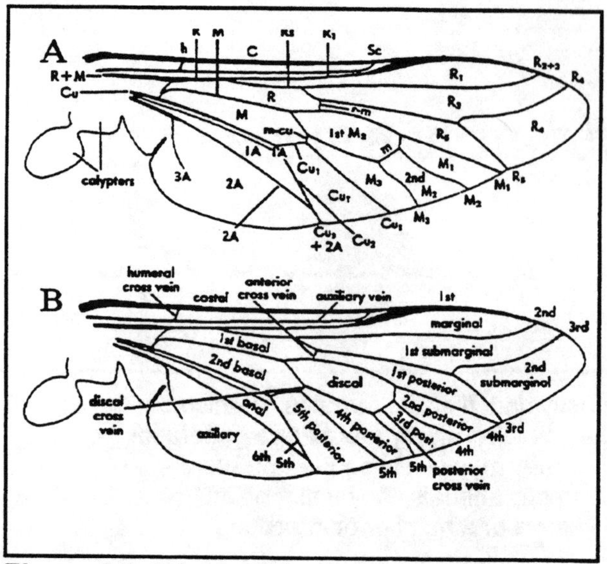


Figure 8.2. Wings of the Tabanidae showing the new (Comstock's, A) and the old (B) nomenclature of veins and cells (from Borror and Whilte, 1970).

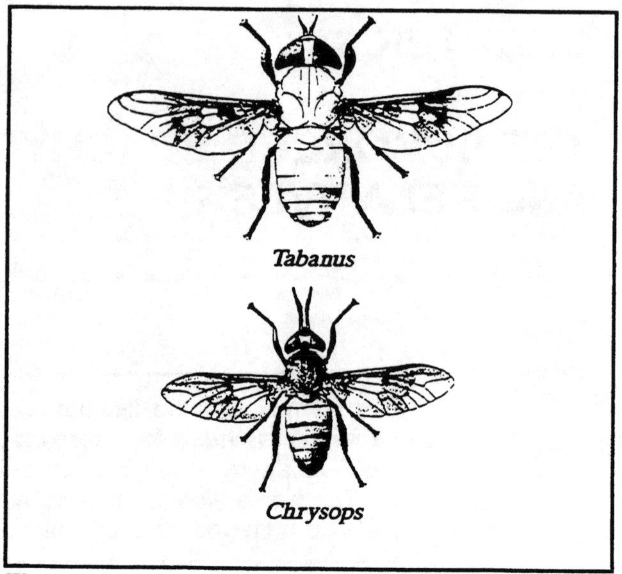


Figure 8.4. Females of *Tabanus* and *Chrysops*.

c) *Haematopota*: rather slender and medium size, dark grey flies. Their winds are held flat over the abdomen but overlapping, and are characteristically mottled grey. Their antennae are as shown in Figure 24. They are particularly common in Africa and the Orient.

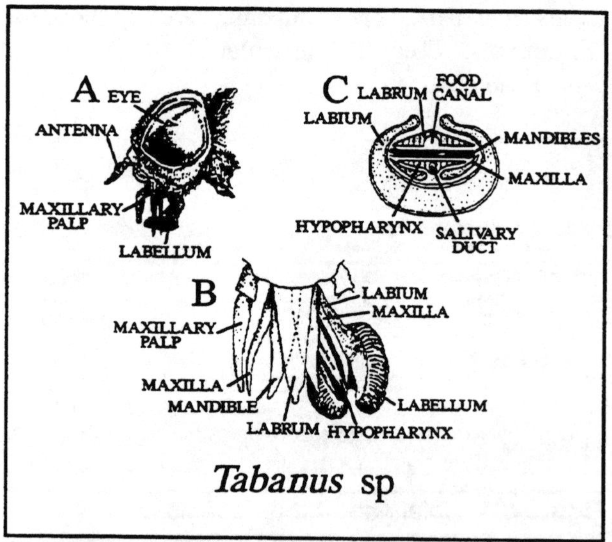


Figure 8.3. General (A), detailed (B), and cross section (C) views of the mouthparts of a horse fly (modified from Furman, 1961).

## 2. Biology

The females lay several hundreds eggs (1-2.5 mm long) at a time, in layered masses. Many species are aquatic or semi-aquatic and deposit their eggs on vegetation overhanging water or moist soil so that the larvae will fall into the proper environment when hatched. In other species, the larvae will grow in drained soil such as that of the forest floor. The time of incubation depends largely on weather conditions but the common range is 4 to 7 days in the summer.

Depending on the species, the larvae are found at the bottom of collections of water, buried in the mud, or in the soil of forest or pastures. In the aquatic or semi-aquatic species, the larvae moves to drier soil to pupate. In most species the larvae grow rapidly during summer and fall but remains dormant during the winter to pupate only during the next spring. The pupae commonly develop in 1 to 3 weeks. Most species, therefore, will produce only one generation per year. In a few species, the larvae will develop in 1 to 6 weeks so they can produce two generations per years. In still others, it takes 2 or 3 years to complete a single generation. It is not

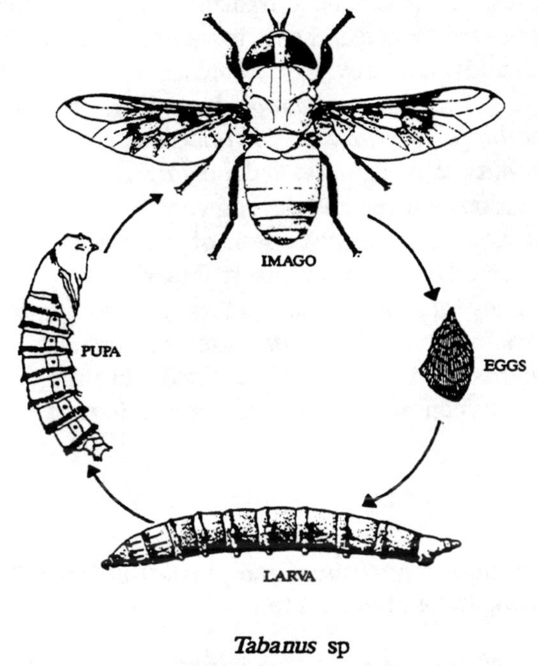


**Figure 8.5.** Life cycle of Tabanidae (from USDA).

clear whether these periods area characteristic of the species of tabanid or a response of the larvae to environmental conditions.

Like in the Nematocera, the adult Brachycera emerge from the pupal case through a straight or T-shaped break on the dorsal aspect, which explains the name Orthorrhapha (Gr *orthos* = straight, *rhaphes* = suture) under which the Nematocera and Brachycera are sometimes gathered. Emergence occurs in the morning and mating takes place shortly afterwards. The males feed on plants and die soon after mating. The females remain fertile for life but must feed on blood before each oviposition.

Emergence is fairly well synchronized for each species in a determined geographic area and the females are believed to remain active for not more than two months. Different species emerge at different times in the season, however, so tabanids may be a problem during the entire fly season (April to September in south-central United States). Most tabanids are active during the day and prefer the warmest hours. During the rest of the day, they relax in bushes, lower part of the trees, and on fences. They often follow moving objects, even cars.

*Tabanus* have a wide range of hosts with certain preference for large domestic animals over humans. *Chrysops* show preference for deer and humans, and *Haematopota* appear to prefer cattle. None of them is too restricted by their preferences, though.

### 3. Medical importance

The tabanids are important because they annoy the animals, cause cutaneous wounds, remove blood, and transmit pathogens.

The mere presence of a few tabanid flies in the vicinity of large animals is enough to disturb grazing. The hosts try to get rid of the pests by tail switching and head slinging which compounds interruption of feeding with expenditure of energy. When the flies are numerous, the animals may completely stop grazing and bunch together for protection, situation that may continue for several days at a time.

During feeding, the female tabanids produce painful cuts in the host's skin with their powerful mandibles and maxillae, and absorb the blood that flows. This leaves sizable wounds that keep ooz-ing blood for a while and attract other pests such as the screwworm, *Cochliomyia hominivorax*. Animals that underwent massive attacks may appear covered with blood. It has been calculated that a single large tabanid may take 0.36 ml of blood and that 320 specimens may feed on a single animal in an 8-hour period.[2] This represents more than 100 ml of blood taken, and possibly an equal or larger amount oozed from the wounds after the fly left.

It has been reported that the sustained attack by tabanids may cause a reduction of milk production of 66% in two weeks and almost 100% in three weeks, and a drop of body weight of 100 lb per cattle during massive outbreaks. Control of tabanids, on the other hand, has produced daily gains of 2.3 lb per head of beef cattle.[3] The US

Department of Agriculture estimated in 1976 that tabanids caused an annual loss of $ 25 million in cattle production.[4]

In addition to causing annoyance, wounds, and blood loss, the tabanids are particularly well adapted for transmission of pathogens.[5] Their obligatory hematophagia, the repeated cutting of the skin that permits the release of tissue parasites, and the large blood meal they take are all factors that facilitate the contact of the fly with pathogens. Furthermore, in part for habit and in part for the defensive movements of the host, the tabanids tend to feed on one animal for a short time and continue their meal on another animal. This **interrupted feeding** facilitates the mechanical transmission of pathogens from an infected host to a susceptible host. Tabanids are proven mechanical vectors of *Besnoitia besnoiti, Trypanosoma vivax, T. evansi, Bacillus anthracis, Francisella tularensis, Anaplasma marginale,* and the viruses of the equine infectious anemia and the hog cholera. Their role in the mechanical transmission of other organisms is suspected but solid proof is still lacking.

They are biological vectors of two important filarial nematodes (*Loa loa* of humans, and *Elaephora schneideri* of deer and other ruminants) and a trypanosome (*Trypanosoma theileri* of cattle).

**Summary**

1. The Brachycera important to veterinary medicine are robust and mostly dark flies. They are easily recognized by their typical wing venation and antennae.

2. Most species need aquatic or semi aquatic environments to breed, and produce only one generation per year.

3. The females have scissor-like buccal parts that cause painful bites and leave an oozing wound.

4. The tabanids attack during the warmest hours. Although the females of each species live only a couple of months, successive species may attack livestock during half the year.

5. The tabanids are feared by livestock which often stop grazing in their presence, inflict painful bites, draw important amounts of blood, and may act as mechanical vectors of a number of infections

## REFERENCES

1. Mackerras IM. 1954-1955. The classification and distribution of Tabanidae. Austr. J. Zool. 2:431-454; 3:439-511, 583-633.

2. Tashiro H and Schwardt HH. 1949. Biology of the major species of horse flies of central New York. J. Econom. Entomol. 42:269-272.

3. Steelman CD. 1976. Effects of external and internal arthropod parasites on domestic livestock production. Ann. Rev. Entomol. 21:155-178.

4. US Department of Agriculture. 1976. Control of insects affecting livestock. Nat. Res. Progr. Publication # 20,480, Agr. Res. Serv., Washington, DC.

5. Foil LD. 1989. Tabanids as vectors of disease agents. Parasitol. Today 5:88-96.

# CHAPTER 9

# THE SUBORDER CYCLORRHAPHA OR TRUE FLIES

**Preview**. The Cyclorrhapha of veterinary importance constitute five distinct groups. The non-biting Muscidae which annoy the host with their presence and constant activity and may transmit pathogens, the biting Muscidae which are hematophagous and may transmit pathogens, the Calliphoridae and Sarcophagidae the larvae of which develop in carrion and occasionally on living tissues, the Oestridae which are abligatory parasites at the larval stage, and the Hyppoboscidae which are obligatory parasites at the adult stage

The **Cyclorrhapha** (Gr *kuklos* = circle, *rhaphes*= suture, see below) are small to fairly large diptera with short antennae formed by three segments. The first segment is buried into a recess of the fly's head and the third segment hangs down (it is pendant) and bears a dorsal bristle (= arista) that is hairy in some species (Figures 7.3, 9.1, and 9.2). With one exception (*Melophagus ovinus*), all

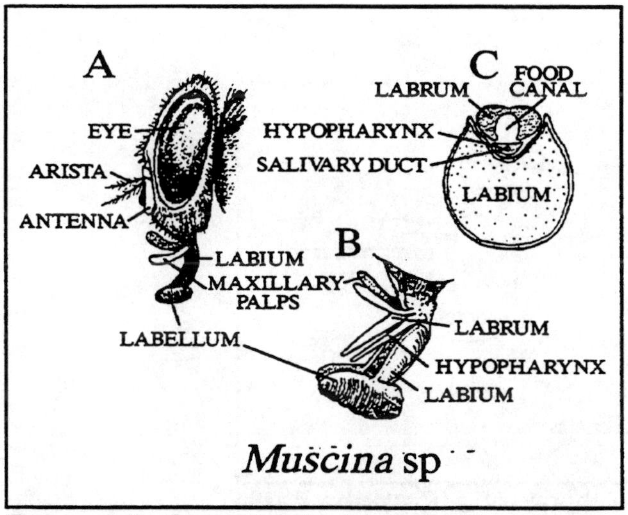


**Figure 9.1.** General (A), detailed (B) and cross section (C) view of the mouthparts of a non-biting Muscidae (modified from Furman, 1961).

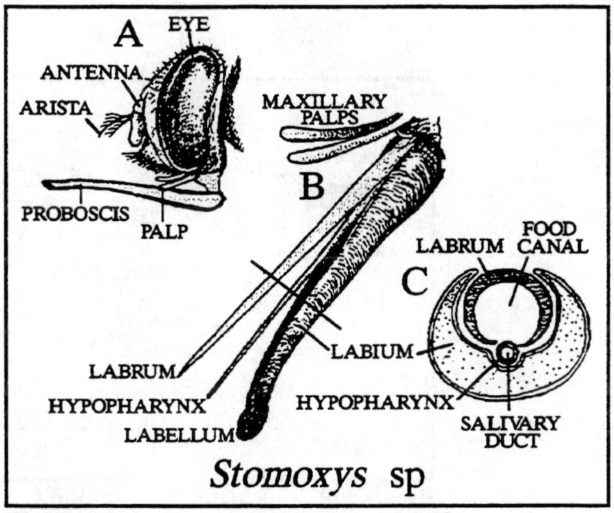


**Figure 9.2.** General (A), detailed (B), and cross section (C) view of the mouthparts of a biting Muscidae (modified from Furman, 1961).

species of veterinary importance are winged. Their mouthparts lack developed mandibles and maxillae and the remaining organs are variable depending on the feeding habits of the specific fly. In some species (e.g., the house fly, *Musca domestica*), the mouth is adapted to take liquid food and the soft labium ends in two expansions called labella (sing. labellum) that act as sponges (Figure 9.1). In others (e.g., the stable fly, *Stomoxys calcitrans*), the mouth is adapted to piercing the skin and sucking blood so the labium forms a long and hard proboscis (Figure 9.2). In still others (e.g., the horse bot flies, *Gasterophilus* spp.), the mouth parts are rudimentary and the adult fly does not eat.

The larvae are worm-like organisms with an evident external segmentation but without a distinct head (e.g., maggots, bots). They possess one or two hooks on the cephalic end that move vertically. These hooks possess a supporting cephaloskeleton the morphology of which is important for the identification of the species. Caudally the larvae end on a flat surface that bears two spiracles and is surrounded by tubercles. The morphology of the spiracles and tubercles is also important larval stage. The adults emerge by pushing out a for classification. Plate VI will assist in the identification of some important species.

The pupae are enclosed in a case (called **puparium**) formed by the hardened skin of the last circular opening at the anterior end of the puparium which earned the group the name of Cyclorrhapha.

The Cyclorrhapha is a very large group with more than 40 families and possibly 70,000 species. Although their typical antennae makes verification of the suborder easy, identification of families and genera is based on subtle details of thoracic and cephalic structures and wing venation (Figures 9.3 and 9.4) that are the province of the specialist. Furthermore, in many cases there is no consensus about number and extension of the diverse families. For our purposes, we will consider only five families of sufficient veterinary importance to merit individual discussion: the **Muscidae** or muscoid flies, the **Calliphoridae** or blow flies, the **Sarcophagidae** or flesh flies, the **Oestridae** or bot flies, and the **Hippoboscidae** or louse flies. They will be discussed individually.

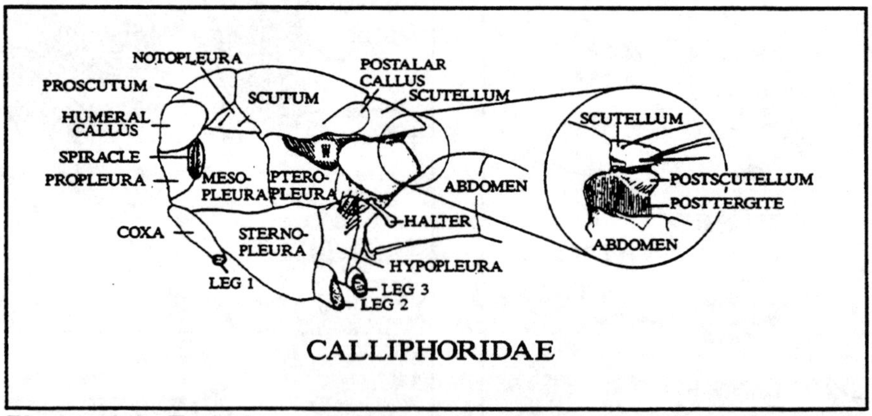


**Figure 9.3.** Typical morphology of the thorax of a Cyclorrhapha fly (modified from Smart, 1948).

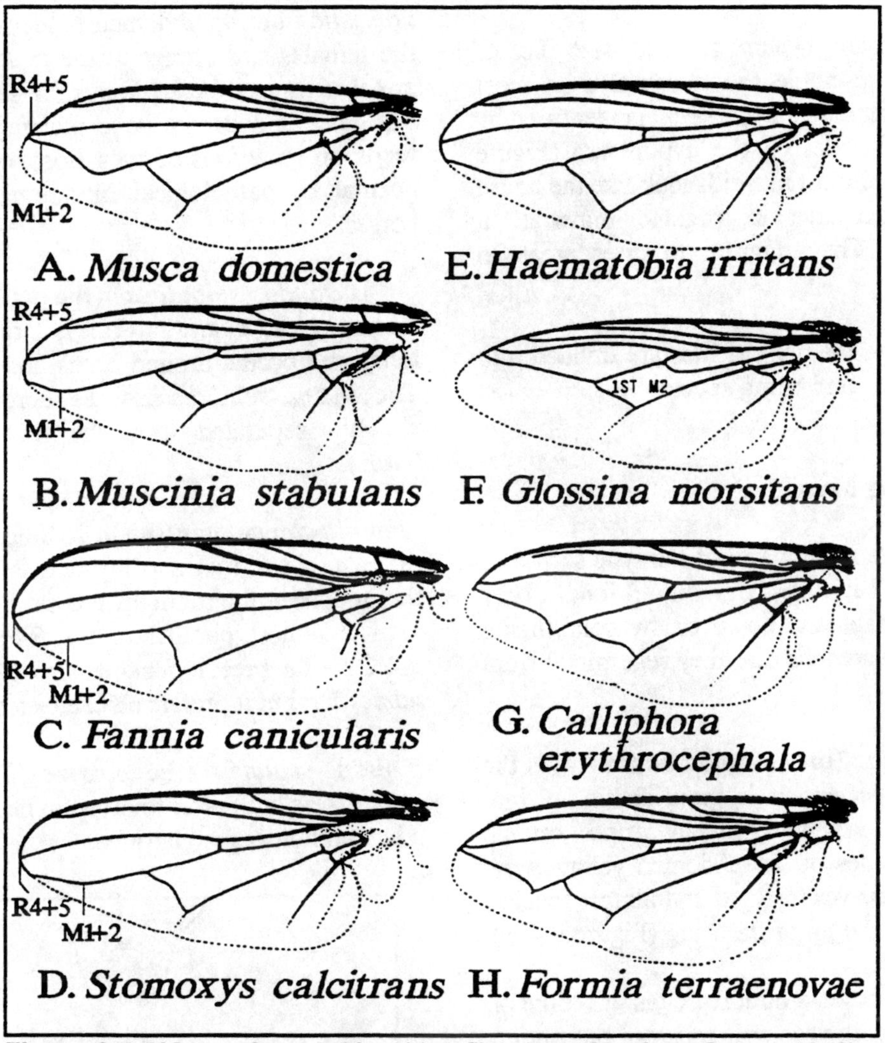


**Figure 9.4**. Wings of some Muscidae flies (modified from Smart, 1948).

## 1. THE MUSCIDAE OR MUSCOID FLIES

The Muscidae are medium to small size flies of dull color that resemble the house fly, its most common representative. This family is identified by the absence of bristles on the hypopleura (Figure 9.3). The larvae of most muscids look like the house fly maggots and live in organic material in decomposition. They migrate to drier areas to pupate.

Conventionally, the muscid flies are divided into non-biting species and biting species.

### a) The non-biting Muscidae

These flies have mouthparts of the type shown in Figures 9.1. and can ingest only liquid food. They may eat solid materials, however, by solubilizing them first with secretions that they regurgitate from their stomaches.

*Musca domestica* (**the common house fly**) is the most common species. It is grey, about 5-9 mm long, with four dark longitudinal stripes on the thorax and the sides of the abdomen yellow-grey. The M1+2 vein curves forward and almost touches the R4+5 vein at the tip of the wing (Figure 9.4.A).

The female lays over a hundred eggs at a time on any kind of decaying vegetable material but prefers fecal materials; horse manure first, and human excreta second. At optimal temperature (25-35C), the eggs hatch in 8-12 hours and the larvae develop through three instars in 4-11 days to reach 10-12 mm in length. The larvae move to drier parts and usually bury themselves in loose soil to pupate. The adults emerge in 4-28 days (Figure 9.5). The egg-to-adult cycle may take only 9-10 days at 30C but it takes 45 days at 16C.

The adult fly may live 1-2 months and lay up to 6 batches of eggs during her life. *M. domestica* is mostly, but not exclusively, an indoor fly that is often found in the house, barns, and stables. It is particularly attracted to human food but also to excrements and any kind of filth.

*Musca autumnalis* (**the face fly**) is similar to *M. domestica* but its abdomen is black on the sides in the females and orange in the males. The face fly appears to need host protein for sexual maturation but since it does not have piercing mouthparts, it feeds on secretions of eyes, nose, or wounds, or on normal or pathological discharges of cattle and horses.

*Muscinia stabulans* (**the false stable fly**) resembles *M. domestica* but is larger (7 to 10 mm long) and occurs around barns and farm-buildings. The M1+2 vein reaches the border of the wing widely separated from the R4+5 vein (Figure 9.4.B).

*Fannia canicularis* (**the little house fly**) is smaller than *M. domestica* and is often found hovering in the middle of the room, or around lights. Its M1+2 vein is almost parallel to the R4+5 vein (Figure 9.4.C). Its breeding habits are like those of *M. domestica* but it prefers chicken excrements.

*Fannia scalaris* (**the latrine fly**) is like *F. canicularis* but prefer to breed in humans excreta so it is common around latrines.

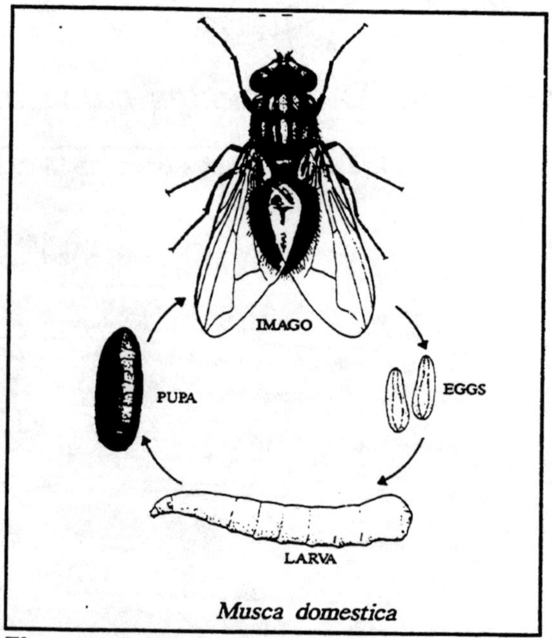


**Figure 9.5.** Life cycle of *Musca domestica*.

**b) The biting Muscidae**

These flies resemble *M. domestica* but have piercing mouth parts of the type shown in Figure 9.2. The probocis projects forward and is clearly visible. Unlike the Nematocera and Brachycera, in the biting Muscidae both males and females are bloodsuckers.

*Stomoxys calcitrans* (**the stable fly**, or biting house fly) is very similar to the house fly but can be differentiated from this by the presence of the forward projecting proboscis, and because the M1+2 vein reaches the tip of the wing well apart from the R4+5 vein (Figure 9.4.D). The proboscis is as long as the head but the palpi are only a fourth as long and scarcely visible. The arista of the antennae has hairs only on the dorsal side (Figure 9.2.)

The females require several blood meals before and between ovipositions. They lay about 25-50 eggs at a time on horse manure, manure of other animals if mixed with straw, or piles of well moist waste vegetables. Under appropriate circumstances, the eggs hatch in 2-5 days, the larvae pupate in 6-26 days, and the adults emerge 5-26 days later. The egg-to-adult cycle may take only 10 days at 30C, or over 2 months at 16C. The females live for about a month and can lay several hundreds eggs in this time. *S. calcitrans* is typically an outdoor fly but will enter buildings (including human dwellings) in bad weather.

*Haematobia irritans* (syn. *Lyperosia stimulans, Siphona irritans*) (**the horn fly**, about 5 mm long) is similar but smaller than S. calcitrans. Its proboscis is shorter, however, and its palps are nearly as long as the proboscis. It breeds preferentially in cattle manure.[1]

*Glossina* spp. (**tsetses**) are brownish, medium to fairly large (8-14 mm) flies, restricted to parts of Africa between the 15N and 15S parallels. They resemble *S. calcitrans* but have long palps that enclose the proboscis. The hairs of the arista that bear small secondary hairs (like a feather, Figure 9.6) and the first $M_2$ (or discal) cell that has the shape of a meat cleaver (Figure 9.4.F) are very characteristic of the genus *Glossina*.

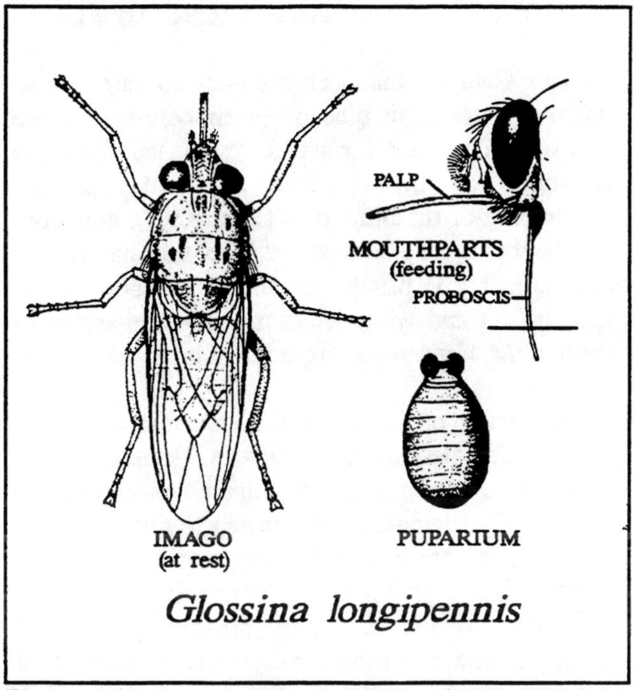


**Figure 9.6.** Imago and puparium of a tsetse, with details of the head (modified from Smart, 1948).

Tsetses are truly viviparous. The larvae are fed by secretions from uterine glands and are deposited when they are ready to pupate. The larva is cylindrical and have two posterior lobes that bear several hundred spiracles. These lobes persist in the pupae although the spiracles are closed in these (Figure 9.6). The adults emerge in 2-6 weeks. The females take a blood meal every 3-4 days and produce a single larvae every 10-20 days for a total of only 8-10 larvae.

Species of tsetses have rather strict requirements for the ecological environments where they can breed, rest, or feed. According to the habitats where they are found most often, tsetses are commonly divided into savanna species (*morsitans* group), forest species (*fusca* group), and riverine species (*palpalis* group). The host specificity of some species is so strict that the fly disappears when its host is removed.

## 2. THE CALLIPHORIDAE OR BLOW FLIES

The Calliphoridae are medium to large flies, usually of metallic blue or green colors (but see below). They are further distinguished from the Muscidae by the presence of bristles on the hypopleura of the blow flies (Figure 9.3), and from the Sarcophagidae because the blow flies have 2 (or, occasionally, 3) bristles on the notopleura. Their mouthparts and wing venation are comparable to those of *M. domestica* (Figure 9.1 and 9.4.A).

The larvae of the calliphorids are carrion eaters and the females lay their eggs in carcasses, meat products, or refuse containing scraps of animal tissues. The females are attracted to the secretions of wounds or inflamed skin and occasionally deposit their eggs on living tissues. In the absence of their favorite breeding medium, they will oviposit, and the larvae will grow, in excreta of humans or other animals, or in vegetable materials in decomposition. The eggs hatch rapidly (6 to 48 hours) and the larvae develop completely in 3-15 days. At that time they are 10-15 mm long and resemble the larvae of *M. domestica*. They drop to the ground and bury themselves until the adults emerge after 3-7 days under optimal conditions. In cold weather, they may hibernate at the pupal stage.

The most common of the many calliphorids described are the following:

*Calliphora* spp. and *Cynomyopsis* spp., **the bluebottle flies**,

*Lucilia* (syn. *Phoenicia*) spp., the **green** and **cupreous greenbottle flies**,

*Phormia* spp., the **black blow flies**, with blue-green reflections,

*Cochliomyia hominivorax* (also called *C. americana* or assigned to the genus *Callitroga* ), and *C. macellaria*, the **primary** and **secondary screwworm flies**, respectively. These are bluish-green flies, 10-15 mm long, with an orange face and three longitudinal dark stripes on the thorax. They are restricted to the American continent. Differentiation of the adults of both species is a task for the specialist.

Whereas *C. macellaria* is a scavenger like the other calliphorids, *C. hominivorax* is an obligatory parasite of warm-blooded animals. The females of *C. hominivorax* are attracted to wounds as small as the bite of a mosquito. In a few minutes they lay batches of up to a couple of hundred eggs in the wound or next to it, for a total of about 3,000 in their lives. Eclosion occurs in less than 24 hours. The larvae penetrate the tissues and eat from them for 4-8 days. They then drop to the ground to pupate and the adults emerge in about a week.

*Chrysomya bezziana* and *C. megacephala* of Africa and southern Asia are very similar in morphology and habits to *C. hominivorax* and *C. macellaria*, respectively, but they do not have the dark stripes on the thorax.

*Cordylobia anthropophaga* (the Tumbu fly or **mango fly**) and *Auchmeromyia luteola* (the **Congo floor maggot**) are non-metallic, dull yellow flies of Africa, that parasitize humans and, occa-sionally, rodents and pigs. In both cases the eggs and larvae are found on the ground. The larvae of *C. anthropophaga* invade the skin but those of *A. luteola* are only temporary bloodsuckers.

## 3. THE SARCOPHAGIDAE OR FLESH FLIES

The Sarcophagidae are medium to large size (10-14 mm long) flies of mate grey color, with three dark longitudinal stripes on the thorax and dark spots on the abdomen. They can be further separated from the Muscidae because the flesh flies have bristles on the hypopleura, and from the Calliphoridae because the Sarcophagidae have 4 bristles on the notopleura.

The sarcophagids are ovoviviparous so they lay a small number of larvae at a time rather than eggs. The larvae, that may reach 17-18 mm, live in and feed on the same materials that support the calliphorid larvae. Like these, they occasionally invade living tissues. The genus *Sarcophaga* have a checkered pattern on the abdomen that changes with the direction of the incident light. The genus *Wohlfahrtia* have black spots on the abdomen that do not change with the light. *W. vigil* of northern United States and Canada invades the healthy skin of rodents, carnivores, and humans.

## 4. THE OESTRIDAE OR BOT FLIES

Entomologists often arrange these flies into three or more families. From the veterinary point of view, it is more convenient to gather them in a single group.

The oestridae are robust and hairy flies that remind one of a bee. They are so highly specialized for parasitism *at the larval stage* that the adults have rudimentary mouthparts, often reduced to a single opening, and most of them do not feed.[2] Because the adults of most species live only a few days, they are rarely seen. The study of their larvae (bots, grubs), collected from infected animals, permits the identification of the insulting species.

The oestrids usually lay their eggs (larvae in the case of *Oestrus ovis*) on the hairs of the host, or in places where the emerging larva can reach the host, in late spring or early summer. In most cases, development of the larvae in the host's tissues proceeds for 8-10 months until they drop to pupate in the ground during the next spring. The new generation of adult emerges about a month later.

*Gasterophilus intestinalis* (**the horse bot fly**, 14 mm long and light brown), *G. nasalis* (**the throat bot fly**, 13 mm long and rusty yellow), and *G. haemorrhoidalis* (the **nose bot fly**, 10 mm long and black with yellow and orange bands) are the common bot flies of equines. Other species exist. The abdomen of the females in prolonged in a narrow and long ovipositor.

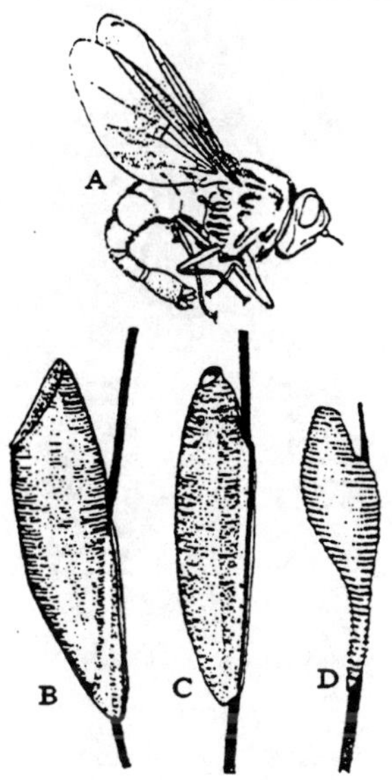


*Gasterophilus* spp

**Figure 9.7**. A female of Gastrophilus (A) with eggs of *G. intestinalis* (B), *G. nasalis* (C), and *G. haemorrhoidalis (D)* (modified from Cameron, 1942).

The eggs (1.3-1.5 mm long, Figure 9.7) are attached to the hairs singly, close to the tip, and parallel to the hair. They have clasps, as long or longer that half the length of the egg, that fit the hair like a muff. The eggs of *G. intestinalis* are attached mostly to the hairs of the forelegs, those of *G. nasalis* to the throat between the jaws, and those of *G. haemorrhoidalis* around the mouth and cheeks. The eggs of *G. nasalis* and *G. haemorrhoidalis* hatch spontaneously in 2-6 days but those of *G. intestinalis* require stimulation by the moisture and warmth of the host's tongue to hatch. By crawling or being taken with the tongue of the host, the larvae reach the host's mouth and penetrate the oral mucosa where they wander for 3-4 weeks, moult, and initiate a mucosal migration down the esophagus to the stomach. Once there, they emerge into the lumen, attach with their cephalic hooks to the mucosa of the stomach or, occasionally, the duodenum, and develop to the third instar. They release their hold and pass with

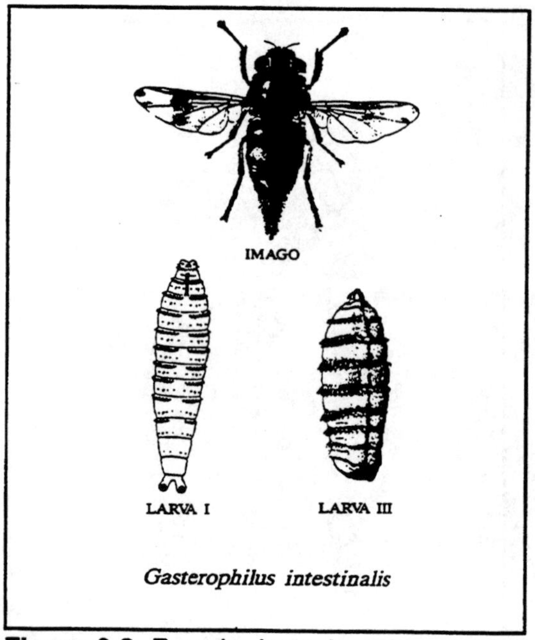


**Figure 9.8**. Female, larva I, and larva III of *Gasterophilus intestinalis*.

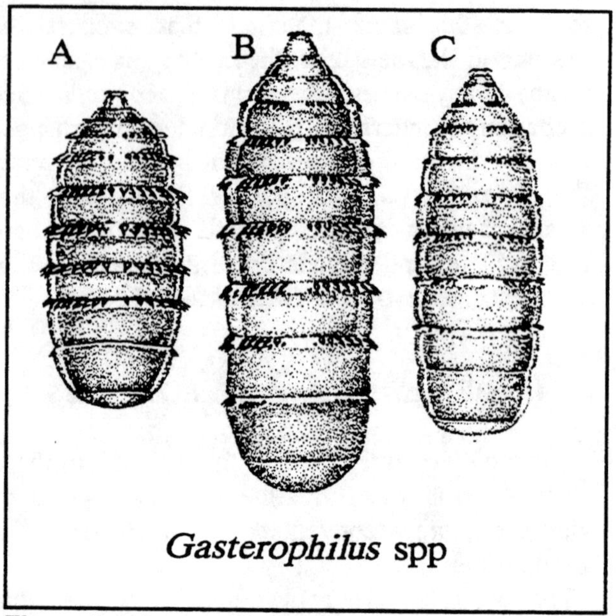


**Figure 9.9.** Larvae III of *Gasterophilus nasalis* (A), *G. intestinalis* (B), and *G. haemorrhoidalis* (C) (from Cameron, 1942)

the feces in late spring or early summer to pupate in the ground for 3-4 weeks (Figure 9.8).

The young larvae in the stomach are yellow to red but the old larvae that pass in the feces are brown and have a number of spines that assist in their identification. *G. haemorrhoidalis* has a double row of pointed spines in all segments except the last two ones, *G. nasalis* has a single row of spines in all segments except the last one, *G. intestinalis* has a double row of blunt-tipped spines in all segmetns except the last one (Figure 9.9).

*Hypoderma lineatum* (**the common cattle grub**, about 13 mm long) and *H. bovis* (**the northern cattle grub**, about 15 mm long) are the most common cattle bot flies, warble flies, or cattle grubs. They are also called heel flies. Other species have a more restricted distribution. They are black with bands of yellow or orange hairs. Occasionally they may infect horses.

The female attaches a row of 5-15 eggs (*H. lineatum*) or a single egg (*H. bovis*) near the base of the host's hairs in late spring or early summer. The eggs are ovoid (about 0.8 x 0.2-0.3 mm), disposed at a 45° angle to the hair, and set by one end on a short stalk of gluing material (Figure 9.10). A larva emerges in 3-6 days, penetrates the skin in a couple of hours, and wanders through the connective tissue until reaching the wall of the esophagus (*H. lineatum*) or the neural canal (*H. bovis*) in late fall or early winter. Shortly afterwards, the larvae migrate to the skin of the back, cut a breathing hole through the skin to the outside, and moult to the second instar. About a month later, a new moult produces a third instar larva that becomes dark with age and forces its way through the hole to drop to the ground in late winter or early spring. The mature larvae may reach 25-28 mm in length (Fgure 9.11). The inflammatory lesions caused by the larvae under the skin are commonly called warbles. Pupation lasts 20-40 days.

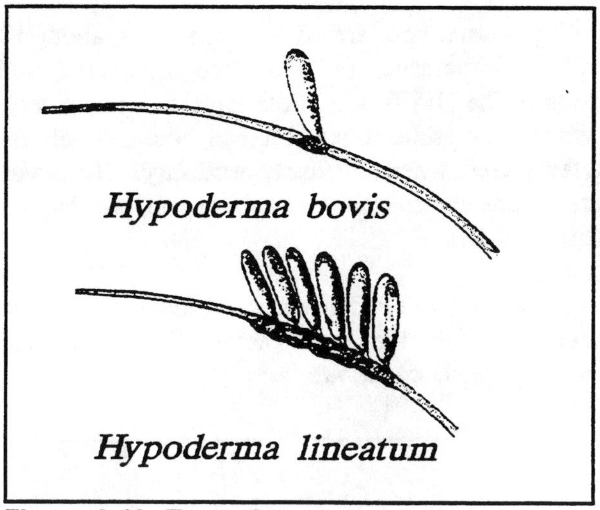


**Figure 9.10.** Eggs of *Hypoderma* spp.

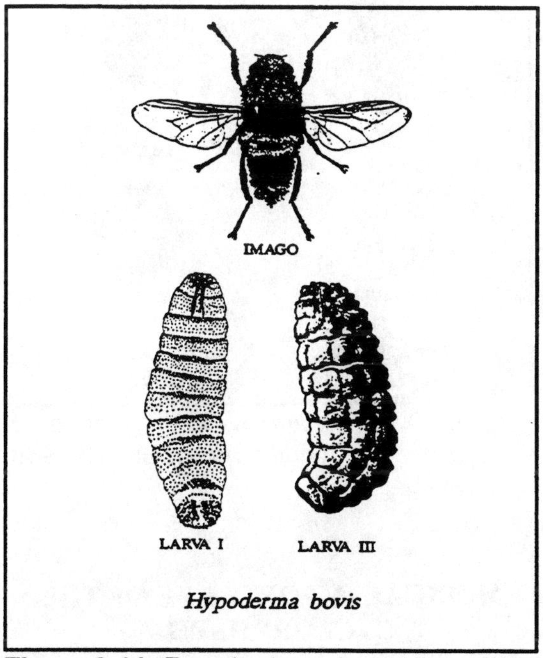


**Figure 9.11.** Female, larva I, and larva III of *Hypoderma bovis* (modified from Smart, 1948).

*Oestrus ovis* is the common **nasal bot fly of sheep**. It may occasionally infect goats. This fly is somewhat smaller (10-12 mm long) and less hairy than the cattle and horse bot flies. It also lives longer than the other blow flies; up to 28 days. The head and thorax are light brown and the abdomen silvery black.

The female is ovoviviparous and deposits her larvae in or near the nostrils of sheep. The larvae move up to the nasal and frontal sinuses, attach to the mucosa, and develop to a third instar larvae in 8-10 months (Figure 9.12). Larvae deposited in early summer in tropical areas may mature in one month and, by exception, two generations may occur in a year. In the spring, the mature larvae (20-25 mm long) work their way out through the nostrils (or are sneezed out), fall to the ground, and pupate rapidly. Pupation lasts 3-6 weeks, or longer in cold weather.

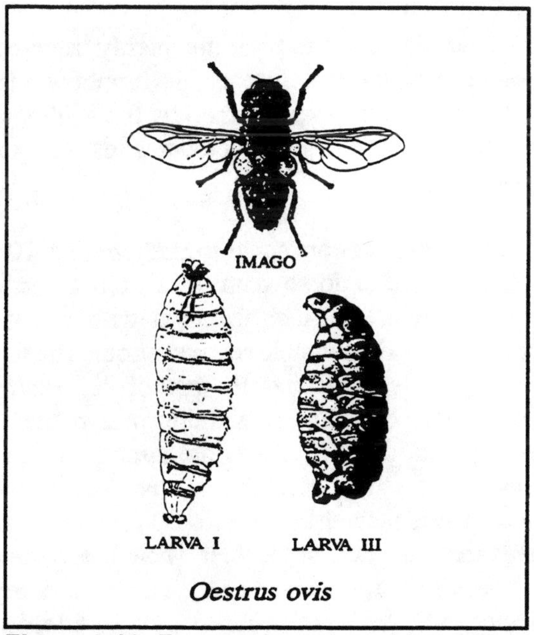


**Figure 9.12.** Female, larva I, and larva III of *Oestrus ovis* (modified from Smart, 1948).

*Rhinocephalus purpureus* is the nasal bot fly of horses in the Old World.

*Cuterebra* spp. are the **bot flies of rodents** or warble flies of rodents and are restricted to North America. These are large (20 mm long), little hairy, black or blue flies that deposit their eggs near their host burrows. The larvae penetrate their host through the natural openings and after a tissue migration appear under the skin of the neck or head. They affect rodents, lagomorphs, domestic carnivores, and occasionally humans. The larvae develop in 3-8 weeks and the pupae overwinter.

*Dermatobia hominis* **(the neotropical warble fly)** is a blue fly, 12 mm long, restricted to Latin America. Although it is called the **bot fly of man**, it causes serious losses in cattle[3] and also infests pigs, horses, carnivores, rodents, and even birds. Because the fly inhabits the forest, her larvae reach their hosts through a carrier (see page 2). The larva does not migrate upon penetration, and matures in 5-10 weeks. Pupation lasts about 2-3 months.

## 5. THE HIPPOBOSCIDAE OR LOUSE FLIES

While the oestrid flies are highly adapted to parasitism by the larval stages, the hippoboscids are highly specialized to parasitism by the adult stages. All are hematophagous ectoparasites of warm-blooded vertebrates.

The hippoboscids are small to medium (2.5-10 mm long) flies with a dorso-ventrally flattened head and thorax, and a sack-like abdomen with a leathery integument and no visible segmentation. The mouth has a proboscis similar to that of *S. calcitrans* (Figure 9.2) but that is withdrawn into the head when not in use. The legs are strong and widely separated at their insertion in the thorax which makes them resemble a louse. Some species have wings that may persist for their whole life, or be cast off when they reach their host. The most common species of veterinary importance, *Melophagus ovinus*, lacks wings and halteres. Like the tsetses, the hippoboscids are truly viviparous since they feed their larvae with uterine secretions. Larviposition occurs when the larva is ready to pupate.

*Melophagus ovinus* **(the sheep ked)** is a reddish-brown, wingless fly, 4-6 mm long, that is often confused with a tick or a louse. It spends all its life on its host and the female glues the larvae to the wool where they pupate in a few hours. The pupa is brown, broadly ovoid, and 3-4 mm long (Figure 9.12). The adults emerge in 3-6weeks. After 2-4 weeks, the females start laying one larvae every 10-12 days for a total of 10-15 larvae during their 4 months of life. Off the host, the adults survive for only 2-8 days.

*Hippobosca* spp. are rusty brown flies, about 10 mm long, parasites of cattle, camels, horses, and dogs in the Old World. Although they retain their wings, they prefer to stay on their host and only fly a few meters when absolutely necessary. The larvae are deposited in sheltered places on the ground (Figure 9.13).

*Pseudolynchia canariensis* is a brown louse fly of pigeons and the biological vector of the protozoan, *Haemoproteus columbae*.

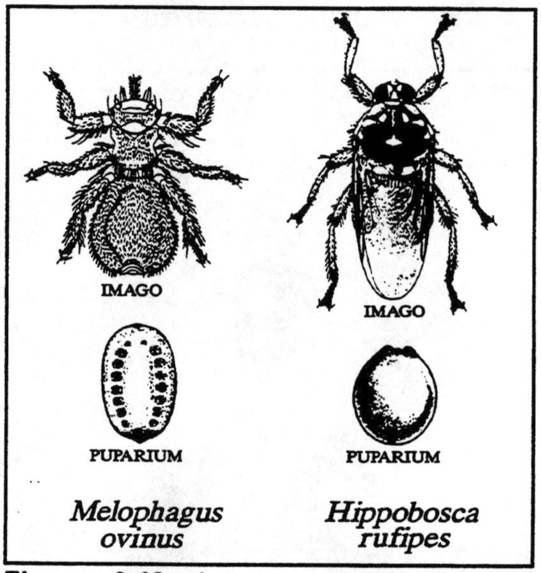


**Figure 9.13.** Imagoes and puparia of Hippoboscidae (modified from Smart, 1948, and Lapage, 1956).

## MEDICAL IMPORTANCE OF THE CYCLORRHAPHA

The Cyclorrhapha are a source of concern because they annoy the grazing animals, bite them, remove blood, parasitize their tissues, and transmit a number of infections.

### A. Annoyance

All cyclorrhapha produce annoyance. It is surprising to see the fright with which livestock respond to the approach of the bot flies, despite the fact that oviposition or larviposition by these flies must be painless for the host. The best example of annoyance due exclusively to the presence of a fly is *Musca autumnalis*, the face fly, that is very persistent but lacks structures to bite the host. The U.S. Department of Agriculture has estimated that this fly produced annual losses of $ 140 millions to the cattle industry and $ 5 million to the pig industry between 1973 and 1975.[4] Reductions of milk production of 25% and of weight gain of 114 g per day have been reported. These losses may include, however, the effect of a keratoconjunctivitis that *M. autumnalis* contributes to transmit mechanically.

**B. Bites**

Because of the annoyance caused by their persistence around the host, their painful bites, and the removal of blood, *Stomoxys calcitrans, Haematobia irritans,* and other biting flies are a source of major losses.

*S. calcitrans* feeds 2-3 times a day, during daylight, and rests off the host when not feeding. The presence of more than 25 flies per animal per day already begins to produce economic effects. Under severe attack, milk production may drop by 40-60% and weight gain by 10-15%. The annual losses have been estimated in $ 398 million per year.[5]

*H. irritans* attacks in large swarms, feeds 24-38 times a day, during the 24 hours, and persists near the host almost constantly. Consequently, it is more harmful than *S. calcitrans*. A single fly may take 0.5-2.0 mg of blood per meal so 5,000 flies (a large but not exceptional number) can removed 50-380 ml of blood per day. Annual losses by *H. irritans* have been estimated in $ 730 million per year.

Like with the lice, the population of *Melophagus ovinus* peaks on the host in winter. The bites and activity of these highly mobile flies produce irritation of the skin and causes the sheep to rub and bite its skin which diminishes the quality of the fleece. The feces of the fly, loaded with digested blood, stain the wool permanently which also reduces its price. Repeated bites produce small, firm, pimple-like nodules that reduce the price of the sheep skins. This condition is known as **cockle**.

When many keds are present (592 per sheep or 363 per lamb, but not with 150 per sheep or 61 per lamb), the host may develop anemia. The infection of lambs with 225 keds from fall to spring reduced carcass weight by 10%, clean wool yield by 20%, and market value of the skins by 18%.[6]

**C. Invasion of tissues by larvae (myiases)**

The blowflies and flesh flies are important because they may infest living tissues with their larvae (= **myiases**). Most blow flies lay their eggs in carcasses and only accidentally infest living tissues,when they are attracted by the secretions of wounds or inflamed skin (**accidental myiases**). *Lucilia* spp. are particularly attracted to oviposit in soiled or wet wool (particularly with feces or urine), or wool with bacterial or fungal growths. They are the primary agents of sheep myiasis or strike. The larvae may remain in the fleece (wool maggots) damaging only the wool, but may also take advantage of minor skin abrasions to invade the tissues. Sheep strike by *L. cuprina* caused $ 41 million in losses in Australia in 1974-75.

Species that require living tissues to breed (like *C. hominivorax* and the oestrids) are the agents of **obligatory myiases**. Obligatory myiases of the skin is a major problem not only because of the annoyance by the adult fly and the wounds by the lavae but also because the secretions of the wound invaded with maggots attract other flies that disturb the animal and may deposit new eggs. Secondary bacterial infections are also common in small ruminants and horses. Animals with cu-taneous myiases that remain untreated for more than two weeks during the fly season often die. A successful campaign of eradication of *C. hominivorax* from the southeast of the United States in 1958-59 cost $ 10 million but it saved annual losses of $ 20 million to the local cattle industry.

Identification of the insulting species is important when repeated instances of cutaneous myiases are found since the significance and strategy for control of accidental myiases is quite different from those of obligatory myiases. Plate VI will assist in this task.

The penetration of *Hypoderma* larvae in the skin causes a painful puncture that becomes inflamed and exudes serum. In severe infections, the larvae in the esophagus or neural canal may cause esophagitis or paralysis and other nervous disorders. The larvae that return to the skin of the back produce a large focus of subcutaneous inflammation that soon develops into a fibrotic cyst that encloses the larva (= **warble**). These cysts are firm and raised over the skin level and crowned by a breathing hole of up to 3-4 mm in diameter. More than 300 warbles have been found in a single animal. When secondarily infected, they may turn into suppurating abscesses. Emergence of the mature larvae is followed by normal healing. If large, the resulting connective tissue scar may fall off during the industrial processing of the hides. Infection by *Hypoderma* is lighter in older animals, presumably by development of immune resistance.

Experimental infections with *Gasterophilus haemorrhoidalis* have caused severe discomfort to horses during its migration in the oral cavity. The same effect is presumed for the other *Gasterophilus* species. The gastric infection is commonly assumed to be apathogenic although the mature larvae produce deep craters in the mucosa with their cephalic hooks, and the presence of a few hundred larvae is not uncommon. Some authors have found gastritis, ulceration, peritonitis, colic, blockage and rupture of the stomach, or esophageal paralysis in heavy infections.[7] The mature larvae of *G. haemorrhoidalis* attach to the rectum before passing outside. Heavy infections have caused proctitis with rectal prolapse in zebras. Presumably, the same may occur in horses.

The damage caused by *Oestrus ovis* depends on the size of the nasal cavities of the host, the size of the larvae (2 mm long for the hatching first larva to 25 mm long for the mature third larva), and the number of larvae. In most infections, there are only about 10 or fewer larvae but cases have been reported with several hundreds. In severe infections the larvae produce a rhinitis with a profuse discharge and sneezing. Continuous activity of the parasites causes a thickening of the mucosa with impairment of breathing. Large larvae that die in the sinuses may induce a purulent inflammation that occasionally involves the brain. Infections in lambs have been reported to produce reduction of weight gain of as much as 4%.

*Cuterebra* infections are occasionally seen by the veterinarian as a growing subcutaneous cyst in the neck or chest of dogs or cats. It causes evident discomfort to the host who licks it or bites it constantly. Left to itself, it usually opens as a suppurating abscess.

### D. Transmission of pathogens

Because of its habit of visiting human food and any kind of filth, *Musca domestica* is a major mechanical transporter of pathogens on its body and its digestive tract. The practice of regurgitating digestive content to solubilize solid food facilitates the contamination of human foodstuff. One to 6 million bacteria have been recovered from the body of a single *M. domestica* and more than 100 different pathogens, including viruses, bacteria, protozoan cysts, and helminth eggs, are known to be carried by it.[8]

Although the significance of the house fly as a vector is mostly based on circumstantial evidence and has been study in regard to human infections, flies with similar habits may be significant in the transmission of infections of veterinary impor-tance. *Fannia canicularis*, for example, transmits by contamination the virus of New Castle disease, and *Musca autumnalis* transmits *Moraxella bovis*, the agent of the infectious keratoconjunctivitis (pink-eye) of cattle.

Mechanical transmission of pathogens that are present in the blood is also facilitated by hematophagia. *Stomoxys calcitrans* is known to transmit *Trypanosoma evansi* and *Trypanosoma vivax*, *Bacillus anthracis*, *Brucella* spp., and the virus of the equine infectious anemia. Its role may be less important than that of the tabanids but still may be substantial.

A number of flies are biological vector or intermediate hosts of parasites. For example, *Fannia* sp. and *Musca* spp. for *Thelazia* spp., *Haematobia irritans* for *Stephanofilaria stilesi*,

*Melophagus ovinus* for *Trypanosoma melophagium*, *Musca domestica* for *Habronema* spp., and *Stomoxys calcitrans* for *Habronema microstoma*. By far, however, the most important biological vector among the cyclorrhapha are the tsetses. Transmission of animal trypanosomes negates the full use of about 10 million $km^2$ (4 million square miles) of African land that could otherwise sustain 125 million cattle. The losses are estimated in $ 5 billion per year. They also transmit human trypanosomes that, despite constant decline, still kill 10,000 people per year in Africa.

**Summary**

1. The Cyclorrhapha flies are recognized for the presence of a three-segmented antenna, the distal segment of which is pendant and carries an arista.

2. There are five families of Cyclorrhapha of veterinary importance: Muscidae, Calliphoridae, Sarcophagidae, Oestridae, and Hippoboscidae.

3. The Muscidae resemble the house fly and are recognized by the absence of bristles on the hypopleura. Their larvae develop in organic material in descomposition, and their pupae in dry soil. Conventionally, the muscids are divided into non-biting and biting species.

4. The non-biting muscids (*Musca, Muscinia, Fannia*) annoy the host with their constant activity and may act as mechanical or biological vectors.

5. The biting muscids (*Stomoxys, Haematobia, Glossina*) suck blood from their hosts and may act as mechanical or biological vectors.

6. The Calliphoridae or blow flies (*Calliphora, Lucilia, Phormia, Cochliomyia*) and the Sarcophagidae or flesh flies (*Sarcophaga, Wohlfahrtia*) have bristles on the hypopleura. The former have shiny, metalic colors and two or three bristles on the notopleura. The latter have dull, gray colors and four bristles on the notopleura.

7. The larvae of the calliphorids and sarcophagids develop in carrion, and the pupae in dry soil. Occasionally, the larvae may invade inflammed living tissues. The larvae of *Cochliomyia hominivorax* and *W. vigil* require living tissues.

8. The Oestridae are bee-like flies the larvae of which are obligatory internal parasites. *Gasterophilus* lives in the stomach of equines, *Hypoderma* under the skin of cattle, and *Oestrus* in the nasal cavity of sheep.

9. The Hippoboscidae are obligatory hematophagous ectoparasites. *Melophagus* infests sheep .

10. The Cyclorrhapha affect their hosts by causing annoyance with their presence and/or bites, sucking blood, producing accidental or obligatory myiases, and transmiting pathogens mechanically or biologically.

## REFERENCES

1. Marchiondo AA. 1987. Biology, economic effect and control of the horn fly. An. Hlth. Nutr. 42(5):6-10.

2. Zumpt F. 1965. Myiasis in man and animals in the Old World. Butterworth, London, 267 pp.

3. Sancho E. 1988. *Dermatobia*, the neotropical warble fly. Parasitol. Today 9:242-246.

4. US Department of Agriculture. 1976. Control of insects affecting livestock. Nat. Res. Progr. Publication # 20,480, Agr. Res. Serv., Washington, DC.

5. Drummond RO, Lasmbert G, Smalley HE Jr, and Terril CE. 1981. Estimated losses of livestock to pests. In CRC, *Handbook of pest management*, vol. 1, CRC Press, Boca Raton, Florida, 111-127.

6. Everett AL, Roberts IH and Naghski J. 1971. Reduction in leather value and yield of meat and wool from sheep infested with keds. J. Amer. Leather Chem. Assoc. 66:118-130.

7. Koehler PG and Butler JF. 1977. External parasite control on horses. Univ. Florida Inst. Food Agric. Sci. Circular 425, 12 pp.

8. Greenberg B. 1973. Flies and disease. Vol. II. Biology and disease transmission. Princeton Univ. Press, Princeton, New Jersey, 477 pp.

# PLATE VI. PICTORIAL KEY TO SOME COMMON SPECIES OF FLY LARVAE

(J. M. Seago)

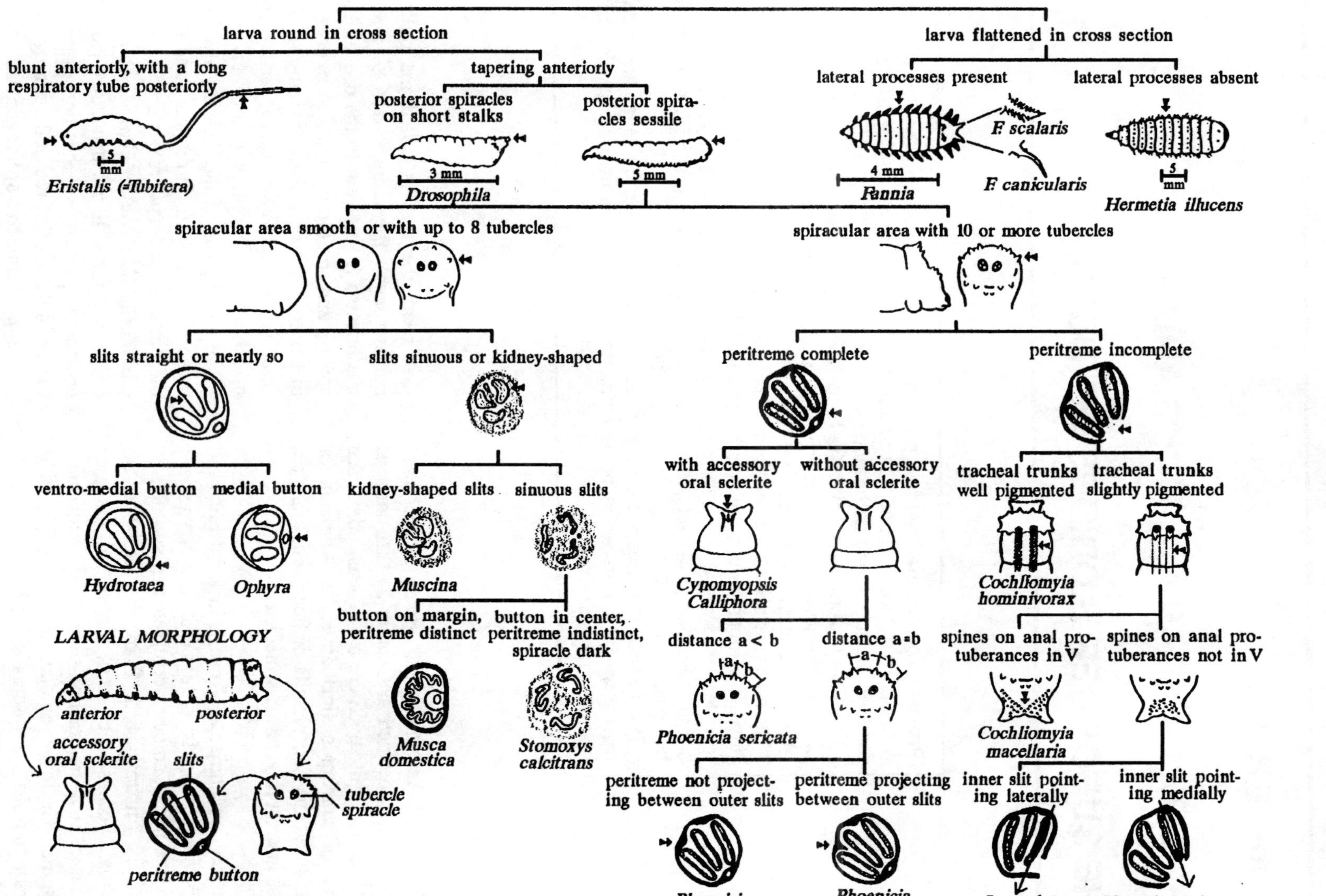


(Adapted from the US Dpt. of Education, Health, and Welfare)

# CHAPTER 10

# THE ORDER ACARINA: TICKS AND MITES.

# THE SUBORDER IXODIDES OR TICKS.

**Preview.** The Acarina have four pairs of legs and no antennae whereas the Insects have three pairs of legs and one pair of antennae. The ticks are distinguished from the mites for their larger size and other features.

There are two groups of ticks: **the hard ticks**, which have a dorsal plate and the mouthparts at the anterior end, and the **solf ticks**, which lack a dorsal plate and have the mouthparts on the ventral surface.

The hard ticks are obligatory hematophagous parasites and each of their mobile stages (larvae, nymphs, adults) takes a blood meal that last several days. Once engorged, the female lays several thousands of eggs and dies. The solf ticks are also obligatory hematophagous parasites but they take short meals and live off the host. The female takes several meals and lay eggs after each feeding.

Ticks annoy their hosts, cause skin lesions, draw blood, may cause tick paralysis, and may transmit a number of pathogens. Hard ticks are more pathogenic for domestic animals than soft ticks.

The order Acarina is the group of the class Arachnida (as defined in Chapter 2) that contains the **ticks and mites**. There are at least other nine orders of arachnids (including the Araneida or Spiders and the Scorpionida or Scorpions) that are of less interest to veterinary medicine.

Like all Arachnida, the Acarina lack antennae and wings, have four pairs of legs (but their larvae have only three pairs), and an incomplete metamorphosis. They are distinguished from the rest of the Arachnida because their head, thorax and abdomen are fused in a single, non-segmented sack called **idiosoma** (Gr *idio*= unique, *soma*= body). The anterior end of the idiosoma bears the buccal parts (rather than a complete head) that are called **capitulum** or **gnathosoma** (Gr *gnathos*= jaw). With purposes of description, the part of the idiosoma that bears the legs is called the **podosoma** (Gr *podos*= legs), the combination of podosoma and gnathosoma (equivalent to the cephalothorax of the spiders and scorpions) is called **prosoma** (Gr *pro*= in front of) whereas the remaining of the idiosoma (that is the equivalent to the abdomen) is called **opisthosoma** (Gr *opisthen*= behind).

The mouthparts of the Acarina are different from those of the insects. In the main and from the top to the bottom, they have two paired appendices called **chelicerae** (Lat *chela*= claw, Gr *keras*= horn) that end in pincer-like structures, a tongue-like **epistome-epipharynx** that constitutes the prolongation of the roof of the oral opening, and a tongue-like **hypostome-hypopharynx** that constitutes the prolongation of the floor of the oral opening. In some mites the chelicerae end in hooks or stylets, and the hypostome is missing.

The proximal end of these structures is encased in a sclerotized ring called the **basis capitulum**. From either lateral side of the basis capitulum, a palpus formed by four segments projects forward. The distal (4th) segment is ventral and very small. The shape of the basis capitulum and the palpi is important for the identification of some genera of ticks (Figure 10.1)

Many Acarina have thickened areas of the exoskeleton at specific locations that are called **plates** or shields. The shape and position of the diverse plates are useful for the identification of some genera or species. Many Acarina have a terminal structure in their legs called **pretarsus**. It is composed of a stalk (= pedicle) and a bell-shaped sucker (= caruncle). The characteristics of the pretarsi are also useful for the identification of some mites.

The Acarina are divided into several suborders. The suborder **Ixodides** includes the ticks, and the suborders **Mesostigmata**, **Trombidiformes**, and **Sarcoptiformes** include the mites of medical importance. They will be discussed separately.

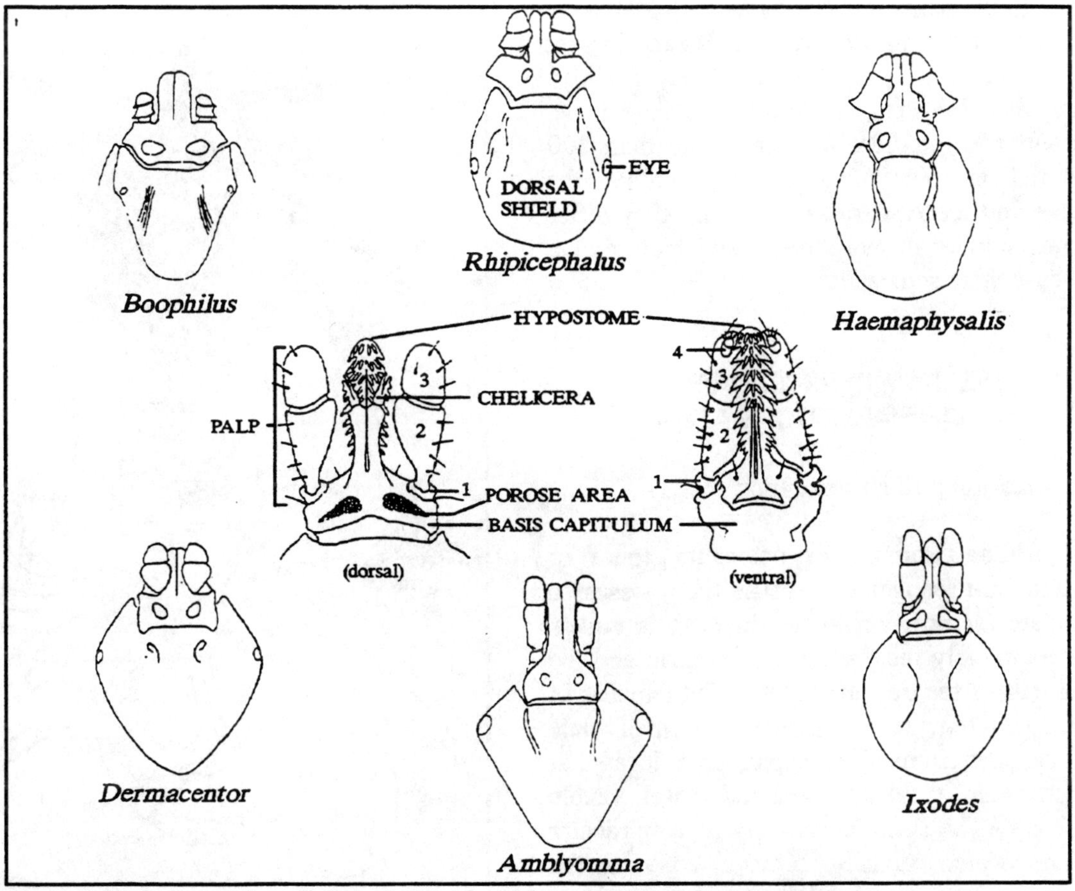


**Figure 10.1.** Capituli and dorsal shields of female ticks of various genera.

# THE SUBORDER IXODIDES OR TICKS

The **Ixodides** possess the characteristics of the Acarina. They are distinguished from the mites because the ticks have a toothed hypostome that anchors the tick during feeding, and possess a Haller's organ. The Haller's olfactory organ is a pit with sensory setae located on the dorsal surface of the tarsus of the first pair of legs. In practice, differentiation is easy because the ticks are clearly visible with the naked eye (the unfed larvae may be about 1 mm but still visible) whereas the largest among the common parasitic mite rarely reach to 1.0 mm when fully fed, and most are microscopic.

The suborder Ixodides contains more than 800 species that are distributed into two families: the **Ixodidae** and the **Argasidae**. Because they differ very substantially in morphology and biology, we will discuss them separately.

## THE FAMILY IXODIDAE OR HARD TICKS

### 1. Identification and classification

The **Ixodidae** (from *Ixodes*, one of its genera) or **hard ticks** are recognized because they possess a dorsal plate (**scutum** or dorsal shield) that covers almost completely the dorsum of the male and the anterior half of the dorsum of the unfed female. In the engorged female, it appears as a small plate behind the capitulum. Their capitulum is located at the anterior end of the idiosoma and is well visible from above. The spiracles, usually on a spiracular plate, are located caudally to the insertion of the fourth pair of legs. The Ixodidae are closely related to the mites of the order Mesostigmata to the extent that some acarologists gather both of them in the suborder Parasitiformes.

The dorsal aspect of the basis capitulum of the adult females presents a pair of oval depressions called **porose areas** (Figure 10.1). In some ixodid ticks, the scutum has colored markings but in others is of a solid color; the first type is described as **ornate** and the second as **inornate**. The males of

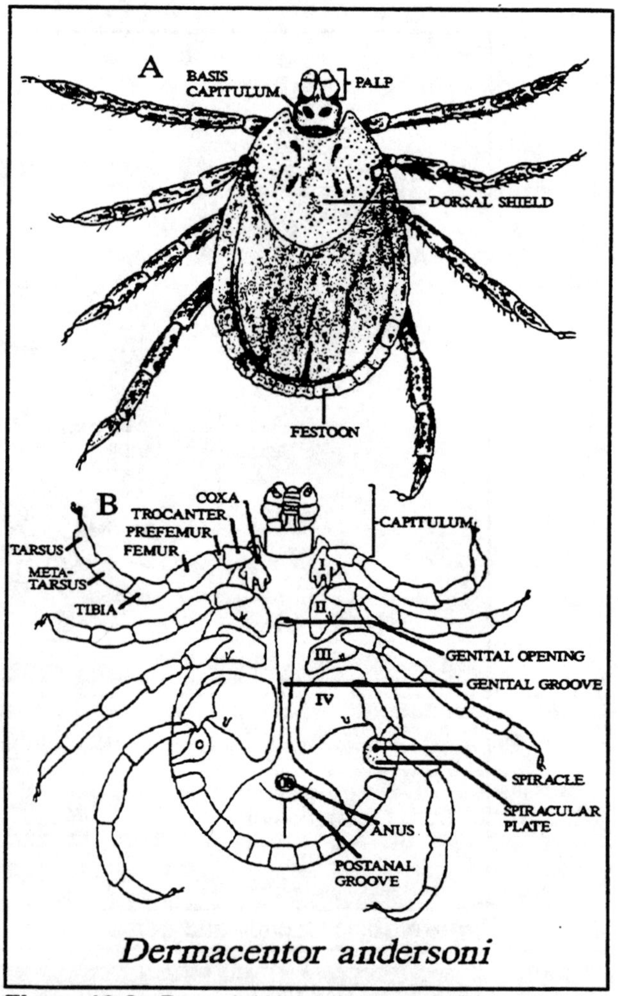


**Figure10.2.** Dorsal (A) and ventral (B) view of a female of *Dermacentor andersoni.*

some genera have some plates at both sides of the anus that are called **adanal plates**. The posterior margin of the idiosome has folds called **festoons** in some genera. The festoons are very distinct in the unfed tick but may disappear in the fully engorged female. Figure 10.2 shows some other morphological structures that are important for the identification of ticks.

The family Ixodidae includes some 14 genera and almost 700 species of ticks the identification of which is a task for the specialist. Figure 10.1 and Plate VII, however, should permit the identification of the adults of the ixodid genera that affect domestic animals. Adult stages are recognized by the presence of the genital opening on the ventral aspect that is absent in larvae and nymphs. Further information can be found in Hoskins[1] and Strickland et al.[2] The most important genera and species of ticks that affect domestic animals are the following:

*Amblyomma*. These are mostly tropical, 3-host ticks (see below), distributed in tropical America, and Africa south of the Sahara. This genus contains about 100 species, the most common in the United States being *A. americanum* (called **the lone star tick** for a whitish spot at the caudal end of the female scutum, Figure 10.3) and *A. maculatum*, **the Gulf Coast tick**. The preadult stages prefer to develop on birds or small mammals and the adults on medium and large mammals. *Amblyomma* are little host specific, however, and any stage may infest a wide variety of mammals, including humans.

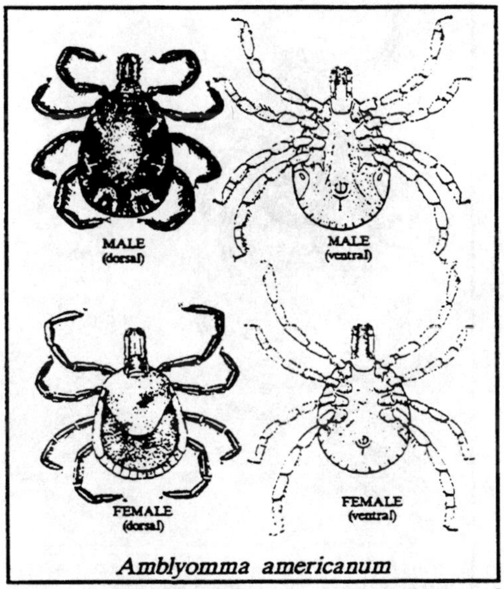


**Figure 10.3.** Dorsal and ventral views of male and females of *Amblyomma americanum* (USDA).

*Boophilus*. This genus contains five species and is distributed in all tropical and temperate zones. They are 1-host ticks (see below) of cattle but may infest horses and, occasionally, other domestic or wild ruminants. *B. annulatus*, **the cattle fever tick** of wide distribution (Figure 10.4), used to be a major pest in the United States but it was eradicated through a massive national campaign between 1906 and 1943. *B. microplus*, **the tropical cattle tick**, is distributed in the tropical parts of the American continent, Asia, and Australia.

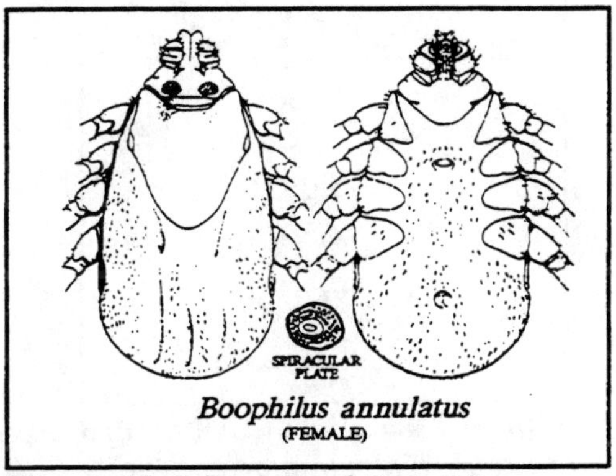


**Figure 10.4.** Female of *Boophilus annulatus* (USDA).

*Dermacentor*. This mostly North American genus contains more than 30 species, most of them 3-host ticks. Species are distributed from tropical areas of Latin America to cool areas of Canada. The preadult stages grow in small mammals, particularly rodents. The adult stages have specific but not too strict host preferences. *D. andersoni* (**the Rocky Mountain wood tick**, Figure 10.2) infests ruminants, horses, dogs, humans, and other mammals mainly in the western part of the United States and Canada. *D. variabilis* (the **American dog tick**) infests dogs, humans, ruminants, horses and other mammals, mainly in the eastern and central part of

North America. *D. albipictus* (**the winter horse tick**) and *D.* (syn. *Anocentor, Otocentor*) *nitens* (**the tropical horse tick**) are 1-host ticks that infest equines but also may be found on ruminants.

*Haemaphysalis*. This genus includes about 150 species and is distributed all over the world. They are mostly parasites of small mammals and birds

*Hyalomma*. This genus consists of more than 20 species Figure 10.5) and is distributed in the Old World south of the 45N parallel. It contains 1-, 2- and 3-host ticks.[1] Adult *Hyalomma* ticks are primarily parasites of domestic animals and, due to their direct effect and their role as vector, they may constitute one of the most important ectoparasites in veterinary medicine.

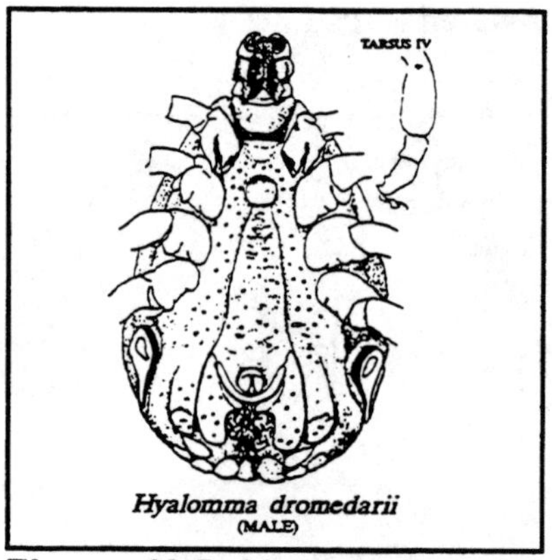


**Figure 10.5.** Ventral view of a male of *Hyalomma dromedarii.*

*Ixodes*. This cosmopolitan genus consists of about 250 species of 3-host ticks, about 40 of them in the United States.[2] The preadult stages prefer birds or small mammals whereas the adult stages may infect a variety of larger mammals, including humans and domestic animals. The American species, *I. scapularis* (**the black-legged tick**, Figure 10.6), feeds on birds, small mammals, and even lizards as a larva or a nymph, and on ruminants, horses, pigs, dogs, and humans as an adult.

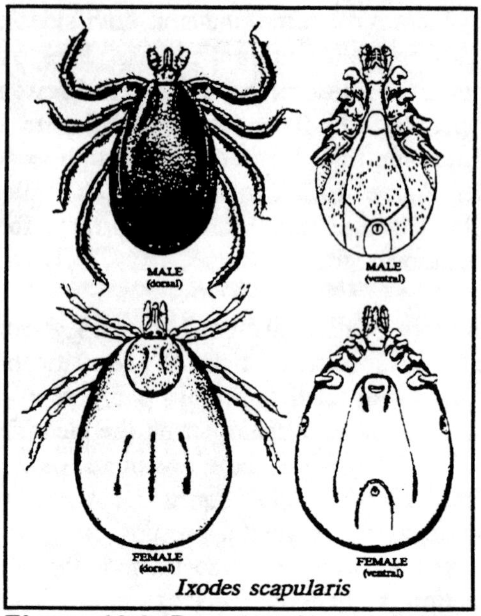


**Figure 10.6.** Dorsal and ventral views of a male and a female of *Ixodes scapularis.*

*Rhipicephalus*. This genus contains more than 60 species, most in Africa and a few in the rest of the Old World. Many are 3-host ticks that infect a variety of mammals. The only cosmopolitan species is *R. sanguineus*, **the brown dog tick** (Figure 10.7). In most of the world, this species is a 3-host tick with the preadult stages on many small

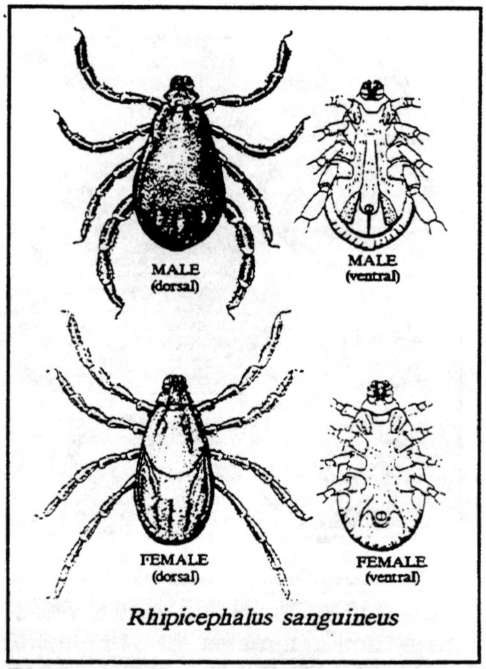


**Figure 10.7.** Male and female of *Rhipicephalus sanguineus.*

mammals and the adults on a wide variety of medium and large mammals (ruminants, equines, carnivores, humans, etc.). In the United States, it behaves mostly as a 1-host tick of dogs. Only rarely it is found on cattle, horses, or humans in contact with dogs.

## 2. Biology

The life cycle of the ixodid ticks consists of four stages: egg, larva, nymph, and adult. The larvae are actually similar enough to the adults as to be considered nymphs. They are called larvae (or seed-tick), however, because, unlike the other moving stages, they have only three pairs of legs (the fourth pair is missing).

Depending on the number of hosts that they require to complete their life cycle, the ixodids are classified as 1-host, 2-host, or 3-host ticks. In the **1-host ticks** development from larva to adult occurs on a single animal. In the **2-host ticks**, the larvae and the nymphs develop on a single animal but the nymphs drop to the ground to moult to adults, and the adults must look for a new host. In the **3-host ticks**, each moving stage develops on a different animal.

All the moving stages of ixodid ticks are obligatory hematophagous parasites. Ticks with long buccal parts (*Amblyomma, Hyalomma*, and *Ixodes*) thrust their capituli deeply into the tissues of the host and rely on their toothed hypostome to hold them in place. Those with short buccal parts (*Boophilus, Dermacentor, Haemaphysalis*, and *Rhipicephalus*) secrete a cement that fixes the arthropod to the host's skin while feeding. In both cases, the tick feeds on the blood pool formed in the lacerated tissues.

The female sucks blood for several days to a few weeks until her size increases a hundred or more times, drops to the ground, and seeks a sheltered place to lay her eggs. Oviposition lasts from a few days to ten or more weeks and results in the production of 2,000 to 20,000 eggs, depending on the species. The female dies shortly after oviposition is completed (Figure 10.8).

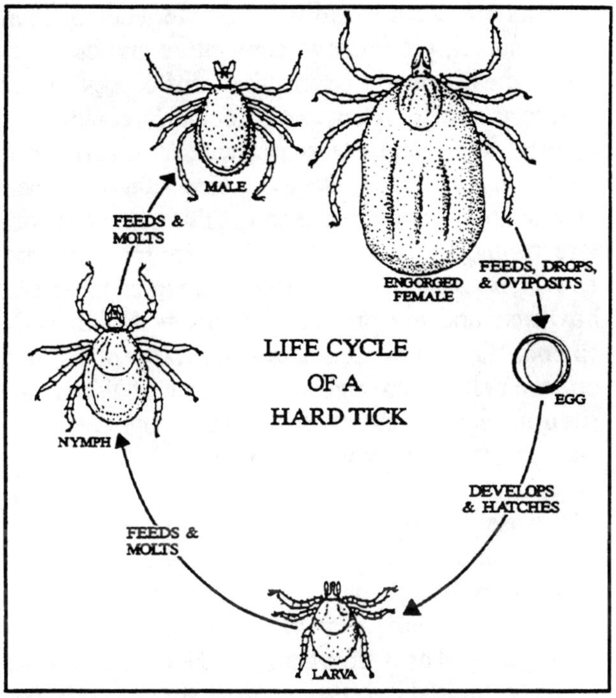


**Figure 10.8.** Life cycle of the hard ticks.

The incubation period depends largely on temperature and humidity, it may range from two weeks to seven months. The larvae that hatch from the eggs have three pairs of legs. After about a week, they climb blades of grass, bushes, or small trees and wait for the approach of an adequate host. They may survive starvation for several months if necessary. After crawling upon their host and engorging for a few days, the larvae moult to eight-legged nymphs. Molting takes place rapidly after the meal when it occurs on the host (in 1- or 2-host ticks), but it may take place after a few days to several months when it occurs off the host (in 3-host ticks). In this last case, its occurrence depends mainly on temperature and humidity.

The development of the nymphs is similar to that of the larvae but they can survive starvation even longer. Adults produced on the host (in 1- host ticks) mate, engorge, and drop to the ground to initiate a new cycle. Those produced off the host (in 2- or 3-host ticks) can survive starvation for many months, even for a couple of years, until they find an appropriate host.

Ticks are sensitive to the characteristics of their environment, particularly temperature and humidity (and the ground cover that influences these characteristics). They are particularly common in tropical and temperate zones, and abound on their hosts during the season that favors their proliferation. In temperate zones, this coincides with late spring, summer, and early fall for most species. *D. albipictus* and *I. scapularis* are adapted to winter, however, and are prevalent from late fall to early spring. In tropical zones, tick are frequently found on their host throughout the year. When the environmental conditions are inappropriate, ticks may proliferate poorly or not at all.

Because 1-host ticks spend most of their lives on the host and are less subjected to the effects of the external environment, they may produce three or four generations per year (e. g., *Boophilus microplus*). The 3-host ticks, on the other hand, are severely limited by the environmental conditions and the fortuitous finding of an appropriate host; they may produce as few as one generation every two or three years (e. g., *Dermacentor andersoni*).

Host-specificity varies widely with the species. Some ticks are almost monospecific (e.g., *Boophilus* spp.) whereas others may feed almost on any vertebrate on sight (e.g., *Amblyomma americanum*). They exhibit clear preferences for specific locations on the host, however. For example, *D. albipictus* is found preferentially in the dewlap and brisket of horses whereas *D. nitens* is found in the ears. These preferences are attributed to differences in the microecology of the skin.

Table 10.I lists some biological characteristics of some common ticks.

### 3. Medical importance

Ticks are important to veterinary medicine as direct cause of damage, agents of tick paralysis, and vectors of infections.

Direct damage occurs as a consequence of the interruption of grazing, the skin trauma due to the bites, and the removal of blood. The insertion of the capitulum in the skin causes an extensive and painful laceration of the tissues that is compounded by allergic reactions to components of the saliva. Animals infested with ticks are not only disturbed by the painful bites but also by the discomfort of the local inflammation and pruriginous allergy that ensues. Furthermore, the lesions attract the attack by parasitic flies, favor secondary bacterial infections, and preclude the industrial used of badly affected hides. Careless removal of a tick often breaks off its capitulum and the pieces left in the wound promote further inflammation. The best way to avoid this is to exert a sustained pull on the tick perpendicularly to the plane of the skin until it relaxes its hold.

Blood removal by itself may be an important factor of disease. A female *A. americanum* can take 0.5-0.8 ml of blood in a 10-day period and several hundreds or thousands ticks may attack a single animal. Aside from the anemia that may develop, replacement of this blood takes away nutrients and energy that the animal could use for growth.

The combined effect on the animals of annoyance, skin irritation, and blood removal is known as **tick worry**. This could be quite significant in severe infestations. Several estimations have concluded that *Boophilus* infestation alone can reduce by about 36 kg (79 lb) the annual weight gain, and by about 180 l (47.5 American gallons) the annual milk production of cattle. The total cost of tick infestations of cattle, including their control, has been estimated in \$ 8 to \$ 21 per animal per year. In 1984 dollars, the 1906-1943 anti-*Boophilus* campaign in the United States cost \$ 500 million but it is believed that the presence of the tick in the United States today would represent annual losses of \$ 1.6 billion to the cattle industry.

It has been recently demonstrated that tick infestation depresses the ability of the host to mount an immune response. This may facilitate the production, or aggravate the course, of concurrent infections in infested animals.

Infestation by ticks sometimes produces an ascending flaccid paralysis that finally kills the host by respiratory arrest.[3] The paralysis begins a few days after the female ticks start to engorge and progresses to death in a week or less. If the ticks are removed, it regresses spontaneously in a few days. Sheep, dogs, and humans are the most susceptible but important mortality has been reported in cattle. Other domestic and wild mammals as well as birds may be occasionally affected.

More than 20 species of ticks have been implicated as agents of **tick paralysis** or tick toxicosis in different countries. *D. andersoni* and *D. variabilis* are the most important in the United States and Canada, *Haemaphysalis, Hyalomma* and *Ixodes* spp. in Europe, *Ixodes* and *Rhipicephalus* in South Africa, and *Ixodes holocyclus* in Australia. *Argas persicus* causes paralysis in poultry. The disease is commonly related to the engorgement of adult females but males ticks have produced cases in humans, and preadult stages in birds. Although it is generally believed that the paralysis is caused by a neurotoxin inoculated by the tick, this has been substantiated only in the case of *I. holocyclus*.

Their obligatory hematophagia, large blood meals, longevity, and wide host range make ticks particularly suitable for **transmission of pathogens**. In this area, they play in veterinary medicine the role that mosquitoes play in human medicine. Hoskins has edited an excellent series of reviews on ticks and tick-borne diseases that is particularly usefull for small animal practitioners.[1]

Many tick-borne pathogens exhibit **transtadial transmission**, this is, they remain in the tick that acquired the infection when it molts from one stage to the next (e. g., the rickettsia *Ehrlichia canis* in *Rhipicephalus sanguineus*). Transtadial (or horizontal) transmission permits the transfer of pathogens from an infected host to a susceptible host by 2- or 3-host ticks.

Since 1-host ticks do not change host within one generation, pathogens transmitted by these ticks exhibit **transovarian transmission**, this is, they infect the ovaries of the tick that acquired the infection and pass with the eggs to the next generation of ticks (e. g. the protozoan *Babesia bigemina* in *Boophilus annulatus*). Transovarian (or vertical) transmission is a strategy that permits effective transfer of pathogens by 1-host ticks. Transovarian transmission is not restricted to 1-host ticks, however, since it also occurs in 3-host ticks (e. g., the rickettsia of the Rocky Mountain spotted fever, *Rickettsia rickettsii*, in *Dermacentor andersoni* and *D. variabilis*).

Table 10.2 lists some of the major infections of veterinary importance transmitted by ticks.

## THE FAMILY ARGASIDAE OR SOFT TICKS

### 1. Identification and classification

The Argasidae (from *Argas*, one of its genera) or **soft ticks** are recognized because they lack a scutum and their dorsum is covered by a leathery integument. The capitulum is located on the ventral surface in the adults and nymphs, and is completely or partially covered by the anterior part of the idiosoma when looked at from above. The spiracles are located anteriorly to the insertion of the fourth pair of legs. Unlike the ixodids, the argasids have only slight sexual dimorphism (Figure 10.9).

The argasid ticks include close to 150 species distributed into the following major four genera.

*Antricola.* These are parasites of bats, of no veterinary importance.

*Argas*. These are flat ticks with the margin of the body thin and a definite sutural line separating the dorsal and ventral surfaces, even on fully engorged specimens. They are primarily parasites of birds, bats, and insectivores. They bite humans or other animals only rarely. *Argas persicus* (the fowl tick, Figure 10.9) is the most widely distributed species. In the United States, the species commonly called *A. persicus* is really a complex of four closely related species.

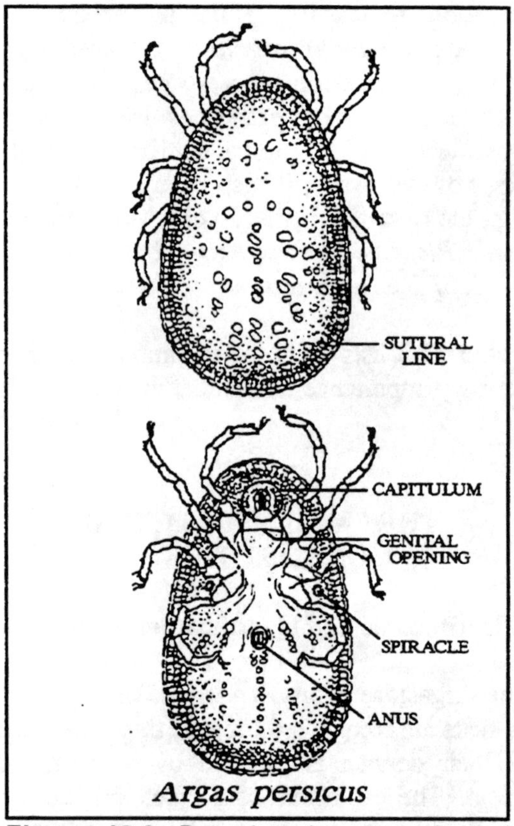


**Figure 10.9.** Dorsal and ventral view of *Argas persicus.*

*Ornithodoros*. These are ticks with the margin of the body rounded and without a definite suture separating the dorsal and ventral surfaces (Figure 10.10). The adults have a well developed hypostome, and the nymphs and adults have a mammillated integument. About 90 species exist in the world and 20 in the United States. Different species feed on birds or a wide variety of mammals. Their host specificity is not strict.

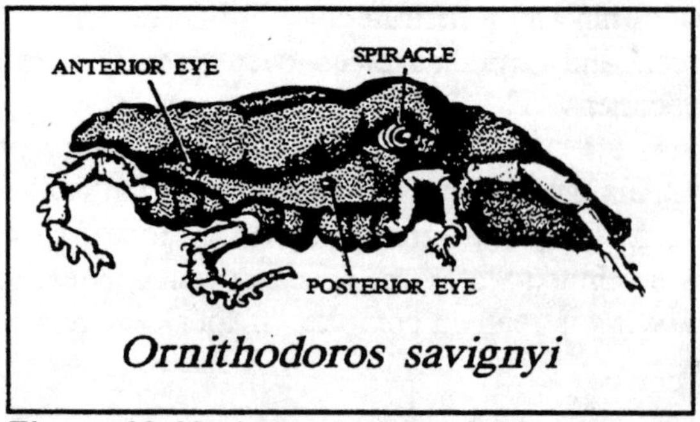


**Figue 10.10**. Lateral view of *Ornithodorus savigniy*

*Otobius*. These are ticks with the margin of the body rounded and without a definite separating suture. The adults have a rudimentary hypostome and a granular integument. The nymphs have an integument covered with spines (Figure 10.11). Of the two species known, only *O. megnini* (**the spinose ear tick**) infects domestic animals. Native of the Americas, this species is now established in parts of Africa and Asia.

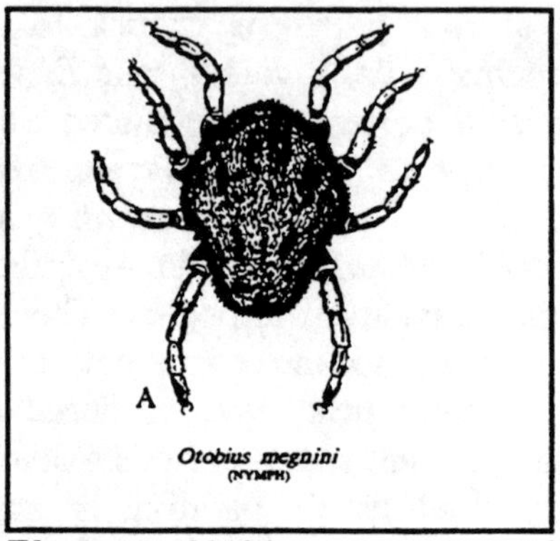


**Figure 10.11.** Nymph of *Otobius megnini.*

## 2. Biology

The argasids are hardy ticks well adapted to arid environments. Differently from the ixodids and with the exception of *Otobius*, (see below) all the moving stages (larvae, up to 8 nymphal stages, and adults) are temporary ectoparasites that live off the host. Between meals they hide in crevices of chicken houses (*Argas* spp.), old livestock bedding (*Ornithodoros* spp.), or under leaves in loose soil.

The females feed on several occasions during their lives, for periods of 1-2 hours each time. They lay batches of 25 to 340 eggs after each feeding, for a total of 500 to 2,000 in their lifespan of 2 to 4 years. The incubation time depends on temperature; it may be as short as 8 days or as long as 107 days. The larva and each nymphal stage commonly takes a blood meal of 15-30 minutes and moult to the next stage. In the absence of a host, all stages can survive starvation for several months. Depending on environmental conditions, the complete cycle from egg to adult may take from 62 to 602 days (Figure 10.12).

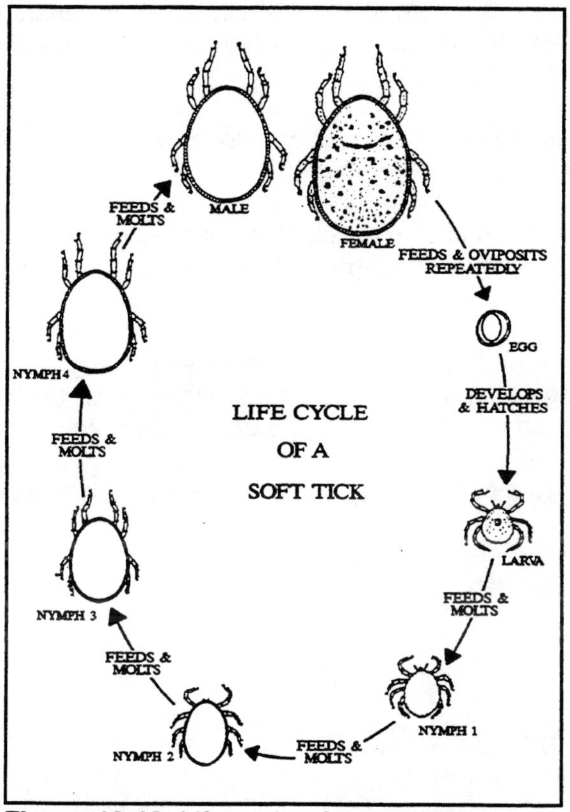


**Figure 10.12**. Life cycle of the solf ticks.

Different from the other argasids that are multi-host ticks, *Otobius megnini* is an aberrant 1-host tick. The eggs hatch on the soil and the larvae crawl upon ruminants, horses, dogs, or, occasionally, other mammals, and work their way deeply into their ears. The larvae and two subsequent nymphal stages remain engorging in the ears for 38 to 220 days. The second nymphs drop to the ground and moult to non-feeding adults that mate and start oviposition.

**3. Medical importance**

*Argas* ticks may produce extensive skin damage, exsanguination, and tick paralysis of birds. Production may be severely affected or stopped altogether when the infestation is intense. They are rarely a serious problem nowadays, however.

Although some *Ornithodoros* species infest domestic animals, they are important as vectors of the relapsing fever (*Borrelia recurrentis*) of humans.

*Otobius megnini* is an important pest of cattle and horses. Affected animals become restless, shake and rub their heads, and may run about until they become exhausted. The tick lesions facilitate the attack by parasitic flies and secondary infections.

In general, the argasids are much less of a problem in veterinary medicine than the ixodids.

## Summary

1. The Acarina are arthropods with four pair of legs (except the larvae) and no antennae.

2. Conventionally, they are divided into ticks (larger, with a toothed hypostome, and a Haller's organ) and mites (smaller and without a toothed hypostoma or Haller's organ).

3. Ticks, in tum, are divided into Ixodidae or hard ticks (with a dorsal plate and the mouth-parts at the anterior end) and Argasidae or soft ticks (without a dorsal plate and with the mouth parts on the ventral surface).

4. The hard ticks (*Amblyomma, Boophilus, Dermacentor, Haemaphysalis, Hyalomma, Ixodes,* and *Rhipicephalus*) have four stages: egg, larva, nymph, and adult. Each mobile stage requires a long blood meal that lasts for days on the host before moulting. After their meal, the females lay thousands of eggs and die.

5. In some cases, each stage develops on a different host (3-host ticks), in others the larvae and nymph develops on one host and the adults on other (2-host ticks), and in still others all stages develop on a same host (1-host ticks).

6. Hard ticks annoy the animals with their bites, cause skin lesions, draw blood, may cause tick paralysis, and are vectors of a number of infections.

7. The pathogens transmitted by ticks may pass from one tick stage to the next within the same generation (transtadial transmission), or from one generation to the next through the eggs (transovarial transmission).

8. The soft ticks (*Argas, Ornithodorus,* and *Otobius*) have several stages: egg, larva, several nymphal stages, and adults. They take short blood meals and hide off the host between meals. The females take repeated meals and lay eggs after each meal.

9. With the exception of *Otobius*, which is a permanent parasite at the pre-adult stages, the soft ticks are multi-host ticks.

10. Soft ticks cause the same damage as hard ticks but are less of a problem among domestic animals.

## REFERENCES

1. Hoskins JD, 1991. *Tick-transmitted diseases*. Vet. Clin. N.A. Sm. An., Pract. 202 pp.

2. Strickland RK, Gerrish RR, Hourrigan JL and Schubert GO, 1976. *Ticks of Veterinary Importance*. Agricult. Hndbk. # 485, USDA, Washington, D.C., 122 pp.

3. Kaiser MN and Hoogstraal H. 1964. The *Hyalomma* ticks (Ixodoidea, Ixodidae) of Pakistan, India, and Ceylon, with keys to subgenera and species. Acarol. 6:257-286.

4. Keirans JE and Clifford CM, 1978. The genus *Ixodes* in the United States: a scanning electron microscope study and key to the adults. J. Med. Entomol. Suppl. # 2, 149 pp.

5. Greson JD, 1973. *Tick paralysis. An appraisal of natural and experimental data*. Canada Dept. Agr. Monograph # 9, 109 pp.

6. Sonenshine DE, 1991. *Biology of Ticks*, 2 vol., Oxford Univ. Press, New York, 447 + 465 pp.

## KEY FOR THE IDENTIFICATION OF GENERA OF ADULT IXODID TICKS THAT AFFECT DOMESTIC ANIMALS

| | | |
|---|---|---|
| 1. | With a visible anal groove in front of the anus | *Ixodes* |
| | Anal groove absent or behind the anus | go to 2 |
| 2. (1) | The second segment of the palpi projects laterally beyond the lateral margins of the basis capituli.(*) Eyes absent | *Haemaphysalis* |
| | The second segment of the palpi does not project as above. Eyes usually present | go to 3 |
| 3. (2) | Basis capituli with six sides (hexagonal) | go to 4 |
| | Basis capituli not hexagonal | go to 7 |
| 4. (3) | Festoons present, spiracular plates triangular or comma-shaped | go to 5 |
| | Festoons absent, spiracular plates oval | go to 6 |
| 5. (4) | With a dorsal spur on the 1st segment of the palpi, adanal plates absent and coxae of fourth legs very large in males. Only in southern and central Africa | *Rhipicentor* |
| | No dorsal spur on the 1st segment of the palpi, adanal plates present and coxae of fourth legs of regular size in males | *Rhipicephalus* |
| 6. (4) | With short palpi that have transverse ridges on the dorsal and lateral aspects | *Boophilus* |
| | Short palpi without transverse ridges. Only in southern Africa and Sudan | *Margaropus* |
| 7. (3) | Short palpi with the second segment triangular, basis capitulum rectangular | *Dermacentor* |
| | Long palpi with the second segment rectangular and twice as long as wide, basis capitulum irregularly triangular or pentagonal | go to 8 |
| 8. (7) | Scutum ornate, festoon well developed, males without adanal plates | *Amblyomma* |
| | Scutum inornate, festoons poorly developed, males with adanal plates | *Hyalomma* |

(*) The shape of the palpi and basis capitulum is determined by examination of the tick from the dorsal aspect (see Figure 10.1.).

**TABLE 10.I. CHARACTERISTICS OF SOME COMMON HARD TICKS (IXODIDAE)**

| SPECIES AND COMMON NAMES | GEOGRAPHIC DISTRIBUTION | ADULT TICKS | | | LIFE CYCLE* | | | | | LONGEST SURVIVAL |
|---|---|---|---|---|---|---|---|---|---|---|
| | | HOSTS | LOCATION | SEASON | # HOSTS | EGGS | LARVAE | NYMPH | ADULTS | |
| *Amblyomma americanum* (Lone Star tick) | SE USA, tropical Latin America | Cattle, horses, dogs, human, others | Ears,dewlap, axillae, escutcheon, groins | Spring and summer | 3 | N= 8300<br>I= 23-117 | E= 3-9<br>M= 8-26 | E= 3-8<br>M= 13-46 | E= 9-24<br>O= 7-23 | Larvae, 346 days |
| *A. cajennense* (Cajenne tick) | S Texas, tropical Latin America | Livestock, dogs, human, others | Between legs, abdomen, ears | Year around | 3 | N= 7700<br>I= 37-154 | E= 3-7<br>M= 10 | E= 3-13<br>M= 12-105 | E= 7-112<br>O= 20 | Adults, 600 days |
| *A. maculatum* (Gulf Coast tick) | Gulf of Mexico & Atlantic Coast, trop. Latin Amer. | Ruminants, equines, dogs, occ. humans | Head | Late summer to early fall | 3 | N= 18000<br>I= 21-142 | E= 3-7<br>M= 7-121 | E= 5-11<br>M= 17-71 | E= 14-18<br>O= 13-75 | Larvae, 71 days |
| *A. variegatum* (Tropical Bont tick) | Puerto Rico, West Indies, Africa | Livestock, wild animals | Brisket, axillae, abdomen, groin, escutcheon | Rainy season | 3 | N= 12000<br>I= 53-86 | E= 5-7<br>M= 14-22 | E= 5-7<br>M= 19-24 | E= 10-12<br>O= ? | Adults, 359 days |
| *Boophilus annulatus* (Cattle fever tick) | Africa, near East, Mediterranean basin | Cattle, occ. horses & deer | Neck, axillae, abdomen, groin, escutcheon | Year around | 1 | N= 4500<br>I= 19-102 | E & M=<br>5-16 | E & M=<br>5-18 | E= 4-14<br>O= 6-70 | Adults, 1053 days |
| *B. microplus* (Tropical Cattle tick) | Puerto Rico, trop. & subtrop. L.A., Afr., Austr., Orient | Cattle, occ. horses & small ruminants | Neck, axillae, abdomen, groin, escutcheon | Year around | 1 | N= 4400<br>I= 14-146 | E & M=<br>5-17 | E & M=<br>7-12 | E= 5-23<br>O= 4-44 | Adults, 588 days |
| *Dermacentor albipictus* (Winter tick) | N & SW USA, Canada, Mexico | Cattle, horses | Dewlap, brisket, axillae, groin | Autumn to early spring | 1 | N= 4400<br>I= 33-71 | E & M=<br>9-20 | E & M=<br>9-12 | E= 8-30<br>O= 19-42 | Adults, 421 days |
| *D. andersoni* (Rocky Mountain Wood tick) | W USA, Canada | Cattle, horses, dogs, humans, others | Head, neck, shoulder, brisket, groin | Late winter to late summer | 3 | N= 7400<br>I= 15-51 | E= 2-8<br>M= 6-21 | E= 3-9<br>M= 11-19 | E= 7-17<br>O= 15-32 | Adults, 27 months |
| *D. nitens* (Tropical Horse tick) | S Florida, S. Texas, trop. L.A. | Equines, occ. ruminants | Ears, mane, abdomen, groin, perineum | Year around | 1 | N= 3400<br>I= 21-28 | E & M=<br>8-16 | E & M=<br>7-14 | E= 9-23<br>O= 15-37 | Larvae, 75 days |
| *D. occidentalis* (Pacific Coast tick) | Pacific coast of USA | Ruminants, horses, dogs, humans | All over the body | Year around | 3 | N= 4500<br>I= 16-38 | E= 3-7<br>M= 6-12 | E= 4-9<br>M= 13-22 | E= 6-17<br>O= 14 | Adults, 2 years |
| *D. variabilis* (American Dog tick) | E & Central USA, Canada, Mexico | Dog, humans, cattle, horses, others | Neck, brisket, axillae, abdomen, groin | Spring to autumn | 3 | N= 6500<br>I= 26-57 | E= 3-13<br>M= 6-247 | E= 3-11<br>M= 24-291 | E= 5-27<br>O= 14-32 | Adults, 14 months |

(*) E = length of engorgement in days, I = length of incubation in days, M = time to molting in days, N = maximum number of eggs per female, O = length of oviposition in days.

TABLE 10.I. CHARACTERISTICS OF SOME COMMON HARD TICKS (IXODIDAE), continuation

| SPECIES AND COMMON NAME | GEOGRAPHIC DISTRIBUTION | ADULT TICKS HOSTS | ADULT TICKS LOCATION | ADULT TICKS SEASON | # HOSTS | LIFE CYCLE* EGGS | LIFE CYCLE* LARVAE | LIFE CYCLE* NYMPHS | LIFE CYCLE* ADULTS | LONGEST SURVIVAL |
|---|---|---|---|---|---|---|---|---|---|---|
| *Haemaphysalis leporis-lacustris* (Rabbit tick) | N & Central America | Rabbits, nymphs occ. on cattle | Ears, head | Spring to autumn | 3 | N= 2400 I= 22-61 | E= 4-11 M= 18-134 | E= 4-11 M= 14-124 | E= 19-25 O= 3-57 | Adults, 588 days |
| *Hyalomma marginatum* (Mediterranean *Hyalomma*) | S Eurasia, N Africa | Ruminants, horses | Dewlap, brisket, axillae, groins, perineum | Spring & summer | 2 or 3 | N= 15000 I= 35 | E= 6 M= 16 | E= 6 M= 20 | E= 6-13 O= ? | Adults, 421 days |
| *Ixodes ricinus* (European Castor Bean tick) | Europe, N Africa, parts of Asia | Ruminants, dogs horses | Face, ears, axillae, groins, escutcheon | Spring to autumn | 3 | N= 3000 I= 42-252 | E= 3-6 M= 28-140 | E= 3-5 M= 56-360 | E= 8-14 O= ? | Adults, 27 months |
| *I. scapularis* (Black-legged tick) | SE, Atlantic coast & N Central USA, Mexico | Livestock, dogs, humans | Head, neck | Autumn to spring | 3 | N= 3000 I= 48-135 | E= 3-9 M= 22-49 | E= 3-8 M= 25-56 | E= 8-9 O= ? | Larvae, 75 days |
| *I. pacificus* (Western black-legged tick) | W USA and Canada | Livestock, dogs, humans | Head, neck | Late winter to summer | 3 | N= 1300 I= 53-55 | E= 4-9 M= 37-38 | E= 7-11 M= 30-33 | E= 7-11 O= ? | Adults, 120 days |
| *Rhipicephalus appendiculatus* (Brown Ear tick) | Humid parts of Africa | Cattle, occ. other ruminants, dogs, others | Ears | Summer & autumn | 3 | N= 5700 I= 28-90 | E= 3-7 M= 10-49 | E= 3-7 M= 10-61 | E= 4-10 O= ? | Adults, 2 years |
| *R. evertsi* (Red-legged tick) | Africa, Arabia | Ruminants, horses | Perineum | Year around | 2 | N= 7000 I= 28-70 | E & M= 10-15 | E & M= 21-56 | E= 6-10 O= ? | Adults, 14 months |
| *R. sanguineus* (Brown dog tick) | Tropical & sub-tropical areas | Dogs, occ. live-stock & humans in USA. Many spp elsewhere | Ears, neck, be-tween toes | Spring to autumn | 1 or 3 | N= 4000 I= 8-67 | E= 3-7 M= 6-23 | E= 4-9 M= 12-129 | E= 6-50 O= ? | Adults, 568 days |

* E = length of engorgement in days, I = length of incubation in days, M = time to molting in days, N = maximum number of eggs per female, O = length of oviposition in days.

**Table 10.II. MAJOR VETERINARY INFECTIONS TRANSMITTED BY TICKS**

| INFECTION (ORGANISM) | VECTOR TICK(S) |
|---|---|
| Anaplasmosis (*Anaplasma* spp.) | *Boophilus* spp.,<br>*Dermacentor* spp.<br>*Rhipicephalus* spp.<br>*Hyalomma* sp. |
| African swine fever (virus of ASF) | *Ornithodorus* spp. |
| Babesiosis or Piroplasmosis (*Babesia* spp.) | |
| - of cattle | *Boophilus* spp. |
| - of sheep | *Rhipicephalus bursa* |
| - of dogs | *Rhipicephalus sanguineus* |
| - of horses | *Dermacentor* spp.<br>*Rhipicephalus* spp.<br>*Hyalomma* spp. |
| East Coast fever (*Theileria parva*) | *Rhipicephalus* spp. |
| Ehrlichiosis (*Ehrlichia* spp.) | |
| - of cattle | *Hyalomma* spp. |
| - of sheep | *Rhipicephalus bursa* |
| - of dogs | *Rhipicephalus sanguineus*<br>*Dermacentor* spp.<br>*Hyalomma* spp.<br>*Ixodes ricinus* |
| Fowl pox (virus of FP) | *Argas persicus* |
| Fowl spirochetosis (*Borrelia anserina*) | *Argas persicus* |
| Heartwater fever (*Cowdria ruminantium*) | *Amblyomma* spp. |
| Lyme disease (*Borrelia burgdorferi*) | *Ixodes* spp. |
| Q fever (*Coxiella burnetti*) | *Amblyomma* spp.<br>*Dermacentor* spp.<br>*Rhipicephalus sanguineus*<br>*Haemaphysalis* sp. |
| Rocky Mountain spotted fever (*Rickettsia ricketsii*) | *Dermacentor* spp.<br>*Rhipicephalus sanguineus*<br>*Amblyomma* spp.<br>*Haemaphysalis* sp. |
| Tularemia (*Francisella tularensis*) | *Amblyomma americanum*<br>*Dermacentor* spp.<br>*Rhipicephalus sanguineus*<br>*Haemaphysalis* sp. |

# PLATE VII. PICTORIAL KEY TO GENERA OF TICKS IN THE UNITED STATES

(Harry D. Pratt)

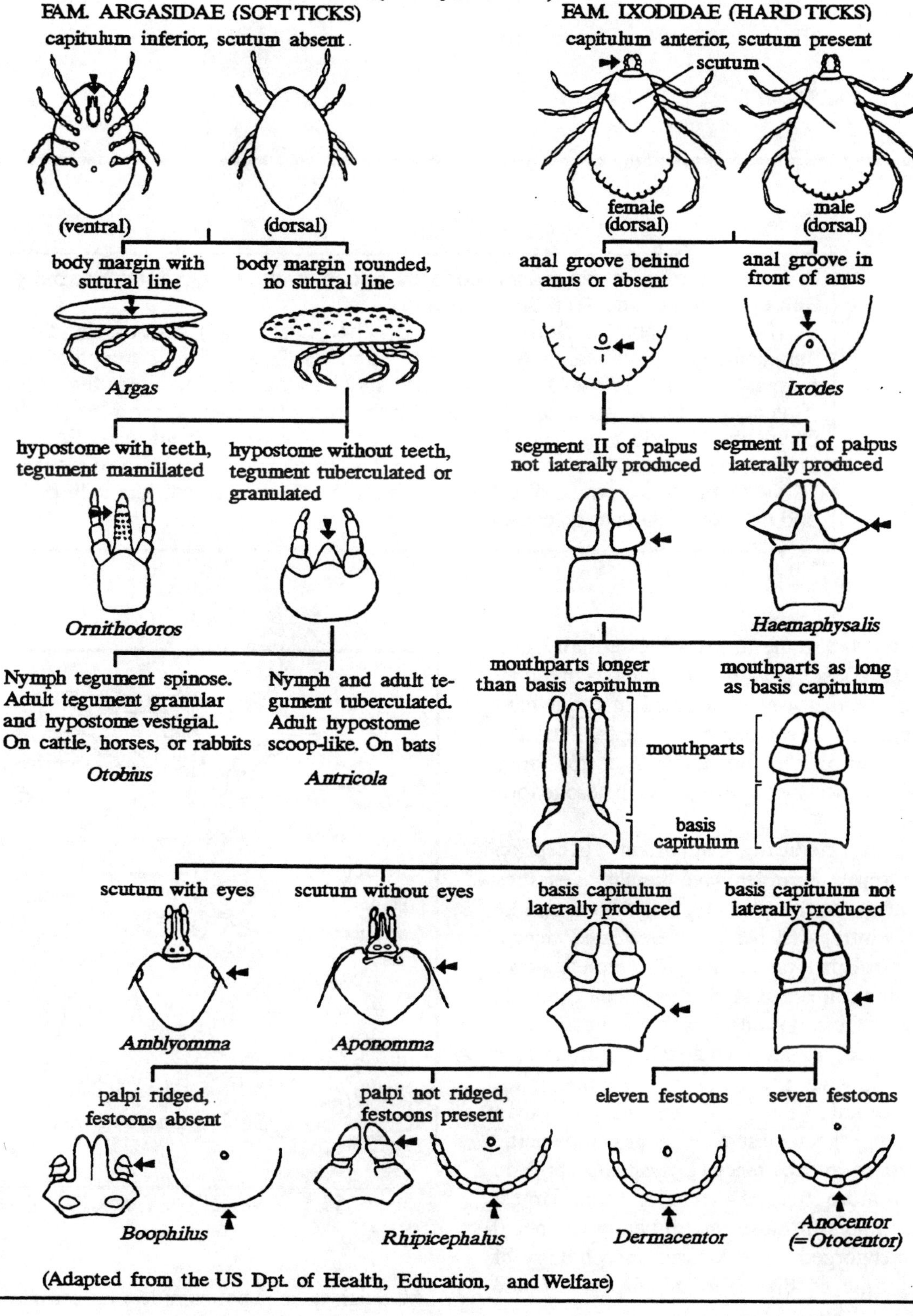


(Adapted from the US Dpt. of Health, Education, and Welfare)

# CHAPTER 11

# THE MITES

Preview. The mites of veterinary importance belong to three suborders: **Mesostigmata**, **Sarcoptiformes**, and **Trombidiformes**.

The Mesostigmata (Dermanyssus, Ornithonyssus, etc.) are mostly temporary hematophagous ectoparasites of birds and rodents. The Sarcoptiformes are permanente ectoparasites that include species that burrow into the epidermis (Sarcoptes, Notoedres, Cnemidocoptes) and others that live on the skin (Psoroptes, Chorioptes, Otodectes). The Trombidiformes (Demodex, Cheyletiella, Psorergates, Trombicula) are quite heterogeneous from the morphologic and biologic viewpoints.

This mites are the cause of cutaneous manufestations that interfere with production and may cause severe disease.

Unlike the ticks, the mites are essentially free living arthropods. Only a few of the more than 30,000 species known, distributed in more than 200 families,[1] have become adapted to the parasitic mode of life. For this reason, the mites of medical importance are a rather heterogenous group.

With one medically important exception (*Demodex* spp.), the mites have the characteristics of the Acarina (see chapter 10), this is, a sack-like body (**idiosome**) that bears differentiated buccal parts (**capitulum**) rather than a complete head. The parasitic mites can be distinguished from the ticks because the mites either lack a hypostome or it is not toothed, do not have a Haller's organ (see chapter 10), and are smaller than the ticks. Whereas the unfed tick larvae are rarely less than 1.0 mm long, the largest permanent ectoparasitic mites of common occurrence (*Cheyletiella* spp.) do not reach more than 0.4 mm and the largest temporary mites (*Mesostigmata*) barely reach 1.0 mm when engorged. The external morphology of a typical mite is discussed in chapter 10 and illustrated in Figure 11.1..

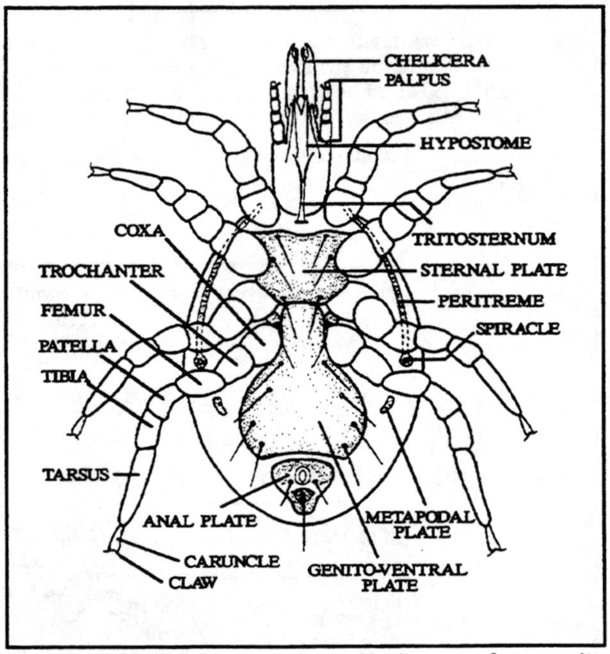


**Figure 11.1.** Typical morphology of a mite (USDA).

Although there is not complete agreement among the specialists,[2] the parasitic mites can be separated into three suborders (the **Mesostigmata**, the **Sarcoptiformes**, and the **Trombidiformes**) that will be discussed separately. Classification of species of mites is based on the observation of subtle structures of well-prepared specimens, and is best left to the specialist. Only in the few cases in which reporting of a given species is obligatory and no specialist is available, the untrained veterinarian should consider going through this task.[3]

## 1. THE SUBORDER MESOSTIGMATA

### 1.1. Identification and classification

The Mesostigmata (Gr *mesos* = middle, and Lat *stigmata* [sing. *stigma*], alternative name for the spiracles or respiratory openings) are recognized because they have a pair of **spiracles** toward the middle of the body (caudal and lateral to the third coxae). An elongated plate, called **peritreme**, runs from each spiracle toward the capitulum (Figure 11.1). The ectoparasitic mesostigmata are quite homogeneous in morphology so they are easy to recognize.

The species most likely to be found by a veterinarian are: *Dermanyssus gallinae*, **the cosmopolitan chicken mite**; *Ornithonyssus sylviarum*, **the northern fowl mite** (Figure 11.2.), and *O. bursa*, **the tropical fowl mite**. The three species are small (up to 0.5-1.0 mm long), quite similar among them, and infest chickens, other poultry, and wild birds. Occasionally, they may bite humans. Separation of the species, rarely needed by the veterinarian, can be done by observation of the chelicerae (needle-like in *Dermanyssus* and pincer-like in *Ornithonyssus*), and the hairs of the sternal plate of the female (two pairs in *D. gallinae* and *O. sylviarum* and three pairs in *O. bursa*).

Other mesostigmata are ectoparasites of rats *(O. bacoti*) or mice (*Allodermanyssus sanguineus*), or affect the respiratory passages or pulmonary parenchyma. For example, *Pneumonyssoides caninum* lives in the nasal cavities of dogs; *Pneumonyssus* spp. in the lungs of monkeys; and *Sternostoma tracheacolum* in the air passages and lungs of canaries.

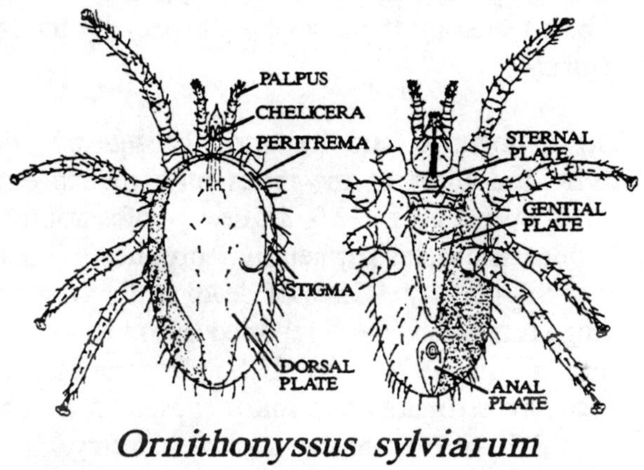


**Figure 11.2.** Dorsal and ventral views of a female of *Ornithonyssus sylviarum*.

### 1.2. Biology

The biology of the endoparasitic mesostigmata is poorly known. The ectoparasitic mesostigmata are hematophagous organisms with five life stages: egg, larva, protonymph (Gr *protos* = first), deutonymph (Gr *deuteros* = second), and adult. With the exception of *O. sylviarum* that spends all its life on the host, the ectoparasitic mesostigmata are temporary parasites. They hide in cracks and crevices or under debris near the host's bed, and climb on the host periodically to feed. They lay a few eggs in their hiding places after each meal. The eggs hatch in 1-3 days to produce non-parasitic larvae. Every 1-2 days the larvae molt to protonymphs, the protonymphs to deutonymphs, and the deutonymphs to adults. Each of these stages (except the deutonymph of O. sylviarum) feeds on blood, particularly at night. Under optimal conditions, the entire life cycle may be complete in little more than a week but the mites may live for up to 2-6 months without food in vacated premises

### 1.3. Medical importance

*D. gallinae* is very dependent on the existence of hiding places, *O. bursa* is less so, and *O. sylviarum* is not dependent at all. Modern poultry operations that provide few places to hide discourage parasitism by the first species but may still be affected by the other two, especially by *O. sylviarum*.

The annoyance and irritation caused by the activity and bites of the mites may reduce egg production by up to 15% in heavy infestations.[4] Fifty thousand mites per hen may produce a blood loss of 6% per day. Cases of death of the host by exsanguination have been reported but must not be common. In 1976, the U.S. Department of Agriculture estimated that mites caused an annual loss of $ 30 million to the poultry industry.[5]

Although the chicken mites do not live permanently on humans, they may bite people in contact with infested birds. Some people develop an allergic dermatitis to these bites. Humans can also be attacked by rodent mesostigmata when infested rodents are exterminated from a house but their mites remain.

*Borrelia anserina* and the viruses of Newcastle disease, fowl pox, Saint Louis encephalitis, Eastern encephalitis, and Western encephalitis have been recovered from chicken mites. Transmission of these infections by these mites is suspected but epidemiological evidence suggests that they are unimportant in the transmission of encephalitides.

The respiratory mites rarely cause health problems but mild rhinitis has been attributed to *P. caninum* of dogs, and respiratory distress to *S. tracheocolum* of canaries.

## 2. THE SUBORDER SARCOPTIFORMES

### 2.1. Identification and classification

The parasitic Sarcoptiformes (from *Sarcoptes*, one of its genera) are recognized because they do not have respiratory openings (they breathe through the skin or swallowing air), and their coxae have strong chitinous supporting structures (= **apodemes or epimera**) that look like dark, thick ridges directed from the base of the legs toward the center of the idiosome (Figure 11.3). They are mostly small (less than 0.4 mm), whitish or yellowish (since they do not feed on blood), weakly sclerotized mites, with well developed pretarsi.

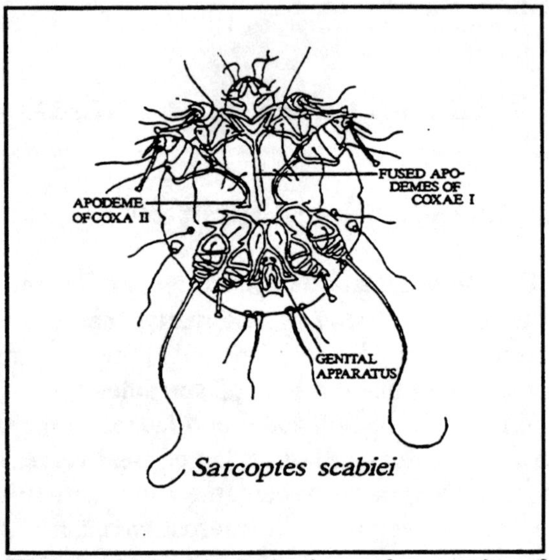


**Figure 11.3.** Ventral view of a male of *Sarcoptes scabiei.*

The Sarcoptiformes most important to veterinary medicine belong to the families **Sarcoptidae** (genera *Sarcoptes*, *Notoedres*, and *Cnemidocoptes*) (Figure 11.4) or **Psoroptidae** (genera *Psoroptes*, *Chorioptes*, and *Otodectes*) (Figure 11.5).

The **Sarcoptids** have a round body with short legs, lack adanal copulatory suckers or abdominal lobes on the males,or genital apodemes in the females. They burrow into the host's epidermis.

The **Psoroptids** have an oval body with long legs, adanal copulatory suckers and abdominal lobes in the males (not very conspicuous in *Otodectes*), and genital apodemes in the females. They live on the surface of the host's skin.

The **adanal copulatory suckers** are a pair of suckers on the ventral side of the males, close to the anus Figure 11.5). The **abdominal lobes** are a pair of tubercles on the posterior margin of the males (Figure 11.5). The **genital apodemes** are a pair of chitinous ridges that arise from either side of the genital opening of the female and run backwards.

Differentiation of *Cnemidocoptes* from *Sarcoptes* or *Notoedres* is rarely necessary in veterinary practice because *Cnemidocoptes* spp. are exclusive parasites of birds whereas *Sarcoptes* and *Notoedres* infest only mammals. Differentiation between the latter two genera can be done by observation of the position of the anus: looking at them from the dorsum, the anus of *Sarcoptes* is terminal whereas the anus of *Notoedres* is dorsal (Figures 11.4).

Differentiation of *Otodectes* from *Psoroptes* or *Chorioptes* is also rarely necessary in veterinary

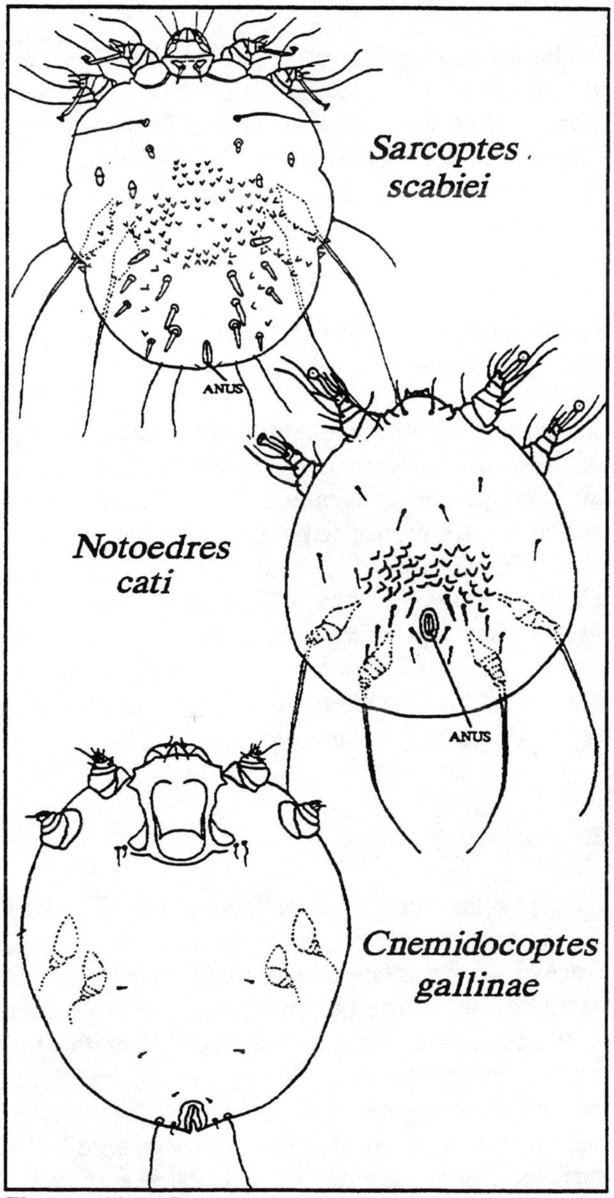


**Figure 11.4.** Dorsal view of the females of some common Sarcoptidae.

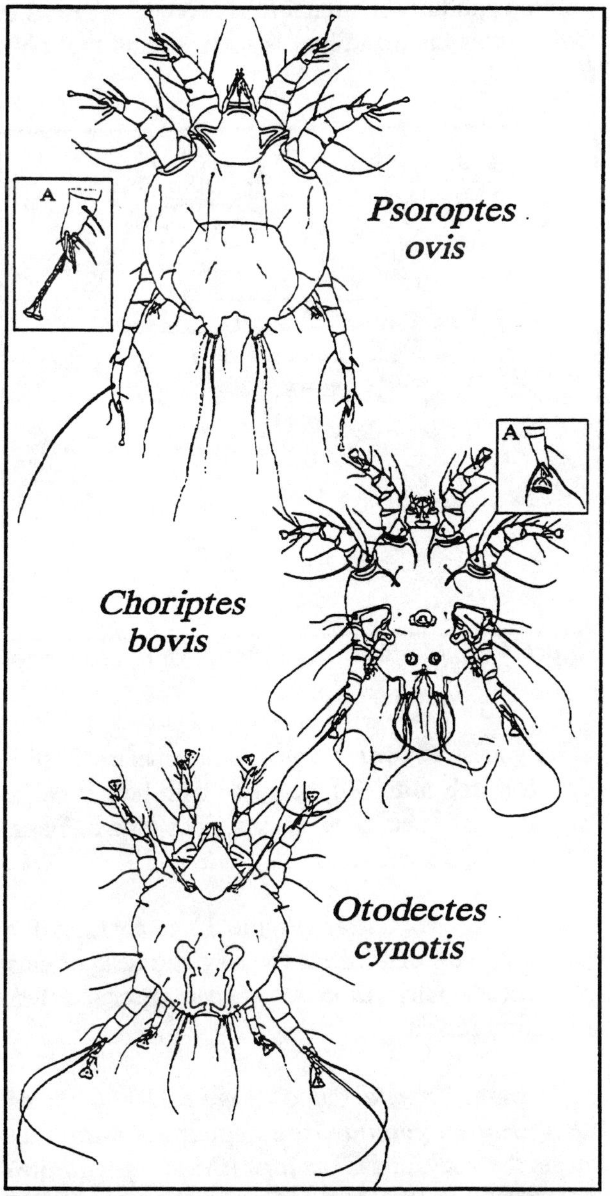


**Figure 11.5.** Male specimens of some common Psoptidae

practice because *Otodectes* is a parasite of carnivores whereas *Psoroptes* and *Chorioptes* are parasites of food animals and equines. Differentiation between *Psoroptes* and *Chorioptes* can be done by observation of the pretarsi: they have long and three-segmented stalks in *Psoroptes* (on legs I, II, and III in males, and I, II, and IV in females) but short, unsegmented stalks in *Chorioptes* (on all legs in males, and on legs I, II, and IV in females) (Figures 11.5). The capitulum of *Psoroptes* is pointed and the abdominal lobes conical whereas in *Chorioptes* the capitulum is rounded and the lobes truncated.

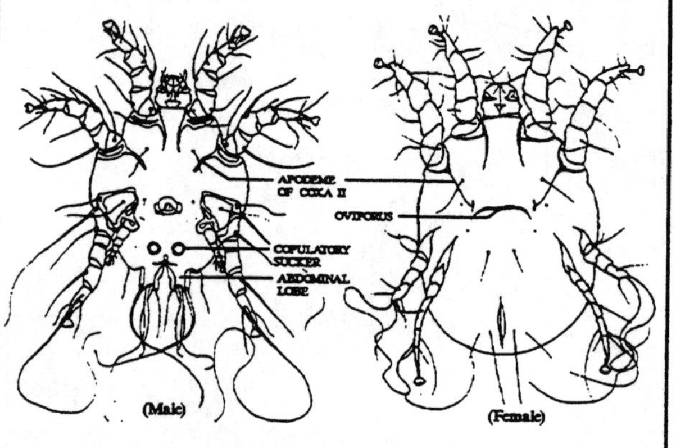


*Chorioptes bovis*

**Figure 11.6.** Morphological details of Psoroptidae.

The genus *Sarcoptes* contains the species *S. scabiei* **(the itch mite**, Figure 11.4) with host specific varieties that affect pigs, horses, dogs, and humans, and less often ruminants.

The genus *Notoedres* (Figure 11.4) contains the species *N. cati* that infects the ears and head of cats and, occasionally, rabbits. Other species affect laboratory rodents.

The genus *Cnemidocoptes* (Figure 11.4) contains the species *C. gallinae* (**the depluming mite**) that infests the body, and *C. mutans* (**the scaly-leg mite**) that infest the legs and beak, of poultry and other birds. Other species infest caged birds.

The genus *Psoroptes* (Figure 11.5) includes a number of host specific varieties. The species recognized as valid nowadays are *P. ovis* (**the sheep scab mite**) that affects sheep, cattle, and horses, *P. equi* that infests equines, *P. cuniculi* that infests rabbits, goats, and equines, *P. natalensis* of bovines and equines, and others of more restricted geographic distribution.[6] In the past, these mites were named after the host species from which they were collected.

The genus *Chorioptes* (Figure 11.5) also includes a number of host specific varieties that used to be named after the host species that harbored them. The only valid species of ample distribution today is *C. bovis* (syn. *C. ovis, C. equi, C. caprae,* etc.) that affects cattle, sheep, goats, horses, and rabbits.[7]

The genus *Otodectes* (Figure 11.5) contains the species *O. cynotis* (**the ear mite**) that infests several species of carnivores.

A number of other Sarcoptiformes infests the skin of laboratory rodents (e.g., *Trixacarus* spp.), or the air passages and air sacs (e.g., *Cytodites* sp.), or the subcutaneous tissues (e.g., *Laminosioptes* sp.), of fowl. Some Sarcoptiformes (e.g., *Acarus* spp., *Dermatophagoides* spp., *Glycyphagus* spp., *Tyrophagus* spp.) proliferate in stored food products. Their incidental bites may cause temporary dermatites in food handlers, and their inhalation may cause respiratory, asthma-type allergies.

### 2.2. Biology

Despite the importance of these mites, their biology is known only for some species and, even in those cases, important details are often missing. All parasitic Sarcoptiformes live permanently on their hosts, feeding on lymph. The females of the sarcoptids penetrate into the epidermis and form tunnels where they deposit their eggs. The remaining stages can be found in the tunnels or on the skin surface. The psoroptids live on the skin surface but are often found under the crusts produced by the infestation.

The females lay one egg at a time, probably 3-5 per day, for a total of 40-90 eggs. The eggs hatch in 1-5 days, and larvae, pronymphs, and deutonymphs are produced. The adults appear 10-14 days after oviposition. The life cycle from egg to egg may take from 10 to 21 days. On the host, the females live for 20-40 days. Off the host and under optimal conditions, they survive for 2-3 weeks at the most.

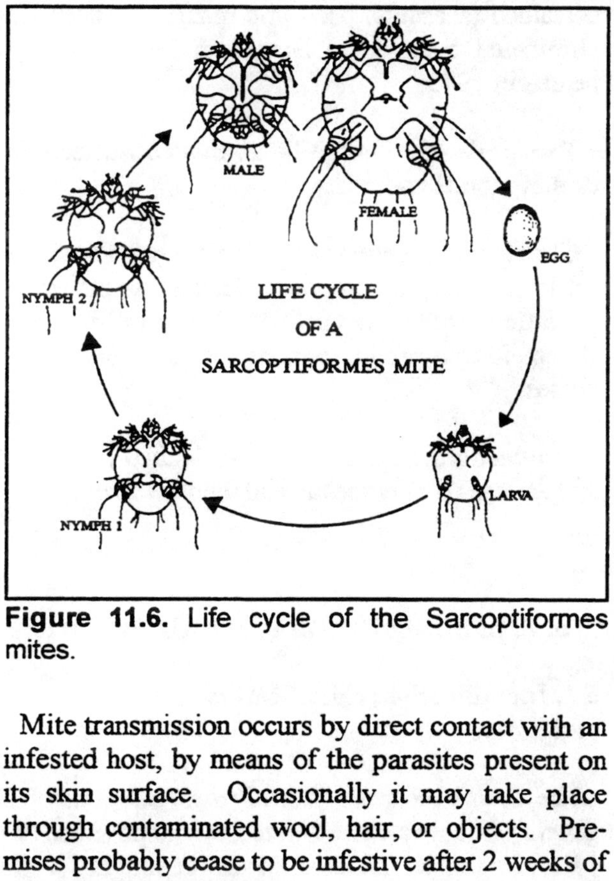


**Figure 11.6.** Life cycle of the Sarcoptiformes mites.

Mite transmission occurs by direct contact with an infested host, by means of the parasites present on its skin surface. Occasionally it may take place through contaminated wool, hair, or objects. Premises probably cease to be infestive after 2 weeks of removing infested animals.

Multiplication on the host is very rapid to the extent that a couple dozens mites may generate over a million in 2-3 months of a primary infestation. The host usually develops some immune resistance so that the number of mites decreases after a few months, and secondary infestations do not grow so fast. Allergic symptoms, however, may still be very important in immune resistant hosts, despite the reduced number of parasites.

Because the sarcoptiformes remain constantly on their host, they are comparatively little affected by weather conditions. They are more abundant in winter, however, and the infestation may regress spontaneously in the summer, although not all parasites die. These mites have preferences for microecological conditions of the host's skin and are often found in specific locations on the host.

### 2.3. Medical importance

Infection or infestation with ticks or mites is generically called **acariasis** but the cutaneous condition caused by permanent skin mites is traditionally called **mange** (scabies in humans).

The **sarcoptids** pierce the tissues to suck lymph and deposit excretions and secretions in the thickness of the epidermis. The host responds to the trauma and inoculation of allergens with an inflammation that progresses to an acute phase with formation of small papules and vesicles. These are rapidly followed by exfoliation and formation of small but numerous yellowish crusts produced by the inflammatory exudate. As the condition becomes more chronic, there is loss of hair or wool, hyperkeratosis and acanthosis of the skin, and edema and proliferation of the underlying connective tissue. As a consequence, the skin looks thickened, folded, crusted, and bare. Pruritus appears very early in the infestation so the biting, scratching, or rubbing by the host aggravate the lesions, and favor secondary infections. Untreated, heavily infested animals may die. Some authors have reported a spontaneous recovery in the summer but the mites do not disappear.

The **psoroptids** puncture the surface of the skin to suck lymph (*Psoroptes*) or gnaw the surface of the skin (*Chorioptes, Otodectes*). The trauma, and probably the inoculation of allergens with the saliva, cause an intense inflammation with formation of small papules and pustules. The rupture of the pustules and the abundant inflammatory exudate produce large and thick yellowish to brown crusts (= **scabs**). The hair or wool becomes matted and discolored and soon begins to fall off, or is pulled off by the host. As the area loses the natural covering, the mites move to the periphery of the lesion, often under the crusts, and the condition extends. Like in the sarcoptic mange, pruritus is intense and may cause the host itself to aggravate the damage. The skin looks more inflamed and with larger and thicker crusts, but less thickened and folded, than in the sarcoptic mange. The difference, however, is not enough for clinical distinction, particularly in acute mange.

Mange may produce important decrease of production due to the torture of a persistent, painful, and pruriginous dermatitis, and the loss of wool. The U.S. Department of Agriculture estimated that during 1973-1975 mites produced losses of \$ 70 million per year to the beef cattle industry, \$ 10 million per year to the dairy cattle industry, \$ 7 million per year to the sheep and goat industry, and \$ 30 million per year to the swine industry.[5]

Animals heavily affected with mange occasionally die. Although the reasons for death are not clear, it has been proposed that loss of heat in cold weather due to denudation of the skin, secondary infections, loss of body fluids and electrolytes, and possibly mite toxins may play a role.

**Sarcoptic mange** is the most severe mange of horses and dairy cattle, the only important in pigs, common in dogs, rather infrequent in beef cattle, and rare in sheep. In this latter, it attacks only the areas of skin free of wool. It is the only mange (= scabies) of humans. Sarcoptes are very host specific; only the dog mite is known to affect heterologous species, it may cause temporary dermatitis in humans.

**Notoedric mange** is the cat mange. It begins at the tip of the ears (**ear kanker**) and may affect the entire head, and even extend to the rest of the body.

**Cnemidocoptic mange** is the fowl mange that affects the feather follicles causing loss of feathers (**depluming mange** by *C. gallinae*), or the skin of the legs causing severe hyperkeratosis (**scaly-leg mange** by *C. mutans*).

**Psoroptic mange** (= **scab mange**) is the most important mange of beef cattle, and very important in sheep in which it causes extensive loss of wool. It also affects horses but is uncommon in dairy cattle. The infestation of any of these host species is notifiable to the Animal Health authorities in the United States. In this country, the horse infestation has not been reported for several decades, the sheep infestation was eradicated in 1970, and programs for the eradication of the cattle infestation are in course. Maintenance of the eradication demands active and sustained measures: psoroptic mange of sheep was eliminated from Great Britain in 1952 but reappeared in 1973.

**Psoroptic ear mange** by *P. cuniculi* affects the ears of rabbits and goats.

**Chorioptic mange** is the most common mange in cattle and sheep but important lesions are infrequent in cattle (particularly beef cattle), and rather rare in sheep. It also produces mange of the hind legs in horses.

**Otodectic mange** or **otocariasis** affects the ears and ear canals of domestic and wild carnivores.

## 3. THE SUBORDER TROMBIDIFORMES

### 3.1. Identification, classification and biology

The Trombidiformes (from *Trombicula*, one of its genera) are mites characterized by the presence of a pair of spiracles situated on the capitulum, at the bases of the chelicerae. Some species lack spiracles, however. The morphology and biology of the parasitic trombidiformes is so heterogeneous that identification of the group is of little use to a veterinarian. It is easier to remember the few species of veterinary importance. There are four genera of trombidiformes that a practicing veterinarian is likely to find: *Demodex, Cheyletiella, Psorergates,* and *Trombicula*.

*Demodex* (**the follicle mites**, Figure 11.6) are very peculiar mites that live in the hair follicles or sebaceous glands of a number of mammals. Rarely, they are found in subdermal tissues or internal organs. They are small (0.1-0.4 mm long) and worm-like. At first sight, their body appears divided like the insects' in head (the capitulum), thorax (the unsegmented podosoma with four pairs of short, stumpy legs), and abdomen (the opisthosoma with transverse striations). The *Demodex* mites found in different hosts are considered to be different species and generally named after the corresponding host (*D. bovis, D. ovis, D. caprae, D. phylloides* of swine, *D. equi, D. canis, D. cati,* and *D. folliculurum* and *D. brevis* of humans). They can be differentiated, mainly by differences in size.[8]

*Demodex* has the typical stages of the life cycle of mites, with two nymphal stages. The females are apparently fecundated on the skin surface and then penetrate the follicles or glands to lay about 20 eggs. The deutonymphs return to the skin surface, mature, mate, and enter the follicles or glands again. The entire life cycle is completed in about 3 weeks. The infection is transmitted by direct contact, and as early as the first hour of life. Transmission must continue through life, however, because the infection is more prevalent in old than in young hosts.

*Cheyletiella* (Figure 11.7) are fairly large mites (about 0.4x0.3 mm) that infest domestic carnivores and lagomorphs. They are recognized by the presence of a large claw on each palpus and a double row of hairs (instead of suckers) on the stalk of the pretarsi. *C. yasguri* infests dogs, *C. blakei* infests cats, and three other species (e.g., *C. parasitivorax*) infest rabbits or hares.

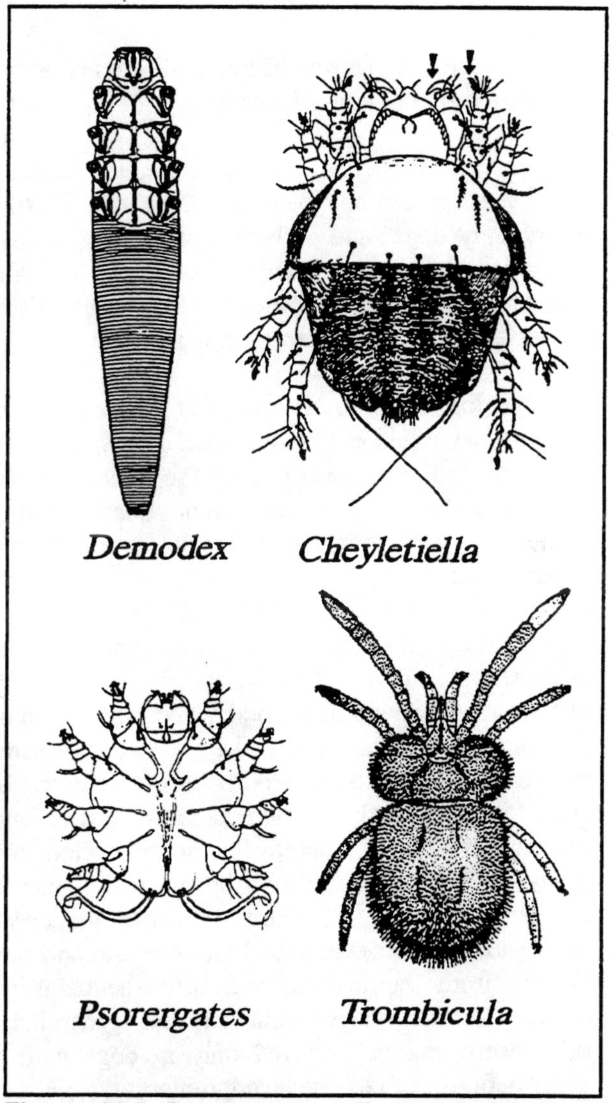

**Figure 11.7.** Some common Trombidiformes.

*Psorergates* (syn. *Psorobia*, **the itch mites**, Figure 11.8) are small (about 0.19x0.16 mm) mites with short and stumpy legs disposed radially and bearing a coiled spine on the femurs. The strong sclerotized support of the legs make the ventral view of the mite appears as if a tiny central body were holding eight massive legs. They are believed to invade the epidermis like the sarcoptid mites. One species infests sheep (P. ovis), another infests cattle (P. bos), and others infest small rodents.

*Trombicula* (**the chiggers**, chigger mites, or harvest mites, Figure 11.9) are free living mites that predate on small invertebrates. Their life cycle includes seven stages. Only the minute red or yellow larva (0.15 mm long when unfed, up to 0.6 mm when engorged) is a parasite of warm-blooded animals. The larva attaches to the skin of a host, injects a fluid that digests the tissues under the skin, and absorbs the lysate. An intense itching often occurs a few hours after the mite began feeding, and the bites and scratching by the host usually aggravate, and may infect, the lesion. Although almost any animal (including humans) may be affected, dogs and cats with lesions in the interdigital spaces or thorax are most often brought to the attention of the veterinarian. Three species of *Trombicula* and some related genera occur in the United States. .

### 3.2. Medical importance

Each of the Trombidiformes discussed above causes a different clinical disease.

*Demodex* is frequently found in healthy hosts; it has been reported in 90% of healthy cattle, 50-70% of healthy dogs, and 20-90% of healthy people. Although demodectic mange may affect virtually any domestic mammal species, it is particularly important in dogs, and secondarily in cattle.

In the dog, **demodectic mange** is not too frequent and may adopt either of two clinical forms: the more common **localized form**, and the less common **generalized form**. The localized or squamous form (red mange of dogs) appears as isolated, non-pruriginous areas of mild inflammation, with hair loss, and usually restricted to the head. This condition tends to regress spontaneously. If not, the skin may become thick, dry, and scaly, and the lesions may extend to other parts of the body. The generalized or pustular form often begins like the localized form but soon extends to large portions of the body. In this form, the inflammation is more intense and causes formation of papules that soon develop into pustules. Secondary infection by pyogenic bacteria is very common. The skin becomes reddened, thickened, and covered with blood, serum, and pus oozing from the lesions, and with the resulting crusts. It was widely believed that generalized demodectic mange occurred only in dogs with a prior deficient of cell-mediated immunity. Now it is known that the immune depression follows, rather than precedes, the disease.[9]

Clinical demodectic mange is infrequent in dairy cattle, and even less frequent in beef cattle. The mites may cause from small papules to small nodules filled with a caseous material containing numerous mites, or even large nodules, sometimes with pus. Only rarely the skin thickens and becomes covered with crusts.

Demodectic mange of horses is rare and may adopt a squamous or a pustular form like the dog's. In other animals it shows a clinical picture like in cattle.

*Cheyletiella* mites are believed to be little host specific so cross infestations between host species may occur. Affected dogs may develop an exfoliative or a crustose form of mange. The **exfoliative form** produces abundant scaling with variable pruritus but little else. Inflammation and alopecia, when present, are usually the result of biting and scratching by the host. The **crustose form** appears like discrete alopecic areas of 2-5 cm in diameter, without an evident inflammatory base. Cats commonly develop the crustose form. Humans in contact with infested pets may develop a temporary dermatitis.

*Psorergates ovis* causes a little contagious, slow-progressing, and very pruriginous mange of sheep. Although the mites produce some inflammation of the deeper layers of the skin, the only external symptom seems to be exfoliation. The biting and rubbing by the sheep to relieve the itching is the main cause of wool loss.

In temperate climates, *Trombicula* larvae attack their hosts in summer and fall. They feed singly or in clusters for a few hours to a couple of days and produce a very pruriginous inflammation that begins a few hours after attachment and continues for several days. Most of the damage derives from the trauma and secondary inflammation caused by host's biting and scratching.

**Summary**

1. The Mites are recognized for the presence of four pairs of legs and no antennae at the nymphal and adult stages. They are distinguished from the ticks because mites do not have a Haller's organ or hypostoma (or the hypostoma is not toothed) and are smaller than the ticks.

2. The Mites of veterinary imporance belong to three suborders: Mesostigmata, Sarcoptiformes, and Trombidiformes.

3. The Mesostigmata have a spiracle by the middle of the body and a peritreme running forward. They are very homogeneous in morphology and biology.

4. The Mesostigmata of veterinary importance are mostly temporary hematophagous ectoparasites of birds (Dermanyssus, Ornithonyssus) or rodents ( Ornithonyssus, Allodermanyssus). Occasionally they attack humans.

5. The Sarcoptiformes do not have spiracles and the coxae of their legs have strong chitinous supporting structures (= apodemes).

6. The short-legged sarcoptiforms (Sarcoptes, Notoedres, Cnemidocoptes) burrow into the epidermis whereas the long-legged sarcoptiforms (Psoroptes, Chorioptes, Otodectes) live on the skin.

7. The sarcoptiforms are the major agents of mange of domestic animals. Sarcoptes causes mange especially in horses, cattle, pigs, and dogs, Notoedres in cats, Cnemidocoptes in birds, Psoroptes in cattle, sheep, and horses (P. cuniculi in the ears of rabbits or goats), Chorioptes in cattle, sheep, and horses, and Otodectes in the ears of carnivores.

8. The Trombidiformes are heterogenous in morphology and biology. Demodex live in the follicles or glands of the skin and may cause mange in dogs or cattle. Cheyletiella live on the skin and may cause mange in carnivores, rabbits, and, ocasionally, humans. Psorergates live in the epidermis and may produce mange in sheep. The larvae of Trombicula may feed on dogs or cats causing pruriginous lesions.

## REFERENCES


1. Baker EW and Wharton GW. 1952. *An introduction to acarology*. Macmillan, New York, 465 pp.

2. Krantz GW. 1978. *A manual of acarology*, 2nd ed. Oregon St. Univ. Book Stores, Corvallis, Oregon, 509 pp.

3. Baker EW, Evans TM, Gould DJ, et al. 1956. *A manual of parasitic mites of medical or economic importance*. Nat. Pest Ctrl. Assoc., New York, 170 pp.

4. De Vaney JA. 1979. The effects of the northern fowl mite, *Ornithonyssus sylviarum*, on egg production and body weight of caged white Leghorn hens. Poultry Sc. 58:191-194.

5. U.S. Department of Agriculture. 1976. *Control of insects affecting livestock*. Nat. Res. Progr. Publication # 20,480, Agr. Res. Serv., Washington, DC.

6. Sweatman GK. 1958. On the life history and validity of the species in *Psoroptes*, a genus of mange mites. Can. J. Zool. 36:905-929.

7. Sweatman GK. 1957. Life history, non specificity, and revision of the genus *Chorioptes* a parasitic mite of herbivores. Can. J. Zool. 35:641-689.

8. Nutting WB. 1976. Hair follicle mites (*Demodex* spp.) of medical and veterinary concern. Cornell Vet. 66:214-331.

9. Barriga OO, Al-Khalidi NW, Martini S and Wyman M. 1992. Evidence of immunosuppression by *Demodex canis*. Vet. Immunol. Immunopathol. 32:37-46.

# CHAPTER 12

# MISCELLANEOUS ARTHROPODS

**Preview.** A few arthropods are of the occasionally concern of the veterinarian. *Linguatula* is a aberrant arthropod that sometimes causes rhinitis in dogs. Spiders or scorpions are periodically blamed for animal diseases. Stings by Hymenoptera (bees, wasps, and ants) may cause cutaneous or general disease in domestic animals.

There is a small number of arthropods that are of the occasional concern of the veterinarian because they may cause sporadic clinical cases or are the object of questions by the client's owner. They are not common enough to deserve an extensive discussion but the veterinarian may need to know a few essentials about them.

## THE PENTASTOMIDA

The **Pentastomida** (from Gr *penta*= five, and *stoma*= mouth, see below)) are believed to be aberrant arthropods distantly related to the crustacea and the mites.[1] The only species found in domestics animals at the adult stage is *Linguatula serrata*. *Linguatula* (from Lat *lingua*= tongue) is an elongated and flat parasite in the outline of a club, with transverse striations, that occurs occasionally in the nasal cavities of canids and, rarely, of herbivores and humans. The males are about 20x3 mm and the females 80-130x8-10 mm. The mouth is at the wider end, ventral, and has one pair of hooks on either side. These hooks can be retracted into small pouches. When retracted, the openings of the pouches resemble four accessory mouths, from where the name pentastomida came.

The eggs (90x70 um) containing a four-legged larva are eliminated with the nasal secretions, or swallowed and passed with the feces. Once ingested by an intermediate host (ruminant, equine, rabbit, rodent, human, etc.), they hatch in the intestine and the larvae migrate to the mesenteric lymphatic nodes, liver, or other viscera where they develop through several molts into a 4-6 mm long nymph (Figure 12.1). The definitive host is infected when it consumes the infected organs.

*Linguatula* attaches to the nasal mucosa with its hooks and sucks blood. Severe infections may cause a prolonged inflammatory rhinitis with all its attendant symptoms. The somatic infection with the larval stages does not produce clinical manifestations. Surprisingly, the infection is rather uncommon in canids but the larvae are found in a large proportion of ruminants. The infection with adults is commonly treated by manual removal of the parasite but probably the organophosphorus insecticides or avermectin may be affective.

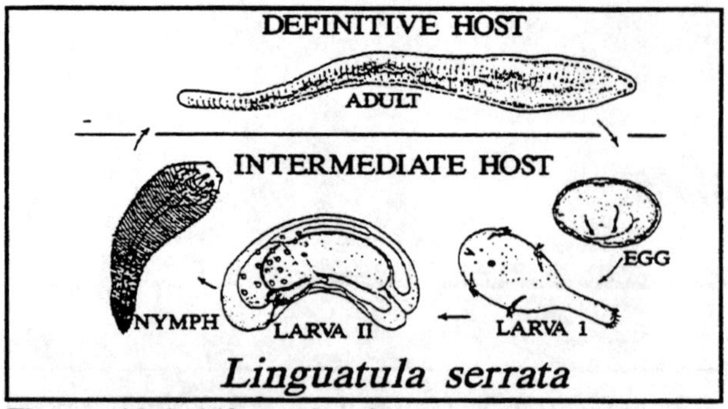


**Figure 12.1.** Life cycle of *Linguatula serrata*.

## THE ARACHNIDA

Veterinarians are occasionally questioned about spiders and scorpions, or presented patients that reportedly were bitten or stung by these arachnida. All spiders and scorpions are venomous but only a few species are able to pierce the mammalian skin, or have a venom powerful or abundant enough to produce disturbances in domestic mammals or humans. Most of them are timid creatures that attack mammals only when they are disturbed.

The **spiders** are recognized as arachnida (see Chapter 2) in which the prosoma (=cephalothorax) and the opisthosoma (=abdomen) are connected by a narrow stalk. Their mouth parts are similar to those on the acarina (see Chapter 9). The venous glands are connected to the chelicerae which are used to bite and inject the venom.

The most common spiders that may cause envenomation in animals or humans are *Latrodectus* spp. and *Loxosceles* spp.[2]

*Latrodectus mactans*, **the black widow** (Figure 12.2), is a complex of several closely related subspecies of the American continent. The female is black, up to 12 mm long, with a red marking in the shape of an hourglass on the ventral surface of the abdomen, and smaller markings on the dorsal surface. The male is black, up to 5 mm long, and with whitish bands and red spots on the dorsum of the abdomen.[3] Other *Latrodectus* species of the New and Old World are black, brown, or whitish.

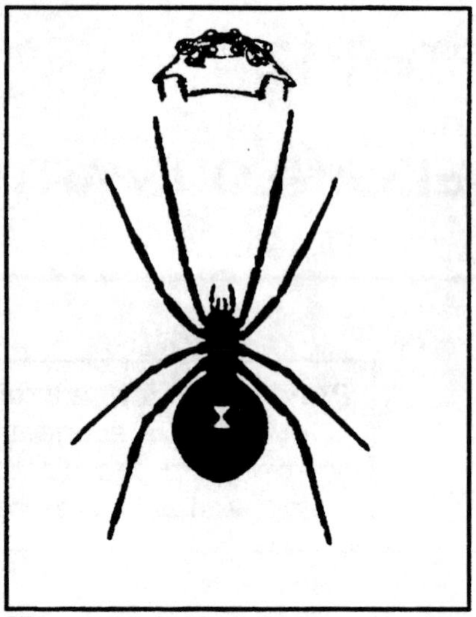

**Figure 12.2.** Female *Latrodectus mactans.* The distribution of its eyes is depicted above (modified from CDC, 1969).

*Latrodectus* are mostly outdoor spiders found under stones or debris near buildings, or in outdoor privies. Their venom is a neurotoxin that causes the release and subsequent depletion of the neurotransmitters from the cholinergic and adrenergic nerve endings.[4] The camel is the domestic animal most sensitive to the venom. The sensitivity decreases in the order cat, horse, dog, sheep, and cattle. The bite often goes unnoticed and leaves only two tiny punctures in the skin. Depending on the amount of toxin injected and the sensitivity of the animal bitten, muscle incoordination and spasms, generalized pain, and excitation may become evident within minutes. Excessive salivation and lacrimation, defecation and vomitation in the carnivores, or dyspnea in the other species soon follow. A flaccid paralysis finally ensues and the animal may die. Mortality is usually below 5% in humans but 90% in cats experimentally bitten by 1-2 spiders. The prevalence of *Latrodectus* bites in domestic animals is unknown. The diagnosis is difficult on purely clinical grounds but it is greatly assisted by a history of spider bite. An anti-venom (prepared in the United States by Merck, Sharp and Dohme Co.) is quite effective but seldom readily available.

Injections of muscle relaxants (e. g., methocarbamol, diazepam), 10% calcium gluconate, or neostigmine have been reported to be effective.

*Loxosceles* spp. are brown spiders up to 15 mm long, of the American continent. They are recognized because they have 6 single eyes whereas most spiders have 8. *Loxosceles reclusa*, **the brown recluse** (Figure 12.3), of the United States has a dark, longitudinal marking in the shape of a violin on the cephalothorax, with the butt by the buccal parts and the handle extending toward the abdomen.

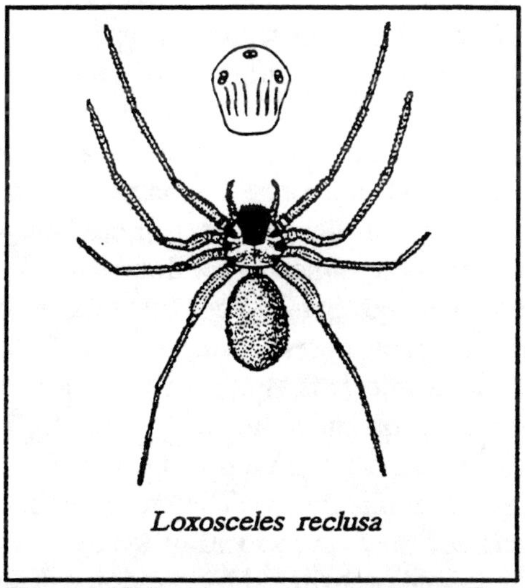


**Figure 12.3.** *Loxosceles reclusa*. The distribution of its eyes are depicted above (modified from CDC, 1969).

*Loxosceles* are mostly indoor spiders that live in protected places such as closets, behind furniture, basements, and undisturbed dark corners. Their venom is a necrotoxin that lyses erythrocytes and endothelial cells. The sensitivity of domestics animals to *Loxosceles* venom has not been determined but dogs and rabbits are known to be quite susceptible. The bite is painful and, depending on the amount of venom injected, it may cause an area of pallor in the skin, that is followed by redness and then a bluish decoloration. Large vesicles with reddish fluid may develop. These appear to be manifestations of damage to the local blood vessels and may develop in a few hours. In the next days, the affected area becomes black and dry, and the skin sloughs. Injectable corticosteroids administered soon after the bite may reduce the damage.

The **scorpions** are recognized as arachnida (see Chapter 2) with large pedipalps that end in massive pincers. The prosoma and opisthosoma are broadly jointed, and the opisthosoma bears a caudal prolongation (metasoma, or postabdomen, or "tail") that ends in a sting (Figure 12.4). The sting is hollow and connected with two venom glands. On the whole, they look like small terrestrial lobsters.

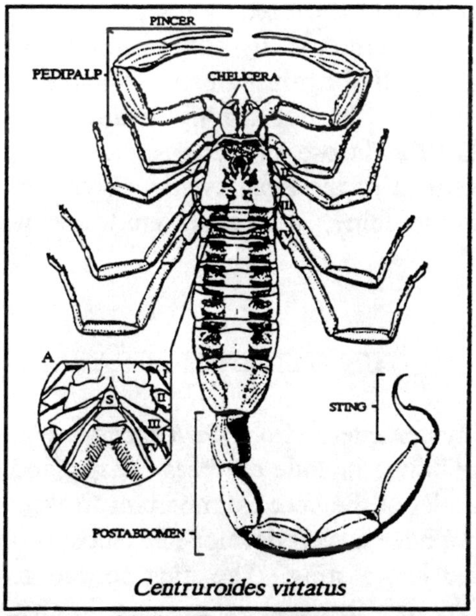


**Figure 12.4.** The common striped scorpion of the United States. The triangular sternum (S) is shown in A.

Virtually all scorpions dangerous to mammals belong to the family Buthidae that can be recognized preliminarily because its members have a triangular sternum (ventral plate between the coxae of the third and fourth pair of legs, Figure 12.4). The classification of scorpions is complex, however, and best left to the specialist.[5] The most venomous species for mammals are some members of the genera *Centruroides* of the states of New Mexico and Arizona in the United States, and of Mexico, *Tityus* of Brazil, Argentina, and Venezuela, and *Androctonus* and *Leiurus* of North Africa and the Middle East. All are rather large scorpions, from 40 to 100 mm long.

Most dangerous scorpions are outdoor creatures that live under stones, loose bark, and other debris, and prowl at night. Their sting is usually painful and injects a venom with components that produce local lesions, or a generalized neurotoxic action. The local phenomena are pain, swelling, and discoloration at the site of the sting, that usually last less than a day. The main general symptoms are excitation, excessive salivation, vomiting, respiratory difficulties, and muscle spasms and cramps. When death ensues, it commonly occurs within a day and is caused by respiratory paralysis or vascular failure. Early administration of anti-venin is effective against the systemic disease but the anti-venin is not readily available. In its absence, 10% glucose intravenously and symptomatic treatment of the manifestations (with corticosteroids, atropine, diazepam, etc.) are recommended.

## THE HYMENOPTERA

The Hymenoptera (from Gr *hymen*= membrane, *pteron*= wing) include the bees, wasps, and ants. The females of the species important to veterinary medicine have a well developed ovipositor that is modified into a sting. The sting appears to be a primitive trait because is missing in the most evolved species.

Because of the greater statistical chance to interact with mammals, the social hymenoptera (those that live in large swarms) are the responsible for most of the medical problems. These are: the honey bee *(Apis mellifera*, Figure 12.5), hornets (*Vespa* spp.), yellowjackets (*Vespula* spp.), paper wasps (*Polistes* spp.), harvester ants (*Pogonomyrmex* spp.), and fire ants (*Solenopsis* spp.). The common species found in the United States are described by Papp and Swan.[3] None of these insects attack mammals spontaneously, but only when they feel threatened. Once one insect attacks, however, the alarm pheromones in the venom induce others to continue the attack.

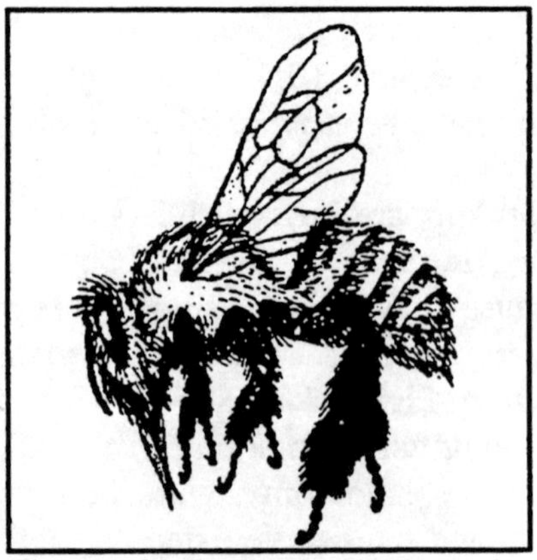

**Figure 12.5.** *Apis mellifera*, the common honeybee (CDC. 1969).

Except for the fire ants, the venom of the hymenoptera contains a number of histamine-like substances, small peptides, and enzymes.[6] The histamine-like substances behave as a venom and cause localized phenomena (sharp pain, a wheal and flare reaction, and edema) immediately upon inoculation. Only when large doses of venom are injected, general symptoms (nausea, vomiting, diarrhea, dyspnea, paresis) may occur. Since each hymenoptera injects at the most 0.1 mg of venom intradermally or subcutaneously and the $LD_{50}$ is 2.5-4.0 mg per kg intravenously, lethal accidents rarely occur in mammals. The enzymes behave as allergens and may cause local or systemic anaphylaxis in animals sensitized by previous stings. The venom of the fire ants contains only necrotizing alkaloids that produce local blisters and sterile pustules within 24 hours.

The lancet of the bee's stinger is barbed so it usually cannot be retrieved from the elastic skin of the mammals and is left behind, with its venom glands, after the sting. Removal of the sting must be done by scraping or with a forceps to avoid squeezing the glands and pumping their content into the skin.

The local symptoms are treated with ice-packs to relieve the pain, congestion, and edema. Compresses of sodium bicarbonate to neutralize the acid fraction of the venom are commonly recommended but it is questionable whether this treatment can reach the venom in the thickness of the skin. The anaphylactic reactions are treated conventionally. In individuals at high risk, desensitization may be achieved by the periodic injection of increasing amounts of venom. This method builds IgG antibodies that combine with the injected allergens before they react with the IgE antibodies responsible for the allergy. The injections must be continued periodically after achieving desensitization, however, to maintain effective levels of IgG.

**Summary**

1. The pentastomid *Linguatula serrata* is occasionally found in the nasal cavity of dogs causing rhinitis.

2. Spiders and scorpions are venomous animals that occasionally may attack domestic animals. The diagnosis relies strongly on the owner of the patient witnessing the accident.

3. Stings by bees or wasps rarely are numerous enough to cause envenomation. Most often they trigger anaphylactic reactions in previously sensitized patients.

## REFERENCES

1. Self JT. 1969. Biological relationships of the Pentastomida: a bibliography on the Pentastomida. Exp. Parasit. 24:63-119.

2. Habermehl GG. 1981. *Venomous animals and their toxins*. Springer-Verlag, Berlin, 195 pp.

3. Papp CS & Swan LA. 1983. *A guide to biting and stinging insects and other arthropods*. 2nd ed. Entomography Publications, Sacramento, 211 pp.

4. Maretic Z & Lebez D. 1979. *Araneism*. Nolit, Belgrade, 255 pp.

5. Keegan HL. 1980. *Scorpions of medical importance*. Univ. Press Mississippi, Jackson, 140 pp.

6. Davis CL. 1979. *Insects. Allergy and disease*. Maracle Press, Oshawa, Ontario, 393 pp.

# CHAPTER 13

# THE NEMATODES OR CYLINDRICAL WORMS

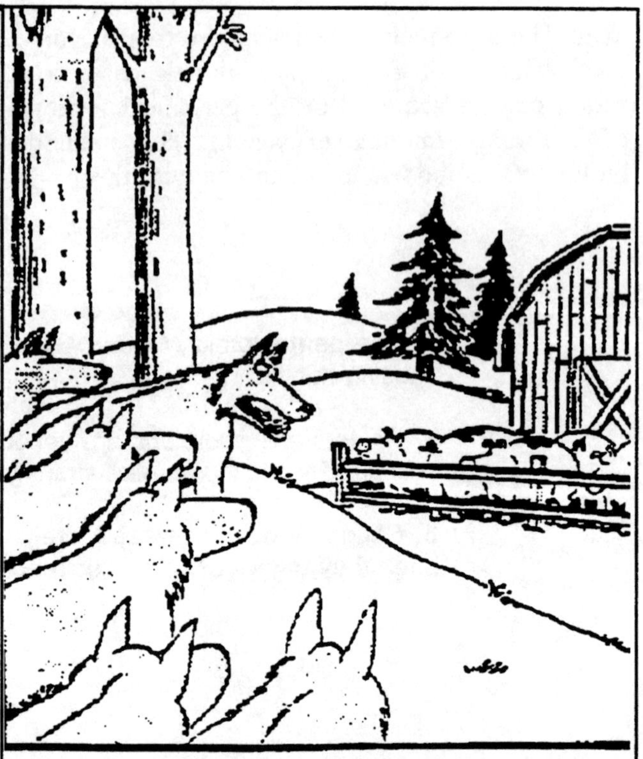

"I say we do it . . . and trichinosis be damned."

**Review.** The Nematodes are cylindrical worms with a morphology and physiology that are rather simple but well adapted to their biological needs. The species parasitic in vertebrates develop in the external environment for part of their life, and move to the host environment for the rest of it. Efficient passage to, and colonization of, each environment, as well as survival in environments that are so dissimilar, are major challenges. Nematodes have developed, however, a number of efficient and varied strategies that allowed them to overcome these difficulties and become very successful organisms.

## 1. Morphology

The Nematodes or **Nemathelminthes** (from Gr *nemas*= thread, and *helmins*= worm) are invertebrates with cylindrical bodies, a body cavity, and a complete digestive tract. Those of veterinary importance may vary from microscopic to about 100 cm long. Conventionally, we will consider them very small if they are microscopic or nearly so, small if they are easily visible but below about 10 mm, medium size if they are between 10 and about 50 mm, large if they measure between 50 and 150 mm, and very large if they are above 150 mm. Whatever their size, the nematodes are much longer than wider so they look like an elongated rod, often with pointed ends. Commonly they are called **cylindrical worms**, or even "round" worms presumably because the section of their bodies is approximately a circle. Chitwood and Chitwood[1] and Bird[2] wrote authoritative reviews of nematode morphology.

### 1.1. External morphology

From the outside the nematodes look smooth, often whitish or yellowish, and with few obvious features. The body is covered by a cuticle that may exhibit microscopic transverse or longitudinal striations. In some species, the cuticle produces expansions along the sides of the body that are called **alae** (sing. ala, from Lat *ala*= wing). Depending on their location, there are **cervical alae, lateral alae**, or **caudal alae**. In the order Strongylida the cuticle of the males expands caudally to form a bell-shaped structure that embraces and holds the female during copulation. It is called the **copulatory bursa**. When present, the structure of the bursa is useful for the identification of genera or species (see Figure 13.1)

The **mouth** is located at the anterior end. Depending on the species, it may be a solitary orifice or be surrounded by lips, papillae, or a number of other structures that will be discussed on the proper occasion. The **esophagus** is often observed from the outside by transparency, particularly in the preadult stages. Although its shape is variable, it readily falls in one of three patterns: **filariform**, when it is long and evenly thin, **strongyliform** (this is, like in the strongylida, see chapter 15), when it is club-shaped, and, **rhabditiform** (this is, like in the rhabditida, see chapter 14), when it has an anterior swelling (= corpus) and a posterior swelling (= bulb) separated by a narrow portion (= isthmus) (Figure 13.2).

The **vulva** opens at different levels of the body depending on the species, and the anus opens near

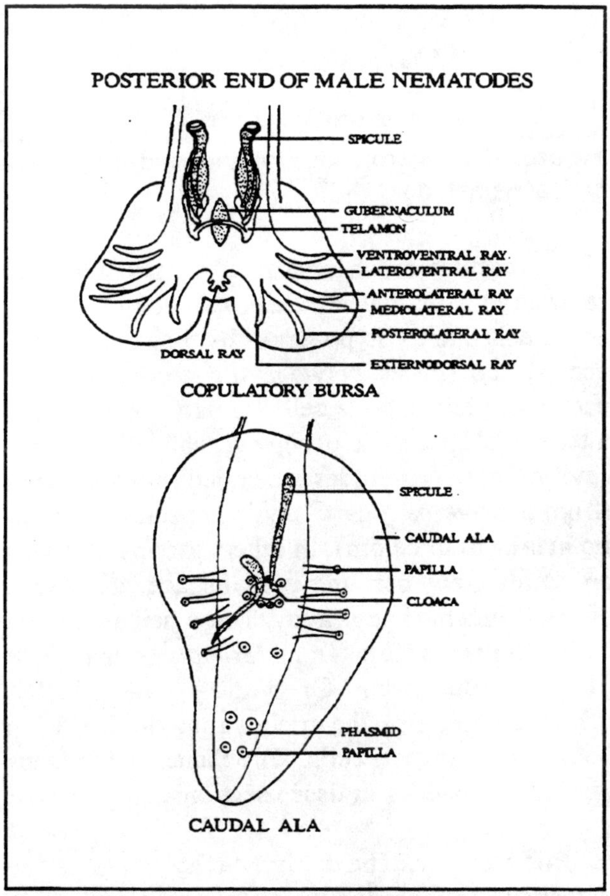


**Figure 13.1.** Morphology of the copulatory bursa and caudal ala of the nematodes.

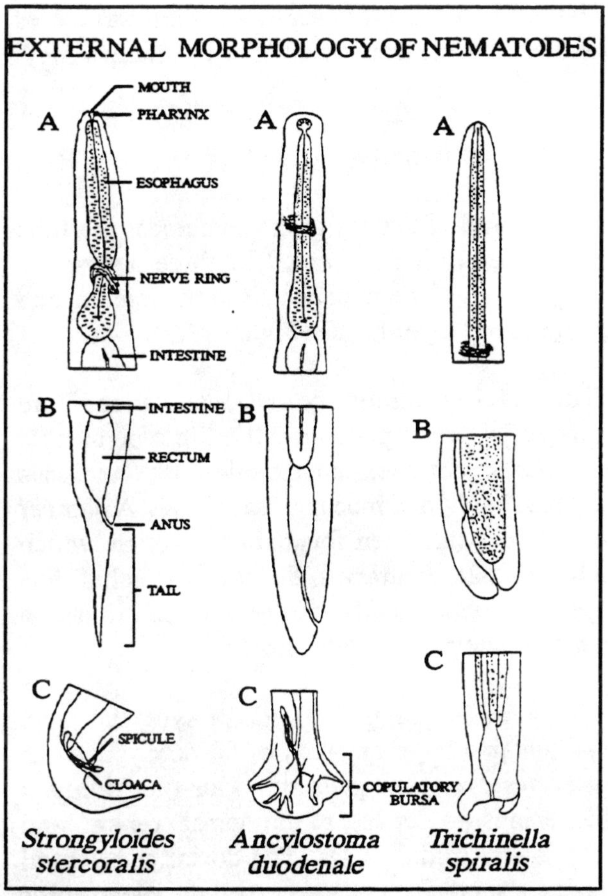


Figure 13.2. Anterior ends (A), posterior ends of females (B), and posterior ends of males of some representative nematodes.

the posterior end. The part of the body posterior to the anus is considered to be the tail. A pair of chemoreceptors (= **phasmids**) in the form of pouches that are virtually invisible in the adult nematode are located at either side of the tail. The male genitalia open together with the anus forming a **cloaca** (= common opening for the genital and digestive apparatuses). The males of many species have one or two needle-like chitinous structures (= **spicules**) in a pouch immediately before the cloaca. When there are two of them, they may be unequal (in size) or dissimilar (in shape). The spicules are protruded and inserted into the vagina during copulation to hold the female and form a bridge for the transmission of the sperms. Some species have a sclerotized plate on the dorsal wall (= **gubernaculum**), or on the ventral and lateral walls (= **telamon**), of the spicular pouch to guide the spicules (Figure 13.1). Like the esophagus, these structures are often studied from the outside by transparency.

### 1.2. Internal morphology

**A. Body wall.** The body of the nematodes is a tube the wall of which is formed by three layers: the cuticle outside, the hypodermis in the middle, and the muscular layer inside (Figure 13.3).

The **cuticle** is a multilayered, acellular structure secreted by the hypodermis. It is little permeable and has a complex composition that includes proteins, lipids, and mucopolysacharides. A number of enzymes has been found in the cuticle which indicates that, contrary to the common belief, this layer is metabolically active and constitutes a dynamic interface with the host.

The **hypodermis** is a cellular or syncytial layer that contains large amounts of fat or glycogen as food reserve. It presents four longitudinal thickenings (= **cords**), at the dorsal, ventral, and both lateral middle lines. The dorsal and ventral cords are small and contain nerves, the lateral cords are larger and contain the excretory canals (when present) and smaller nerves.

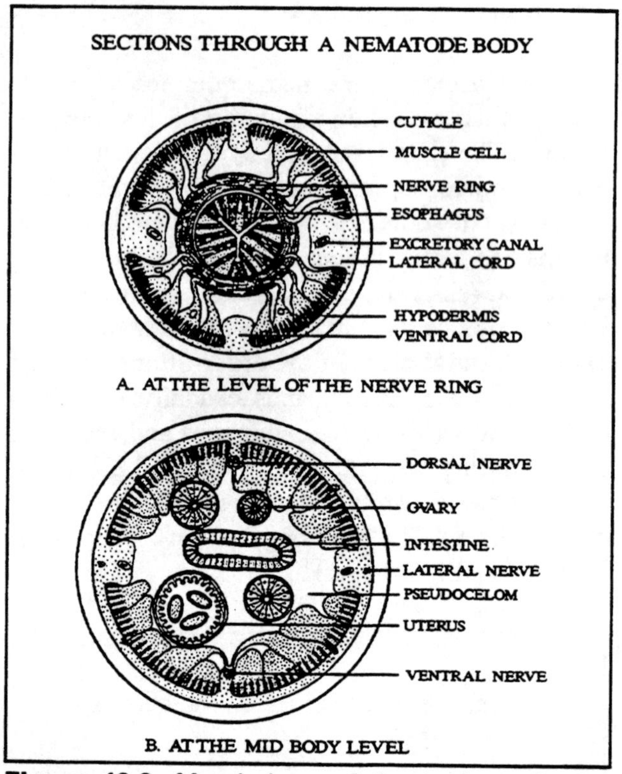


**Figure 13.3.** Morphology of the body wall of a typical nematode.

The **muscular layer** is formed by spindle-shaped contractile cells that are disposed longitudinally and attached to the hypodermis by their sides. They occupy the spaces between the cords. In some nematode groups, these cells are large, only 2-5 per inter-cordal space, and occupy virtually all the body cavity. These nematodes are called **meromyarian** (from Gr *meros*= part, *mys*= muscle) or **celomyarian** (from celom). In others groups, the cells are small, many per inter-cordal space, and do not protrude into the body cavity. These nematodes are called **polymyarian** (from Gr *polys*= many) or **platymyarian** (from Gr *platys*= flat). Finally, others groups, like the trichostrongyloidea, have both types of muscle cells. This characteristic helps identify nematodes in tissue sections.

**B. Body cavity.** The body cavity contains the digestive and reproductive apparatuses, and a few cells of unknown function (Figure 13.3). It is called a **pseudocelom** (from Gr *pseudes*= false) because it does not have a serosal lining. The pseudocelom is filled with a fluid rich in proteins, fats, carbohydrates, enzymes, hemoglobin, nitrogenous compounds, and inorganic ions. This fluid serves the functions of a circulatory system, and keeps a high hydrostatic pressure in the body that operates as a physiologic skeleton to permit the action of the muscle cells.

**C. Digestive system.** The digestive system is a straight tube that begins in the mouth at the anterior end and ends in the anus, near the posterior end (Figure 13.4). The **mouth** is a simple orifice that, depending on the species, may or may not be followed by a **buccal cavity**. Then it comes the esophagus that is often muscular to pump the food into de amuscular intestine, and has a triradiate lumen. In or around the esophagus there are several glands that produce enzymes involved in feeding or molting. The external cuticle reflects on the borders of the mouth and continues inside to line the buccal cavity and the esophagus. In many species, this cuticle forms a number of structures accessory to the mouth or buccal cavity that will be described in the appropriate places. Because this lining changes during the molts, these structures may vary from one nematode stage to the next.

The **intestine**, that follows the esophagus, has a wall formed by a single layer of cells with microvilli to the inside, and a round (but often collapsed) lumen. The total number of intestinal cells may be just a few in some larvae to many thousands in some adults. In non-feeding nematodes (e.g., the infective L3s, see below), the intestinal cells may be filled with stored glycogen, lipids, and proteins so the lumen disappears. The cells in the anterior portion of the intestine secrete enzymes whereas those in the posterior part are absorptive. Finally, a short rectum opens into the anus in the females or into the cloaca in the males.

**D. Reproductive system.** The reproductive system is formed by some long, white, convoluted tubes that fill most of the body cavity (Figure 13.4). The vast size of the female reproductive system is the

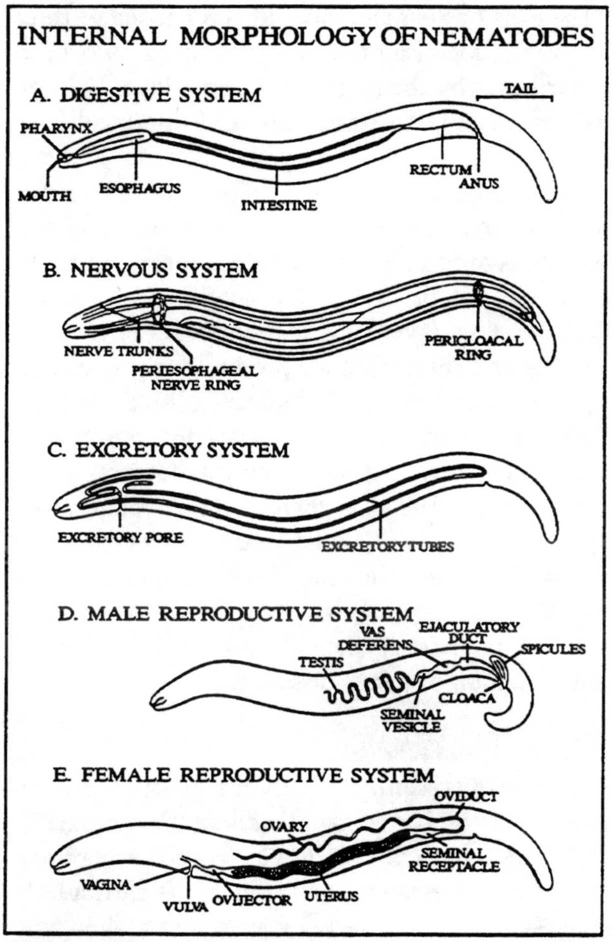


**Figure 13.4.** Internal morphology of a typical nematode.

main responsible for the female nematodes being much larger than the males. In the **male**, there is commonly a single tube that begins with the testis packed with spermatocytes, it follows a seminal vesicle that stores the sperm, and a long vas deferens, often ended in an ejaculatory duct, that takes the sperms to the cloaca during copulation. The nematode sperms are ameboid.

In the **female**, there are commonly two tubes. Each begins with an ovary that is solid in the zone of oogonial germination but shows a small lumen in the zone of oocyte growth. It follows an oviduct that leads to a seminal receptacle, and from there to a tubular uterus. The uterus often leads to a muscular ovijector and from there to a single vagina that opens to the outside through the vulva.

The **eggs** of the nematodes are composed of three layers produced by the zygote, and a fourth layer contributed by the uterus. The inner layer is lipoidal, permeable to gases, but little permeable to water. The middle membrane is a moderately permeable hard shell composed of chitin and tanned proteins. In some species it is interrupted at one or both ends to form an orifice called **operculum**. The outer layer is the lipoproteic vitelline membrane. Outside this layer, many nematode eggs have another protein membrane produced by the uterus. Because of its strength and impermeability, the egg shell is an effective protection for the zygote against the physical and chemical factors of the environment. The size, shape, color, thickness and structure of the wall, and the stage of development of the egg when leaving the host, can be quite varied among the nematodes. The observation of these characteristics often allows a veterinarian the identification of genus or species.

**E. Nervous system.** The nervous system is constituted by a number of ganglia about the esophagus. They are connected by nerves in such a way that they form a periesophageal ring that is particularly conspicuous in the larval stages. From this ring, nerves pass to the anterior and posterior parts of the body, included in the hypodermal cords. Many nerves end in tactile papillae or chemoreceptors (= sense organs) distributed about the head and the rest of the nematode's body.

**F. Excretory system.** In some nematodes, the excretory system consists of a canal running inside each of the lateral hypodermal cords. They join each other and one or two excretory cells about the level of the periesophageal nerve ring, and open to the outside through a ventral excretory pore. There are several variations of this basic pattern, however. In other nematodes, there is only a large excretory cell but not canals. Apart from excretion, this systems is involved in osmotic regulation and production of digestive and molting enzymes.

## 2. Classification

The nematodes are very abundant animals. Estimations put the number of species in perhaps 500,000. About half of the roughly 15,000 species described are free living, the rest are parasites of plants or every kind of animal. Only a little more than a couple hundred species are common parasites of humans or domestic animals.

The nematodes are defined as bilaterally symmetrical invertebrates with a cylindrical body and a pseudocelom. The presence of a complete digestive tract (with a mouth and an anus) and their typical body wall distinguish the nematodes from other pseudocelomate animals. In veterinary medicine, their non-segmented and elongated cylindrical body, and the presence of a body cavity with a digestive tract is enough to separate them from other parasites. An acanthocephalan species, *Macracanthorhynchus hirudinaceus*, looks like a nematode but lacks a digestive tract. A few arthropod parasitic larvae are roughly cylindric but show a distinct transverse segmentation.

The diagnosis of families or genera of nematodes is often based on subtle details of difficult detection. Furthermore, ever since systematic moved from the recognition of organisms by the observation of arbitrary characters to its current emphasis on evolutionary relationships, it became more and more difficult to prepare simple keys for identification. Verification of the genus of the common nematodes of veterinary importance is rather simple if one knows the host and location from where the worms were obtained. This information restricts greatly the alternatives that one must consider. In the absence of this information, or for uncommon parasites, or for the accurate determination of species, the assistance of a specialist may be necessary. The work by Anderson, Chabaud and Willmott[3] is a modern review of nematode classification full of drawings that greatly facilitate the task of inexperienced workers.

Still there are discrepancies among specialists in regard to the proper classification of the parasitic nematodes. Here we will adopt a rather pragmatic classification that is simple, and fits the purposes of a veterinary practitioner (see Chart 3). Customarily, the nematodes are divided into two large groups: the class **Phasmidia** or **Secernentea**, the members of which have phasmids and lateral excretory canals, and the class **Aphasmidia** or **Adenophorea**, embracing the nematodes that lack both. This classification is of little use for the parasites of the higher vertebrates, however. The phasmidia include the orders Rhabditida, Strongylida, Ascaridida, Oxyurida, and Spirurida. The aphasmidia embrace the orders Trichinellida and Dioctophymatida. The brief explanations of these orders that follow are applicable only to the nematodes of veterinary or medical importance.

The **Rhabditida** are very small nematodes, mostly free-living, or parasites of plants or invertebrates. Only the genus *Strongyloides* is an obligatory parasite of the intestine of mammals but a few free-living genera may act as facultative parasites. The adults of the parasitic forms have a long and cylindrical esophagus whereas the free-living forms have a rhabditiform esophagus. Only parthenogenetic females, no males, are known among the parasitic species. They are recognized by their small size, long esophagus, the presence of a transverse vagina without sphincter, and their weakly developed ovijector.

The **Strongylida** of veterinary importance are small to large nematodes of the digestive tract or respiratory apparatus, more rarely of the urinary system. They are easily recognized by the presence of a copulatory bursa supported by muscle rays on the males . This has earned them the common name of **bursate nematodes**. Their esophagus is club-shaped.

The **Ascaridida** are large to very large nematodes of the small intestine, with three prominent lips and a club-shaped esophagus. They are recognized by their presence in the small intestine, their relative large size, their characteristic lips, and the lack of prominent external structures such as copulatory bursae or large buccal cavities.

The **Oxyurida** are small to large nematodes of the large intestine. They are recognized by their typical esophagus with a well developed bulb.

The **Spirurida** are medium size, a few very large, nematodes of the extradigestive tissues (bopdy cavities, body fluids, or connective tissue), or the anterior part of the alimentary tract (esophagus or stomach). Their esophagus is cylindric and often consists of a short, anterior muscular part, and a longer, posterior glandular part.

The **Trichinellida** are small to medium nematodes with a filariform esophagus embedded into a column of glandular cells.

The **Dioctophymatida** are medium to very large nematodes with glandular cells inside a cylindrical esophagus. The males have a single spicule and a muscular copulatory bursa that is not supported by rays. There is only one species of veterinary significance.

## 2. Biology

The most outstanding characteristic of the biology of the parasitic nematodes (and one of the most important to a veterinarian) is their ability to change back and forth from a parasitic condition (the host environment) to a free-living condition (the external environment) to infect new hosts and persist as a species. Through many million years of evolution, they have selected a number of successful strategies to achieve this goal. The changes that a nematode experiences from one generation to the next are commonly referred to as the **life cycle**. Although a number of variations to fulfill particular needs exist, the basic life cycle consists of six phases: fecundation, oviposition, hatching of the egg, formation of an infective larva, infection of a new host, and development to adult. Lee and Atkinson,[4] Croll and Matthews[5] and Wharton[6] have written lucid accounts of nematode biology and physiology.

### 2.1. Fecundation

All nematodes of veterinary importance have separate sexes (= dioecious). With few exceptions (e.g., *Strongyloides*), the females must be impregnated by the males to lay viable eggs. Parthenogenesis is uncommon among parasitic nematodes, possibly because it denies the genetic plasticity needed by organisms that must adapt to changing environments. The sexes find each other with the assistance of chemical attractants equivalent to the pheromones of the insects. Although it has not been tried yet, it is plausible that man-generated interference with these substances could prevent the reproduction of parasites and deter new infections. After copulation, the ameboid sperms are stored in the female seminal receptacle where they survive from several days to a few weeks and fertilize the eggs as they pass by. The entire sperm fuses with the ovum to form a zygote. Further development proceeds through the conventional stages of morula, blastula, gastrula, and tadpole. The final product is a juvenile nematode that, although morphologically not too different from the adult, is conventionally called a larva.

### 2.2. Oviposition

Like the arthropods, most nematodes are oviparous, this is, they lay eggs containing a zygote or a morula. A few species are ovoviviparous (e.g., *Strongyloides*), this is, the females retain the eggs in the uterus and lay eggs containing a juvenile. Even fewer species are described as viviparous (e.g., *Dirofilaria, Trichinella*) because they lay juveniles already hatched. There is no evidence, however, that the female contributes to the nourishment of the juveniles in uterus like the truly viviparous organisms do.

### 2.3. Hatching of the eggs

Depending on the species, the new generation of a nematode may leave the host as a zygote or a morula in the eggshell. Less commonly, they do it as a juvenile in the eggshell, or, infrequently, as a free juvenile. In the first case, the zygote or morula must develop to a juvenile before hatching takes place. In the last case, hatching took place in the uterus.

In all cases studied, hatching is an active process that depends on the production of a **hatching fluid** by the juvenile nematode inside the eggshell.[7] This fluid contains an esterase, a chitinase, proteases, and glycosidases that, with the help of movements of the larva, break down the lipoid membrane of the egg and weaken the middle membrane. The water that penetrates as a consequence of the damage to the membranes is taken up by the larva that enlarges and exerts pressure on the eggshell until it ruptures it.

Production of hatching fluid is believed to be an endocrine phenomenon triggered by stimuli (= signals) from the environment. Nothing is known about these signals for the eggs that hatch in uterus, and little is known about them for the eggs that hatch in the external environment. In this latter case, it has been shown that hatching requires an appropriate range of temperature and moisture, and the presence of a sufficiently developed larva. The eggs of *Nematodirus battus* of the sheep, for example, require a period of chilling followed by an increase in temperature to hatch. This is probably an adaptation to surviving winter and hatching during the spring, when the new generation of lambs is available for infection.

More is known about the signals required by the eggs that hatch in the digestive tract, after being ingested by the definitive host. Specific ranges of temperature, pH, $CO_2$ concentration, redox potential, and, possibly, enzyme activity, in the proper sequence and combination, have been shown to stimulate the hatching of embryonated eggs of ascaridida or oxyurida in vitro. Not all factors are equally important for all nematode species, however. $CO_2$ concentration is the most critical factor for the ascarides but high redox potential (oxidizing conditions), pH, and temperature are the most important determinants for the oxyurids. Since the appropriate combination of stimuli for hatching are likely to be found only in certain regions of the alimentary tract of certain hosts, the biochemical specificity of hatching helps decide which host species will be infected, and in which part of their gut the infective larvae will be released.

### 2.4. Formation of an infective larva

The embryologic development of the zygote results in the formation of a **juvenile** nematode customarily called larva of the first stage or, simply, **L1**. In most nematodes, the physiology of this stage is not ready yet to stand the biochemical conditions of the final host and to develop to an adult. If the L1 penetrates the final host, it is destroyed or passes out unchanged. Before continuing its development in a new definitive host, the L1 must develop into an **L2**, and then into an **L3** or infective larva.In a few nematodes (e.g., the trichinellida, *Filaroides* spp.), the L1 is already infective for the final host. Like in the arthropods, passage of one stage to the next implies growth and change of the external covering. The development of the nematodes is being seen more and more as a process akin to the metamorphosis of the insects to the extent that some authors have proposed to also use the term instar for the stages of the nematodes.

In some nematode groups (e.g., ascaridida, oxyurida), the juveniles remain inside the eggshell while developing to the infective stage. In this case, the L1s develop to L3s under stimulation by appro priate ranges of temperature, humidity, and oxygen supply, and supported by the food reserves existing in the egg. Prolonged exposure to the infrared and ultraviolet radiations from the sunlight is lethal to the egg. Customarily, an egg enclosing an infective juvenile is called an **embryonated egg**. Despite the limited food supply available to the larva, embryonated eggs can survive for many months to several years in a humid, shaded, and cool environment.

In other groups (e.g., strongyloidea, trichostrongyloidea), the L1 leaves the eggshell and proceeds to develop in the external environment. In this case, the L1s feed on bacteria or organic materials in the environment, grow, and molt to free-living L2s. The L2s repeat the same performance, and molt to L3. The L3s, however, retain the cuticle

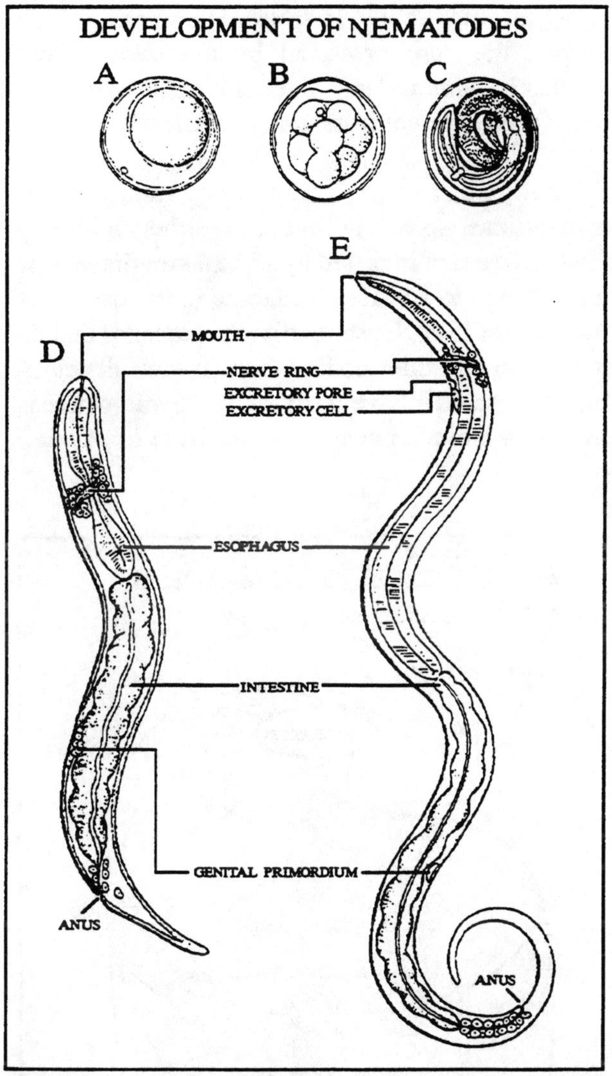


**Figure 13.5.** Eggs with a zygote (A), a morula (B), and a juvenile or larva (C). Larvae of the first (D) and the third (E) stages.

of the L2 as a sheath over their own cuticle (*Strongyloides* spp. is an exception). For this reason, they are called **ensheathed larvae**, term that is used almost as a synonym of infective larvae. The L1s and L2s have a rhabdtitiform esophagus whereas the L3 of most species have a club-shaped esophagus. The former are rightfully called **rhabditiform larvae** but, inexplicably, the latter are called **filariform larvae**. This last term is also commonly used as a synonym of infective larvae. Since the sheath prevents the L3s from eating, they must subsist on food reserves accumulated by the free-living stages in the intestinal cells. In spite of this limited food supply, they are protected by the sheath from weather hazards and may live for months when kept under moderate environmental conditions.

Finally, in a third group (e. g., many metastrongylidae, spirurida), the L1s, either in an egg shell or free, are ingested by an **intermediate host** and develop to an infective larvae in the tissues of this (Figure 13.6). Customarily, the parasites that do not include an intermediate host in their development are said to have a **direct life cycle** whereas those that include one have an **indirect life cycle**.

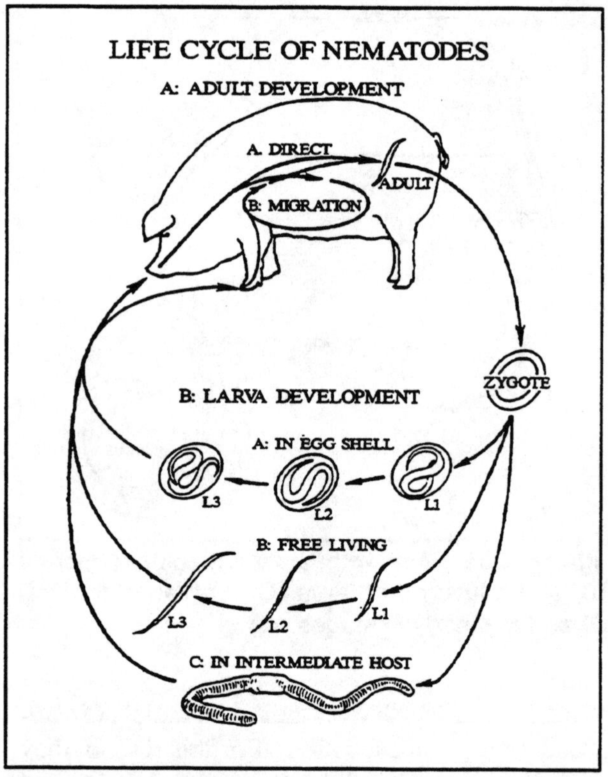


**Figure 13.6.** Common alternatives to the development of a nematode inside and outside its host.

Little information exists on the process of molting in the nematodes. Like in the insects, it consists of the formation of a new cuticle, and loosening and rupture of the old cuticle. Like hatching, this process is thought to be an endocrine phenomenon in which environmental signals bring about the formation of a **molting fluid** which is the responsible for the changes that occur. Only the rupture of the outermost cuticle of the infective larvae, process usually called exsheathment (see below), is known with some detail.

**2.5. Infection of the definitive host**

In nature, the definitive host is generally infected by ingestion of an infective larvae in an eggshell, free, or in an intermediate host. In some cases, the infective larva may penetrate the skin by itself (e.g., *Strongyloides* spp., hookworms) or helped by a vector (e.g., filarioidea). In few cases, infection occurs transplacentally (e.g., *Strongyloides, Toxocara canis, Ancylostoma caninum*) or with the colostrum or milk (e.g., *Strongyloides, Toxocara vitulorum, Ancylostoma caninum. T. canis*).

The L3s that remain in the eggshell are ingested by the new definitive host with its food or water so they must rely on sheer luck to meet the appropriate host. The extraordinary prolificacy of the nematodes that use this strategy (a female of *Ascaris suum* lays up to one million eggs per day) and the long survival of the infective eggs in the environment (up to 5 years for *Ascaris lumbricoides*) maximizes the odds of a successful encounter, however. Human intervention, that keeps large numbers of potential hosts together, also increases the probability that the embryonated eggs will eventually find a new host.

The free-living infective larvae are generally more susceptible to the factors of the environment (extremes of temperature, dryness, solar radiation) than the infective larvae in an eggshell. The former (e.g., *Trichostrongylus, Ostertagia*) live only for several weeks or a few months, and rarely survive the summer of tropical or temperate regions, or the winter of temperate or cool regions. In compensation, the free-living L3s can move into the ground to escape the rigors of the weather, or high on the vegetation where the chances to be ingested by a grazing host are greater. In some cases, (e.g., *Strongyloides*, the hookworms), the infective larvae can penetrate actively through the host's skin. These strategies must be quite effective because the nematodes that use them are only moderately prolific (a female *Ostertagia* or *Trichostrongylus* lays only 100-200 eggs per day, a female *Strongyloides* only 50, and the female hookworms only 4,000-20,000) but they endure well in nature.

The infective larvae that develop in intermediate hosts generally occur in situations in which the intermediate and definitive hosts are members of a same alimentary chain and, therefore, have easy access to each other (e.g., earthworms and pigs for the swine lungworms, *Metastrongylus* spp.). In some cases, the intermediate host is drawn to the definitive host by physiological needs and constitutes a biological vector (e.g., mosquitoes and dogs for the dog heartworm, *Dirofilaria immitis*). As a result, the odds that the definitive host infects the intermediate host and vice-versa are rather high. The use of intermediate hosts not only provides a reasonable assurance that the parasite will reach the final host, but also protects the juveniles from the vicissitudes of the climate, and concentrates the infective stages in one source, which will eventually produce more reproducing parasites once in the final host.

Transplacental and transmmary infections will be discussed with the specific parasites.

The success of these strategies is certainly not serendipitous but the result of million of years of natural selection that eliminated those systems that were inefficient to persist in nature.

### 2.6. Development to adult

Once the L3 penetrates the definitive host it gets rid of its sheath, grows, and molts to an L4. The L4, in turn, grows, and molts to an early adult. The juvenile adults develop their reproductive systems to become fully functional adults, males and females mate, and a new generation begins. The presence of detectable eggs or larvae in the feces or fluids of an infected host is called **patency**, and the period from infection to the beginning of patency is called **prepatency**.

**Exsheathment** occurs after the infective larva is ingested by the definite host and appears to be a phenomenon of the same nature as hatching. Actually, exsheathment partakes of the same signals that stimulate hatching, although in this case $CO_2$ concentration and pH seem to be the main factors. Also, the activity of host's enzymes is necessary for some nematodes. As a result of this stimulation, the infective larva produces an exsheathment fluid that contains a leucine aminopeptidase and other enzymes specific for the species of nematode that produced them. These enzymes digest a thin ring of the sheath close to the anterior end, the resulting cap of cuticle falls off, and the parasite wiggles out of the sheath.[7,8]

In the digestive nematodes that do not migrate through the host's body, exsheathment occurs in the digestive compartment anterior to their definitive location: in the rumen for the gastric nematodes (e.g., *Haemonchus, Ostertagia, Trichostrongylus*), in the stomach for the nematodes of the small intestine (e.g., *Nematodirus*), and in the small intestine for the nematodes of the large intestine (e.g., *Oesophagostomum*).

It is known that the free living and the parasitic stages of the nematodes exhibit metabolic disparities that result from their different environments and purposes. Whereas the metabolism of the former is geared toward growth and survival, that of the latter is directed to reproduction. Little information exists about the metabolism of the preadult parasitic stages but there is some evidence that the change from the free-living type to the parasitic type metabolism is gradual. This suggests that the biochemical requirements of the preadult parasitic stages may be different from those of the adult parasite, and explains the fact that they develop in different parts of the host's body. Barret[9] has reviewed the metabolism of the nematodes and the biochemical characteristics of different host tissues.

Development to the adult stage usually requires some intimate contact with the host tissues. In some species (e.g., *Trichuris* spp., oxyurida, most trichostrongyloidea), the pre-adult stages move steadily to the definitive location of the adult parasite, spending brief periods in the surrounding tissues during their journey. In others, the pre-adults perform extensive migrations through tissues seemingly unrelated to the final location of the adult (e.g., most ascaridia, *Strongylus* spp. (Figure 13.6). Some authors have speculated that extensive migrations is an atavic trait of nematodes that originally possessed intermediate hosts. If this were the case, however, one would expect that the migration occurred before rather than after reaching the infective stage.

It seems obvious, nevertheless, that the developing parasitic stages require environmental biochemical conditions that are present only in some specific host's tissues. These requirements not only include nutrients but also biochemical stimuli. There is a consensus among the specialists today that all phases of the nematode development in the definitive host are directed by biochemical signals from the host, which is the parasite's environment. These signals stimulate hormones or derepress genes, in the proper and necessary sequence. The migrations of de preadult parasitic nematodes, then, are viewed as a search for the appropriate signals.

### 2.7. Adaptation to the host environment

Although living in a host represents a number of benefits for the parasite (such as a reasonably constant environment, a permanent supply of food, and many host's functions that can be used for the regulation of its own biology), it also means a drastic change of metabolism upon penetration, and the confrontation with an often hostile environment. Some of the most obvious problems faced by the parasite is the need to keep its place in a moving locale (intestinal content or blood current), elude the action of the digestive enzymes in the gut, and avoid the effect of the host's immunity.

Some nematodes keep their position by constantly swimming against the current, others embed themselves in the mucus or thread themselves in the mucosa, others anchor themselves by biting the mucosa, and others secrete acetylcholinesterase that inhibits the peristaltic movements in the vicinity of the nematode.

Avoidance of digestion in the digestive tract of the hosts must be an active mechanism residing in the cuticle because the nematodes are digested as soon as they die or their tegument is damaged. Peptides that inhibit host proteases have been reported from several parasitic nematodes but it is not clear whether they are the responsible for their resistance to digestion.

Host's immunity would appear to be a formidable obstacle to parasitism, but parasites arouse in evolution before the inception of immunity. They had the chance to develop and incorporate into their biology a number of strategies to elude immunity. A major strategy was to discard the strongly antigenic substances that were critical to the survival of the parasite. In today's parasites, the antigens that elicit protective reactions are only weakly antigenic, and easily inhibited by other more powerful antigens that do not induce protection (antigenic competition). The parasites that failed to achieve this goal must have been eliminated by their host's immune responses early in evolution. Other strategies to elude host's immunity are also known. Some nematodes hide in sites inaccessible to the immune system (e.g., inside the host's cells, like the larvae of *Trichinella*), others shed cuticular antigens constantly so the effectors of immunity (T cells and antibodies) are diverted to the circulating antigens before reaching the parasite, others disguise themselves by adsorbing host's proteins on their cuticle, and other simply depress the antiparasite responses by diverse mechanisms.[10]

On the other hand, host's immunity provides the parasite with a handy tool to regulate its own biology. For example, Dineen[11] speculated that parasites might use host's immunity to adjust the size of their population to levels compatible with the well-being of the host. The weak parasite antigens that induce protective reactions would be effective only when they reach a certain concentration in the host. Small populations of parasites would be ignored by immunity but larger populations (that may endanger the life of the host) would trigger anti-parasite reactions that would eliminate part of the parasites until the concentration of antigens produced falls again below the reactive level. Host's immunity is also used by some parasites to induce a waiting period at the juvenile stage for the most appropriate opportunity to infect the new generation of hosts (see chapters 19, Trichostrongyloidea, and 21, Ascarides).

### 2.8. Regulation of the life cycle

It has been said that the essence of parasitism is to be in the proper place at the proper time. Since the infective stages of most nematodes have little (if any) mobility, they must simply wait in the place where they happened to occur for the proper time to infect a new host. Through evolution, many nematodes developed the capacity to arrest their development to extend their life and maximize the opportunity of encountering a new host. This arrest may also take place in the host while the parasite waits for the most appropriate time to lay its eggs. **Arrested development**, also called dormancy or hypobiosis, is a period of metabolic inhibition with suspension of growth that is comparable to the diapause of the insects. It can occur at different times in the life cycle of the worm: in the egg, in the external environment, in an intermediate host, in a transport host, or in the definitive host.

The evidence suggests that arrested development is largely an automatic phenomenon that takes place spontaneously after each of several stages of growth. Resumption of development occurs only if and when some stimuli (or signals) external to the nematode trigger the next stage. The prolonged survival of the L3s despite their limited food supply suggests that this stage enters in dormancy automatically upon formation, like the larvae of some mosquitoes, until they are activated by stimuli from the new host. Among the free-living stages of many nematodes, there is a range between the temperature that stimulates their development and the temperature that kills them. This simply stops them from growing. Dormancy in the definitive host will be discussed with the trichostrongyloidea and with the ascaridida.

### 4. Medical importance

Most nematodes are only moderately pathogenic. A long evolutionary process appears to have eliminated those species that endangered the life of their hosts and, therefore, their own existence. Overt disease by nematodes is generally the result of excessive accumulation of parasites in single hosts, often brought about by the need of civilization to have many animals together in a restricted space. Although moderate nematode parasitism is rarely a medical problem, still it can affect in subtle ways the growth and productivity of the host as to become an economic problem. This is a concept particularly relevant to veterinarians working with food animals.

In a few cases, the **pathogenic mechanisms** of the nematodes are obvious: the large strongyles of horses (*Strongylus* spp.) and the hookworms (Ancylostomatidae) bite and digest the intestinal mucosa and suck blood, the dog heartworm (*Dirofilaria immitis*) physically interferes with the contraction of the heart and the function of its valves, the cattle lungworm (*Dictyocaulus viviparus*) occludes the air passages. In other cases, the pathology and its consequences are obvious but its mechanisms of production are more subtle and not completely understood: we still do not know how the hookworms cause atrophy of the intestinal villi, or *Dirofilaria* produces its typical villous endarteritis, or *Dictyocaulus* induces such a severe bronchial inflammation. In still other cases, the pathology appears remote to the activities of the parasite and its pathogenesis is obscure: infections of sheep with *Trichostrongylus colubriformis* consistently depress the appetite and the production of thyroxine, and enhance the levels of corticosteroids. It is not known how the parasite generates these changes.

It seems clear, however, that the pathophysiologic phenomena that operate in parasitic infections respond to the same general and well established principles of homeostasis that rule other diseases. Elucidation of the corresponding details is only a matter of time and effort. In the following chapters, we will discuss what is known about the pathogenesis of the different nematodiases.

Immune responses against helminths occur in the fashion predicted by general principles of immunology: strong in the case of parasites in close or prolonged contact with the host's tissues, and weak in those cases in which the contact is superficial or brief; predominantly IgG production against tissue parasites but mainly IgA production against parasites of the mucosas. Because helminths are biochemically complex organisms, they produce many antigens, some generated by their metabolism (metabolic, excretory-secretory, or ES antigens) and some derived from the body components of specimens that die (somatic or structural antigens). Determination of relevant anti-helminth immune reactions is complex because it requires selection of the proper antigen, understanding of the abundant instances of antigenic competition, and sorting among antigens common to diverse species.

Although the knowledge of anti-parasitic immunity has lagged behind that of bacteria and viruses and much work is still necessary, it is known that it can contribute to the pathogenicity of some parasitic infections, or used for diagnosis or control of the infections. Specific examples will be discussed in the following chapters.

Protective immunity against helminths is much less dramatic than against viruses or bacteria although the immune responses to all three are fully comparable. Unlike viruses or bacteria, most helminths cannot hide inside host cells or multiply rapidly inside the host. Helped by their greater biochemical complexity, however, they developed different strategies than viruses and bacteria to elude host immunity. We mentioned some examples above.

## 5. Epidemiology

The transmission of parasites from one host to the next depends on the production of parasitic elements by an infected host, the development and survival of these elements in the external environment, and the acquisition of the infective stages by the next host. The corresponding details will be discussed with each parasite group. Here we will mentioned only some basic concepts.

In our discussion of nematode biology we mentioned some of the hazards that the parasite must overcome to reach a new host. Now we will examine some of the influences of the external environment on the ability of the parasite to pass from one host to the next.

Once the elements of parasite transmission (eggs or larvae) reach the external environment, they are subjected to aging and to the factors of the climate and weather. **Aging** depletes the food reserves of the L3s and deteriorates the activity of their enzymes. As a consequence, the infective stages lose infectivity with time, and ultimately die.

Climate are the meteorological conditions that prevail in a geographic area. Weather is the climate at a particular time. Whereas the climate indicates whether a parasite can exist in a region, the weather determines its prevalence at a given time. Of the many factors of the climate, only the influence of temperature and humidity upon the transmission of nematodes has been studied with some detail.

**Temperature** acts on nematodes in several ways: it influences the aging process, regulates development, and affects the activity of the free-living stages. Temperature influences the longevity of the infective larvae through its effect on the metabolism: in the laboratory, L3s of *Haemonchus contortus* survive 35 weeks at 24C (75F), 49 at 15C (59F), 83 at 10C (50F), and 87 at 4C (39F). Through regulation of development, temperature dictates to a large extend the geographic distribution of parasites. For example, the eggs of the dog hookworms, *Ancylostoma braziliense*, *Ancylostoma caninum*, and *Uncinaria stenocephala*, develop best between 27 to 32C (81-90F), 23 to 30C (73-86F), and 15 to 25C (59-77F), respectively. This explains that the first predominates in the tropics and subtropics, the second prevails in the temperate zones, and the third occurs from the northern parts of the temperate zones to the subartic regions.

The effect of temperature on the preparasitic stages of the nematodes is complex. The optimal range of temperature is that that produces the greatest proportion of infective larvae. Temperatures above it accelerate development but increase mortality. Temperatures below it prolong survival but may fail to produce infective larvae. Furthermore, the optimal ranges for development of eggs, survival of the free-living stages, or infection of the host may be different. For example, eggs may benefit from a higher temperature that causes a reasonably rapid development and avoids environmental hazards (desiccation, direct sunlight, predators, fungal infections), free-living stages may benefit from somewhat lower temperatures that prolongs survival and the chances to find a host, L3s may benefit from medium temperatures that keep the larva active (so they may climb the herbage to be eaten) but does not exhaust its food reserves.

**Humidity** is another essential factor for the survival of the free-living stages of the nematodes. Laboratory studies have demonstrated that nematodes generally need over 80 to 90% relative humidity for development, and die rapidly below about 60%. Because of the difficulty of measuring relative humidity at the location of the eggs or larvae, in the practice the humidity required for development of nematodes of food animals is expressed as rainfall. For example, the optimum for development and survival of the free-stages of *Cooperia*, *Trichostrongylus*, and *Oesophagostomum* of cattle is 13 to 26C (55-79F) mean monthly temperature and 5-12 cm of total monthly precipitation whereas the optimum for larval survival alone is 8 to 26C (46-79F) of temperature and 5 to 17 cm of precipitation. Precipitation is also a complex factor since too little would desiccate the parasite but too much would wash them away.

The fact that the weather conditions are generally measured at shelters one meter above the ground whereas the free-living parasite stages exist in the soil adds to the complexity of predicting contamination with parasites. Measurements taken in Columbus, Ohio, in June 1983 registered 30.8C (87.5F) and 25.6% relative humidity at a weather station, but 26C (77.8F) and 82.1% in the ground litter layer. Furthermore, the quality and cover of the ground greatly influence the retention and evaporation of water and creates microenvironments that may have little relationship with the general weather conditions. With air temperatures of 13 to 25C (55-77F), larvae of *Ancylostoma caninum* survived 1 day on concrete, 2 on pea gravel, 2-3 on bare ground, but 24 on bluegrass plots.[12]

It is fair to say that little solid information exist on the ecological conditions that permit the development and survival of the nematode infective elements in the field, and this knowledge is difficult to apply with accuracy in practical situations. Experience and careful observations of the conditions in a particular area, however, generally permit educated guesses.

**Summary:**

1. Nematodes are cylindrical worms with a complete intestine and a body cavity.

2. External features like their size, the shape of their mouth, esophagus, spicules, or eggs, or the presence of alae, copulatory bursa, labial structures, etc., in combination with the host and location of the parasite, permit a veterinarian to identify genus or species.

3. The nematode parasites of humans or domestic animals belong to the orders Rhabditida, Strongylida, Ascaridida, Oxyurida, Spirurida, Trichinellida, and Dioctophymatida.

4. In most species, there are four preparasitic stages (egg, L1, L2, and L3), and three parasitic stages (L3, L4, and adult). The L3 is normally the transition stage.

5. The infective stage is commonly an L3 which, depending on the species, may enter a new definitive host in an eggshell, as a free living larvae, or in an intermediate host. Each alternative has biotic advantages and disadvantages.

6. The most common entry into a host is through the mouth but some species can enter transcutaneously (directly or assisted by a vector), in uterus, or with the mother's milk.

7. Once in the host, the parasite needs contact with the host's tissues to develop to adult. Depending on the species, this is achieved through brief stages in the digestive mucosa or extensive systemic migrations.

8. Parasites often find hostile environments (dryness, extremes of temperature, and sunlight outside the host, a moving locale, digestive enzymes, and immunity inside the host) but they have developed ways to deal with them.

9. The pathophysiology and immunology of parasites follows the standard and well known rules of each discipline. The biological complexity of parasites, however, permits them alternatives that are denied to protokariote organisms.

## REFERENCES

1. Chitwood BG & Chitwood MB. 1974. *An introduction to nematology,* consolidated edition, with revisions, University Park Press, Baltimore, 334 pp.

2. Bird AF. 1971. *The structure of nematodes*. Academic Press, New York, 318 pp.

3. Anderson RC, Chabaud AG, and Willmott S. (eds.). 1974-1983. *CIH keys to the nematode parasites of vertebrates*, Nos. 1-10. Commonwealth Agricultural Bureau, Slough, England.

4. Lee DL & Atkinson HJ. 1976. *The physiology of the nematodes*. 2nd ed., Freeman, San Francisco, 215 pp.

5. Croll NA & Matthews BE. 1977. *Biology of nematodes.* J. Wiley, New York, 201 pp.

6. Wharton DA. 1986. *A functional biology of nematodes*. Croom Helm, London, 192 pp.

7. Rogers WP & Summerville RI. 1967. The infectious process and its relation to the development of early parasitic stages of nematodes. Adv. Parasit. 6:327-348.

8. Lackie AM. 1975. The activation of infective stages of endoparasites of vertebrates. Biol. Rev. 50:285-323.

9. Barret J. 1981. *Biochemistry of parasitic helminths.* MacMillan, London, 308 pp.

10. Barriga O.O. 1984. Immunomodulation by nematodes. A review. Vet. Parasit. 14:299-320.

11. Dineen JK. 1963. Immunological aspects of parasitism. Nature (London) 197:268-269.

12. Mark DL. 1975. Survival of *Ancylostoma caninum* on bluegrass pasture. J. Parasit. 61:484-488.

# CHART 13.I. CLASSIFICATION OF THE NEMATODES

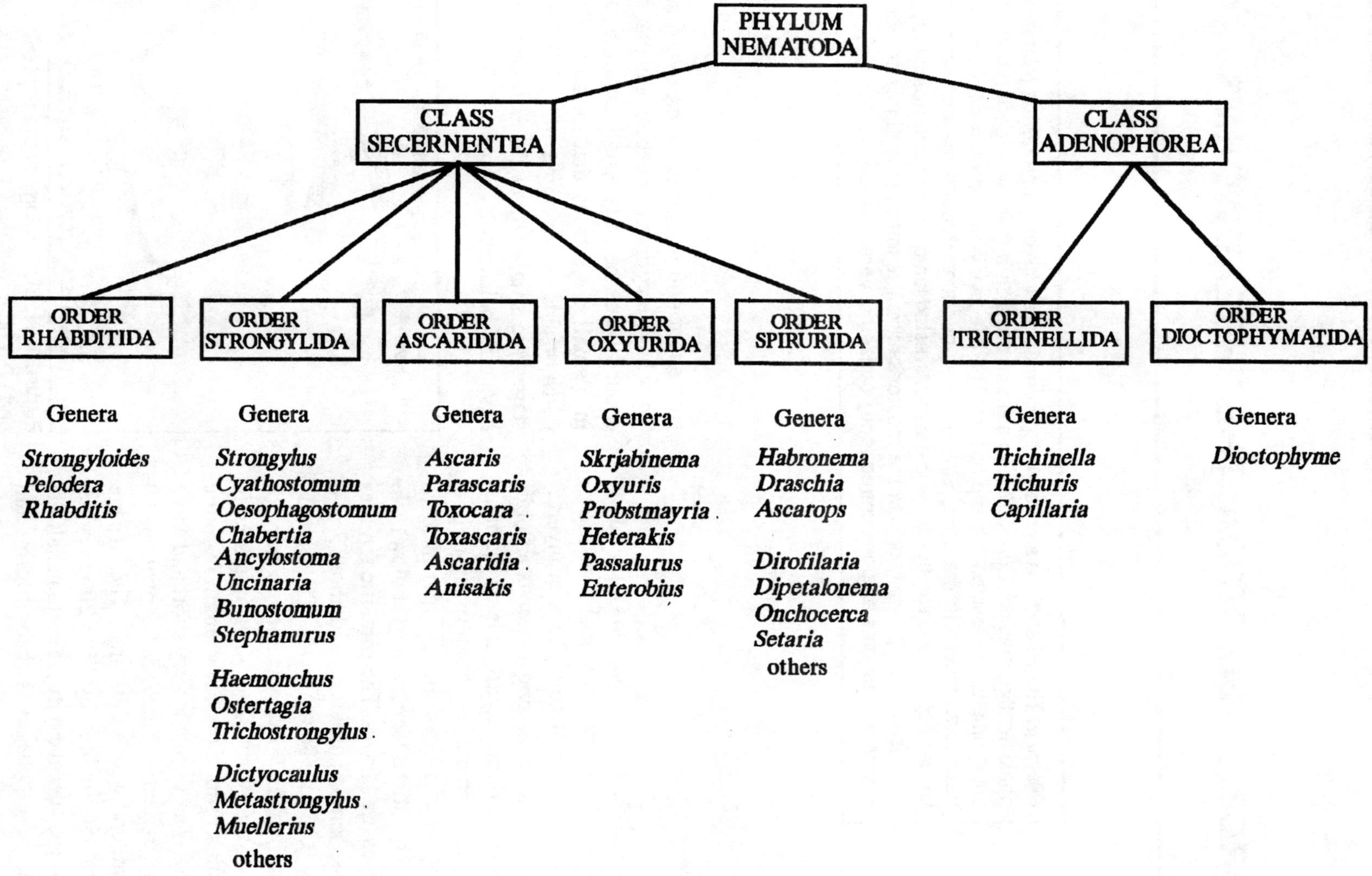

# CHAPTER 14

# THE ORDER RHABDITIDA: THE THREADWORMS

**Preview.** The Rhabditida are free living nematodes with only one genus (*Strongyloides*) consistently parasitic. *Strongyloides* still can develop a free living generation when the environmental conditions are appropriate. The infective larvae enter the host by mouth or transcutaneously. In the host, *Strongyloides* migrates through the circulation and the tissues before reaching the small intestine. Arrested larvae in immune hosts may pass to the offspring congenitally or with the mother's milk. The infection is highly prevalent only in young ruminants and only infrequently causes severe disease .

## 1. Morphology

The **Rhabditida** (from *Rhabditis*, one of its genera) are free-living water or soil nematodes, with some species parasitizing plants or invertebrates. Only the genus *Strongyloides* is an obligated parasite of domestic animals or humans. Unlike the other nematodes of veterinary importance, *Strongyloides* goes through parasitic or free-living generations (see Biology, below). No parasitic males are known. The parasitic females are colorless, semi-transparent, and about 2 to 6 mm long by 0.05 to 0.06 mm wide. The esophagus is cylindrical and occupies about a third of the length of the worm. The vulva is a simple transverse slit a third of the body length from the posterior end. The vagina is very short and there is no evident ovijector. The eggs are oval, 40-60 by 20-40 um, and with a thin shell. The L1s are about 150 to 350 um long by 15 to 20 um wide. The depth of the buccal cavity is less than half the body width, the esophagus is rhabditiform, and the genital primordium is as long as the body is wide. The infective L3s lack a sheath, and measure about 400 to 700 um long by 16 um wide. They have a cylindrical esophagus that occupies about 40% of the body length, and their tail ends in 4 small projections that look like a terminal notch on side view (Figure 14.1). The free living stages are smaller than the parasitic ones, and have a rhabditiform esophagus.[1]

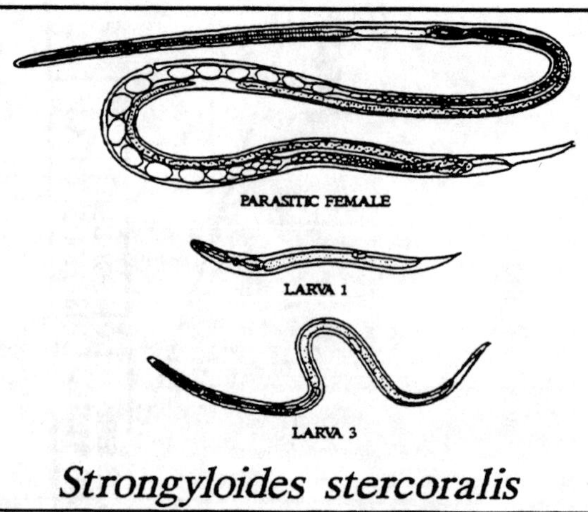


**Figure 14.1.** Morphology of the parasitic female and L3, and free-living L1, of *Strongyloides stercoralis.*

## 2. Identification and classification

The *Strongyloides*, commonly called **threadworms**, live buried into the mucosa of the small intestine. Because of their size and location, they are invisible to the naked eye during necropsy. The only other common nematodes of a comparable size in the small intestine are *Trichostrongylus* and *Trichinella*. The males of *Trichostrongylus* have a prominent copulatory bursa, the females have a shorter esophagus (a fifth or less of the body length), a prominent muscular ovijector, and 85-125 by 37-50 um eggs. The males of *Trichinella* end in a pair of distinct tubercles, the females have a shorter esophagus (a fourth or less of the body length) which is thin and embedded into a stichosome, the vulva is located at the end of the esophagus, and the females contain embryos rather than eggs. Differentiation of the L1s of *Strongyloides* from those of hookworms or lungworms is sometimes necessary (see Diagnosis, in the chapter 16). Identification of the free-living stages is a task for specialists.

Close to 40 species of *Strongyloides* are known, most of them in mammals. The species of veterinary importance are: *S. papillosus* of ruminants, *S. westeri* of equines (up to 9 mm long and 0.1 mm wide), *S. ransomi* of swine, and *S. stercoralis* of dogs, cats, and humans. Accurate identification of species is based on buccal and ovarian characteristics of difficult determination.[2] Because *Strongyloides* are fairly host-specific, preliminary identification can be done on the basis of the host from where the parasite was obtained.

## 3. Biology

### 3.1. Homogonic and heterogonic life cycles

No parasitic males are known among *Strongyloides* but the females are parthenogenetic, this is, their ova develop without fecundation. The parasitic female produces three kinds of eggs[3] that are indistinguishable morphologically: haploid eggs that originate free-living males, diploid eggs that probably generate free-living females, and triploid eggs that presumably produce parasitic females.[4] It is believed that initially all eggs develop into L1s but the further survival of the different kinds of L2s and L3s depends on an environment that supports their specific biological needs. Adverse environmental conditions (low pH, temperatures outside the 20-37C range, non-porous soil, lack of food, abnormal host) favor the development of those L1s that will become filariform, infective L3s. The contrary conditions will select for the L1s that will develop into rhabditiform, free-living L3s.

The life cycle that results in the production of infective larvae is called **homogonic** (from Gr *homos*= same, *gonos*= offspring, generation). In this case, the infective L3s proceed to enter a new host and develop into parasitic females. The life cycle that results in the formation of free-living L3s is called **heterogonic** (from Gr *heteros*= other, different). The rhabditiform L3s molt to rhabditiform L4s and these to rhabditiform males and females. The adults mate and the female lays eggs that develop through free-living L1s and L2s to infective L3s. These infective larvae initiate a new parasitic cycle when they enter a new host (Figure 14.2).

### 3.2. Development outside the host

The female deposits her eggs in the thickness of the mucosa where they embryonate rapidly to leave the host containing an L1 already (in the case of *S. stercoralis*, the L1 hatches when it is still in the intestine). Hatching outside the host occurs in about 6 hours at 27C (80.6F) and the L3s appear in 26-28 hours in the homogonic or heterogonic cycle. In the latter, adults appear in 20-24 hours at 37C (98.6F), 24-28 hours at 30C (86F), or 50-60 hours at 20C (68F). There is no heterogonic development at 15C (59F) or below.

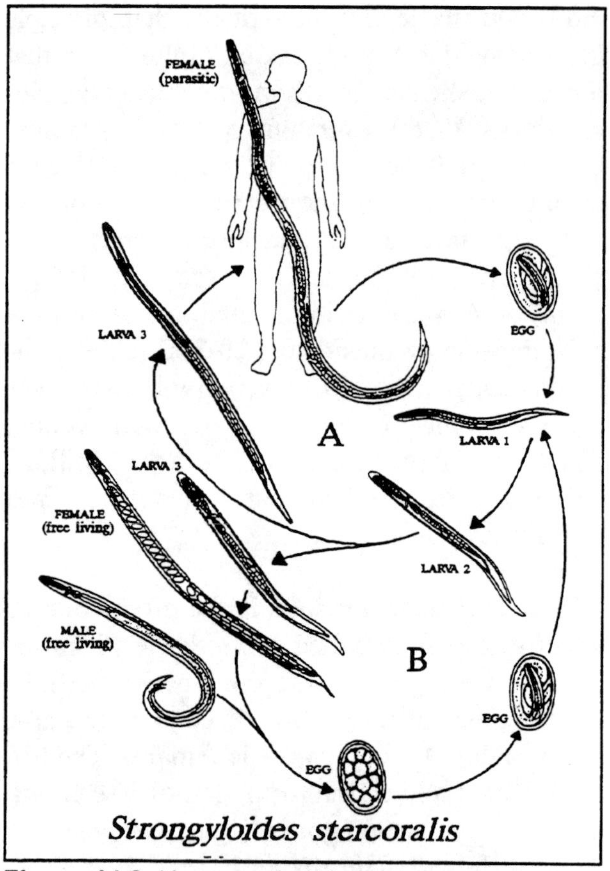


**Figure 14.2**. Homogonic (A) and heterogonic (B) life cycles of *Strongyloides stercoralis.*

### 3.3. Infection and development in the host

Infection can occur by skin penetration or oral ingestion of infective larvae from the external environment, ingestion of larvae with the mother's milk or colostrum, or prenatally.

The transcutaneous infection is more efficient than the oral infection. The infective larvae penetrate the skin with the assistance of enzymes, and enter a lymphatic or blood vessel in a mater of minutes. Within 24 hours, they accumulate in the lungs where they break the walls of the vessels and the alveoli, and start crawling up the air passages. Once they reach the pharynx, they are swallowed and are found in the intestine by the 3rd or 4th day of infection, where they develop into parthenogenetic females. The first eggs appear in the feces at 7-9 days of infection for *S. papillosus*, 6-14 days for *S. westeri,* and 3-7 days for *S. ransomi*. The first larvae appear at 8-16 days for *S. stercoralis*.

When infective larvae are ingested, they may penetrate the oral mucosa or be swallowed to the stomach and intestine. In the first case, they behave as in the transcutaneous infection. In the second, they are believed to develop directly to parasitic females without extraintestinal migration.

Prenatal infections have been reported in calves, piglets, and humans. Lactogenic infections are known to occur in ruminants, swine, horses, rats, and humans. In these cases, the infective larvae mature in the gut of the fetuses or new born animals without extraintestinal migration.

Hyperinfections and autoinfections have been reported in humans but not in domestic animals. In the first case, the L1s develop into infective larvae while in the intestine and these larvae penetrate the intestinal wall to initiate a new infection without leaving the gut. In the second case, the L1s retained around the anus develop into infective larvae which penetrate the perianal skin to initiate a new infection.

In humans, host immunity inhibits the development and pathogenesis of the parasite but does not terminate the infection. When immunity wanes, the parasite resumes development. Asymptomatic patients that presented no larvae in their feces became symptomatic and started passing larvae again upon immunosuppressive treatment. This phenomenon has not been reported from domestic animals but there is little doubt that it must occur. Prenatal and lactogenic transmissions only make biological sense if the larvae are able to wait in the tissues of the mother until advanced pregnancy or lactation to pass to the offspring. The frequency of the lactogenic transmission in ruminants, swine, and equines advocates for the existence of *Strongyloides* immunity-mediated hypobiosis in these species.

### 4. Medical importance

Except in ruminants, and possibly swine, *Strongyloides* infections are not very prevalent. As a rule, they are not very pathogenic either. In all cases, the infection is more common and pathogenic in young hosts. The infection commonly peaks at about 2-3 weeks of age in pigs or 4-6 weeks of age in horses, and disappears spontaneously in 5-6 weeks in pigs or 20-25 weeks in horses. The same must occurs in ruminants because *Strongyloides* is very common in young lambs and calves but very rare in animals older than a year. An infection protects against subsequent infections but older animals that have not suffer prior infections are still susceptible, although not as much as younger animals.

We mentioned above that anti-*Strongyloides* immunity probably causes inhibition of development (like in *Ancylostoma caninum* and *Toxocara canis*) rather than death of the parasites. The high frequency of prenatal and lactogenic infections in ruminants, swine, and equines could not be explained otherwise.

*Strongyloides* can cause pathology during skin penetration, tissue migration, pulmonary passage, or intestinal invasion. Skin penetration usually proceeds rapidly and asymptomatically prior to the development of effective immunity. When immunity is well established, the host responds to the presence of larvae in the skin with a leukocytic-eosinophilic inflammation that is clinically expressed as an erythematous pruritic dermatitis. This sign is more common in humans and carnivores but it has been reported in the other species.

The presence of larvae in the lungs may produce traumatic lesions (when it is massive) or allergic phenomena (when the host has developed immunity previously). Both may translate clinically as pneumonia or bronchopneumonia. This manifestation is uncommon and usually seen only in humans or carnivores.

The parasite in the intestine may produce a catarrhal inflammation with erosion of the mucosa. In severe cases, there may be necrosis and sloughing of the mucosa. The infected animals show anorexia, diarrhea sometimes with blood or mucus, and loss of weight.

In **ruminants**, strongyloidosis is very common in young animals, but usually asymptomatic. When diarrhea is present, it is often intermittent. The main route of infection is believed to be lactogenic in cattle and transcutaneous in sheep. In sheep, the infection may cause lesions that resemble foot rot and facilitate the invasion by the organisms of foot rot.

In **pigs**, strongyloidosis is not very prevalent or severe. It is acquired particularly by the piglets while nursing but also from the contaminated environment. Skin lesions are sometimes seen. In cases of massive infections, the piglets develop a protein-losing enteropathy and many may die.[5]

In **horses**, symptomatic strongyloidosis, manifested by a watery diarrhea, may occurs in foals about 10-14 days of age, resulting from lactogenic transmission from the mare.

In **carnivores**, strongyloidosis may go from asymptomatic to quite severe. The clinical signs commonly appear after the infection has been building up for a few weeks during hot, humid weather. Emaciation despite conservation of appetite and bloody and mucous diarrhea are very characteristic signs. Pneumonia is common in severe infections.

### 5. Diagnosis

Strongyloidosis is suspected by the clinical symptoms and epidemiological circumstances, and verified by the finding of the characteristic larvated eggs (L1s in *S. stercoralis*) in the feces of the patient. Standard flotation methods are adequate to recover eggs but inappropriate to recover larvae. L1s will float only in high density solutions (like 33% zinc sulfate) but they become so crenated and distorted that the procedure is not recommended. They are best demonstrated by some of the larval migration methods described later (see Methods of Parasitological Diagnosis) In fresh feces, the L1s of *S. stercoralis* must be distinguished from the L1s of the lungworms of carnivores (*Filariodes, Aelurostrongylus,* and others). The esophagus of the *S. stercoralis* larvae is about 25% of the body length and the straight tail tapers into a point whereas the esophagus of the lungworm larvae is over 40% of the body length and their tails are undulated or bear a dorsal spine (see Figure 14.1. and chapter 18).

Hatched L1s of the other species of *Strongyloides* can be expected in feces that have been at room temperature (23C or 73.4F) for more than 6 hours, and hatched L1s of hookworms in feces left at room temperature for more than 24 hours. In these cases, it may be necessary to distinguish among *Strongyloides*, lungworm, and hookworm L1s. Differentiation with lungworm larvae is done by comparison of the esophagus length and the tail shape, as indicated above. Differentiation with hookworm larvae is done by comparison of the depth of the buccal cavity (less than half the body width at the nerve ring in *Strongyloides*, and longer than the body width in hookworms), and the length of the genital primordium (longer than the body width in *Strongyloides*, and less than half the body width in hookworms) (see chapter 16).

**Summary:**

1. *Strongyloides* are tiny nematodes of the small intestinal mucosa of ruminants, carnivores, pigs, horses, or humans.

2. Depending on environmental conditions, the larvae leaving the host may develop immediately into infective larvae (homogonic cycle) or develop into a generation of free living worms first (heterogonic cycle).

2. The infective larvae enter the host through the skin or mouth, migrate through the lungs, and develop to adults in the intestine.

3. Migrating larvae may arrest in resistant hosts and later pass to the offspring congenitally or with the mother's milk.

4. *Strongyloides* infects particularly young hosts and is highly prevalent only in lambs and calves.

5. Except when heavy, most primary infections cause mild disease and leave protection against reinfections.

## REFERENCES

1. Georgi, J.R. 1982. Strongyloidosis. In Steele, J. (ed.), *Handbook Series in Zoonoses, Section C: Parasitic Zoonoses,* Vol. II., CRC Press, Boca Raton, Florida.

2. Little, M.D. 1966. Comparative morphology of six species of *Strongyloides* (Nematoda) and redefinition of the genus. J. Parasit. 52:69-84.

3. Chang, P.C.H & Graham, G.L. 1957. Parasitism, parthenogenesis and polyploidy; the life cycle of *Strongyloides papillosus*. J. Parasit. 43 (Suppl.): 13.

4. Little, M.D. 1962. Experimental studies on the life cycle of *Strongyloides*. J. Parasit. 48 (Suppl.): 41.

5. Ekigk, K. & Dey-Hazra, A. 1975. Intestinal plasma and blood loss in piglets infected with *Strongyloides ransomi.* Vet. Parasit. 1:69-75.

# Chapter 15

# THE ORDER STRONGYLIDA OR BURSATE NEMATODES

## THE SUPERFAMILY STRONGYLOIDEA OR LARGE-MOUTHED BURSATE NEMATODES

**Preview**. The Strongylida are medium to small nematodes characterized by the presence of a copulatory bursa on the males. They are divided into three superfamilies of veterinary importance: the Strongyloidea, with a large buccal capsule and a bursa, and most often living in the intestine; the Trichostrongyloidea, with a small bucal capsule, a large bursa, and living in the gastro-intestinal tract; and the Metastrongyloidea, with reduced buccal capsule and bursa, and living in the respiratory system.

The Strongyloidea, in turn, are distributed into three families: the Strongylidae, with a leaf-crown around the mouth opening; the Ancylostomatidae, with teeth or cutting plates around the mouth; and the Syngamidae, with a thickened rim around the mouth. Most lay eggs that are oval, with a thin and transparent eggshell, and containing a few blastomers. They are called strongyle-type eggs.

The **Strongylida** are small to medium size nematodes of the digestive or respiratory tract of mammals. The most characteristic structure of the Strongylida is the presence of a **copulatory bursa**, a bell-shaped caudal expansion of the cuticle of the males, which is restricted to this order. The bursa consists of a dorsal and two lateral lobes supported by muscular rays that receive individual names. Because of the bursa, the Strongylida are commonly called **bursate nematodes**. The males also have two spicules of equal size. In some groups, the spicules are guided by a thickening on the posterior wall of the spicular pouch called **gubernaculum**. Less commonly, there is a similar thickening of the anterior and lateral walls of the pouch called **telamon** (Figure 15.1).

The females are more difficult to identify (one normally relies on the identification of the males) but most lay fairly large (about 85x50 um), oval eggs, with a thin and transparent wall, that leave the host containing a few blastomeres. Eggs like these are conventionally called **strongyle-type eggs** (Figure 15.2). The buccal cavity of the Strongylata is from very large to non-existent, and their esophagus is club-shaped. The name Strongylida came from the greek word *strongylos* which means round. This explains the popularity of the prefix *strongyl-* in the names of nematodes.

The Strongylata of veterinary importance are divided into three superfamilies:

**A. Superfamily Strongyloidea**. It includes nematodes that are mostly parasites of the digestive tract. They are characterized by the presence of a medium to large buccal cavity, always well evident. For this reason, they are commonly called the **large-mouthed bursate nematodes.**

**B. Superfamily Trichostrongyloidea**. It includes nematodes that are parasites of the digestive system. They have a minute or no buccal cavity and are commonly called the **small-mouthed bursate nematodes.**

**C. Superfamily Metastrongylidae.** It includes nematodes that are parasites of the respiratory system. Their buccal cavity is minute and their copulatory bursa is poorly developed. They are commonly called the **lung worms**.

The Trichostrongyloidea and Metastrongyloidea of veterinary importance are fairly homogeneous nematodes that can be conveniently discussed as individual groups. The Strongyloidea, on the contrary, comprise three families that exhibit differences important enough to merit individual discussion. The three families of veterinary importance are as follows:

**a. Family Strongylidae** (from *Strongylus*, one of its genera). In this group, the cuticle around the oral opening divides into fringes that form a circle of leaf-like structures called corona radiata or leaf crown.

**b. Family Ancylostomatidae** (from *Ancylostoma*, one of its genera). In this group, the cuticle forms teeth or cutting plates, but not a corona radiata, around the oral opening.

**c. Family Syngamidae** (from *Syngamus*, one of its genera). This group exhibits a thickened rim around the oral opening but lacks corona radiata, teeth, or cutting plates.

In the remaining of this chapter, we will discuss the Strongylidae that parasitize equines.

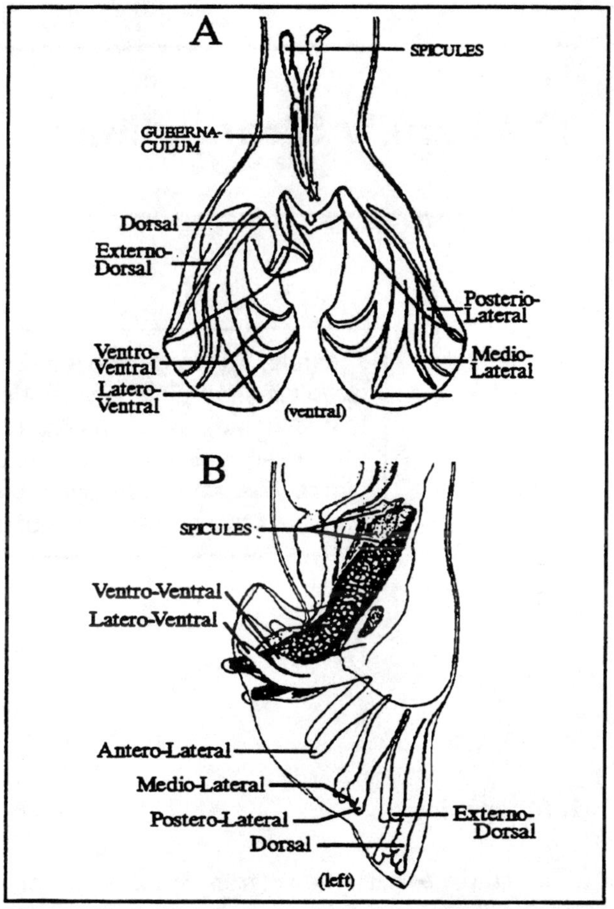


**Figure 15.1.** Morphology of the copulatory bursa of Strongylata in ventral (A) and left (B) views.

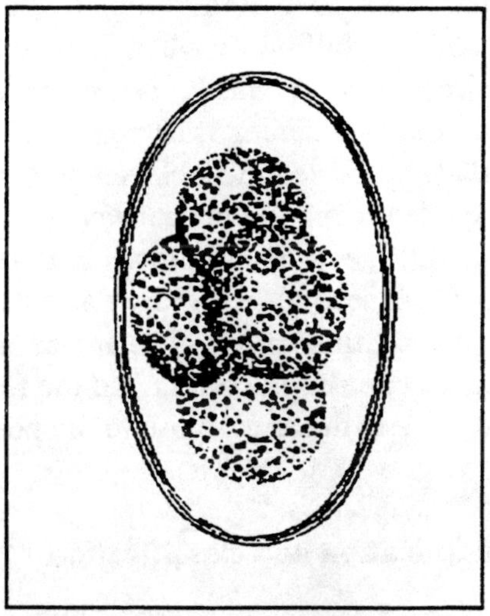

**Figure 15.2.** Typical Strongylata egg (strongyle-type egg).

# The Family Strongylidae. I. The Strongyles of Equines

**Preview.** The large and small strongyles of equines are medium size nematodes of the large intestine. They are very common in horses. The eggs develop into free-living L3s that enter the host by mouth. The parasitic states of the large strongyles migrate outside the intestine, invade the intestinal wall, and later bite the intestinal mucosa and suck blood. The small strongyles only invade the intestinal mucosa and later browse on its surface. Strongyles is a major source of concern for horse lovers.

## 1. Morphology

The family **Strongylidae** (from *Strongylus*, one of its genera) is a fairly homogeneous group of nematodes that parasitize the large intestine of equines and, less frequently, other mammals. They measure about 10 to 50 mm long by 0.5 to 2.0 mm wide and are dull white when starved to dull red, sometimes almost black, when engorged with blood. The oral opening is surrounded by a **corona radiata** (see above) and lacks teeth, cutting plates, or an evident rim. The buccal cavity is globular or cylindrical, deep or shallow, but always very apparent. A second leaf crown and teeth may be found inside this cavity. The males have a well developed **copulatory bursa** and the females have the vulva near the anus, close to the posterior end.

## 2. Identification and classification

The Strongylidae are divided into three subfamilies:

**a. The Subfamily Strongylinae.** Most members of this group are medium size nematodes with a globular or funnel-shaped buccal cavity. The dorsal esophageal gland opens at the oral opening through a channel (= **dorsal gutter**) located on the dorsal wall of the buccal cavity (Figure 15.3). The Strongylinae consists of four genera, *Strongylus, Triodontophorus, Craterostomum*, and *Oesophagodontus* of the large intestine of equines. Only the first two are common.

**b. The Subfamily Cyathostominae** (synonym Trichoneminae). Most members of this group are small nematodes with a cylindrical buccal cavity that may be deep or shallow. The dorsal gland does not reach the oral opening so the dorsal gutter is reduced or absent. This subfamily contains 8 genera and about 50 species that have been the object of numerous arrangements.[1] The most common genera are *Cyathostomum, Cylicocyclus*, and *Cylicostephanus* of the large intestine of equines.

Because of their size, members of the Strongylinae are commonly called **the large strongyles of**

**equines** whereas the Cyathostominae are usually referred to as **the small strongyles of equines**. Some authors restrict the name large strongyles to species of the genus *Strongylus*, and expand the term small strongyles to all other Strongylidae of the equines. Here we will follow the former criterium.

**c. The Subfamily Oesophagostominae.** This group has a cylindrical or globular buccal cavity and a ventral cervical groove near the location of the nerve ring (Figure 16.1). The most important genera are *Oesophagostomum* and *Chabertia*. They are nematodes of the intestine of ruminants, pigs, and lower primates. This subfamily will be discussed in the next chapter.

The accurate identification of the strongyles of equines demands careful observations of the cephalic structures of well prepared specimens. Veterinarians are usually interested in identifying the presence of species of the genus *Strongylus* which are the most pathogenic of the horse strongyles. The descriptions below and figures 15.3, 15.4, and 15.5 should suffice for this purpose. Identification of other genera or species is probably beyond the needs and skills of clinicians without special training. The monograph by Lichtenfels[1] will be a valuable help to those who may want to attempt it.

The genus *Strongylus*, also known as palisade worms or blood worms, is recognized by the presence of a globular buccal capsule that is deeper than wide.

*Strongylus equinus* is the largest of the horse strongyles. It occurs in the cecum and, rarely, the colon. The males are 26-35x1.1-1.3 mm with spicules 2.6 mm long. The females are 38-55x1.8-2.3 mm with the vulva at 12-13 mm from the posterior end. The eggs are oval, 75-92x41-54 um, with a thin and transparent shell, and contain a few blastomeres when leaving the host. The buccal cavity is oval, 1.1 mm deep by 0.9 mm wide, and has two pairs of teeth at the bottom. The dorsal pair is fused at the base (Figure 15.3).

*Strongylus edentatus* is a little smaller. It occurs in the cecum and colon. The males are 23-28x1.3-1.5 mm with spicules 1.9-2.2 mm long. The females are 33-44x1.6-2.2 mm with the vulva 9-10 mm from the posterior end. The eggs are like in *S. equinus*. The buccal cavity is almost spherical, 0.8-1.2 mm in diameter, and had no teeth (Figure 15.3).

*Strongylus vulgaris* is considerable smaller. It occurs in the large intestine, particularly the cecum. The males are 14-16x0.7-1.0 mm and the females 20-25x1.0-1.4 mm. The eggs are like in *S. equinus*. The buccal cavity is funnel-like, 0.5x0.6 mm and with a pair of circular teeth at the bottom (Figure 15.3).

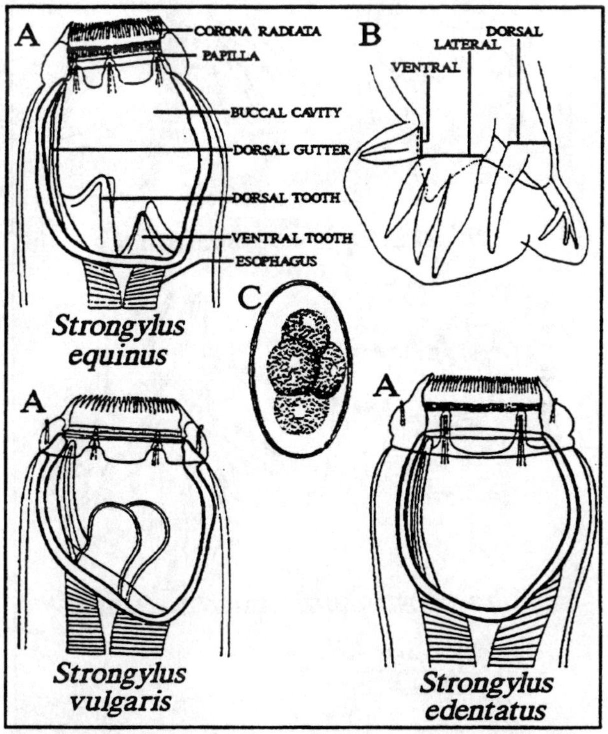


**Figure 15.3.** Cephalic ends (A), caudal end of the males (B), and egg (C) of *Strongylus* spp. of horses.

The genus *Triodontophorus* is recognized by three large teeth, each composed of two plates, that project from the esophageal funnel into the buccal cavity, and an external leaf crown composed of numerous but small fringes (Figure 15.4). These worms are about 9-25 mm long and have a well developed dorsal gutter.

The genus *Craterostomum* is recognized by three small triangular teeth in the esophageal funnel, which do not project into the buccal cavity, and an external leaf crown composed of few but large fringes. These worms are 6-10 mm long and have a well developed dorsal gutter (Figure 15.4).

The only species of the genus *Oesophagodontus* is recognized by the presence of three lancets in the esophageal funnel which do no project into the buccal cavity, and by the lack of a dorsal gutter (Figure 14.4). It is 15 to 24 mm long.

The Cyathostominae may be distinguished from the Strongylinae because they are smaller (4-15 mm, rarely up to 20 mm long), have a smaller buccal capsule which is cylindrical or annular and lacks a dorsal gutter, and in most species the males have an elongated dorsal lobe in the bursa that makes them look tapered at the posterior end, particularly from the side view (Figure 15.5). Identification of genera or species of Cyathostominae is rarely necessary in veterinary practice and normally it requires a specialist.

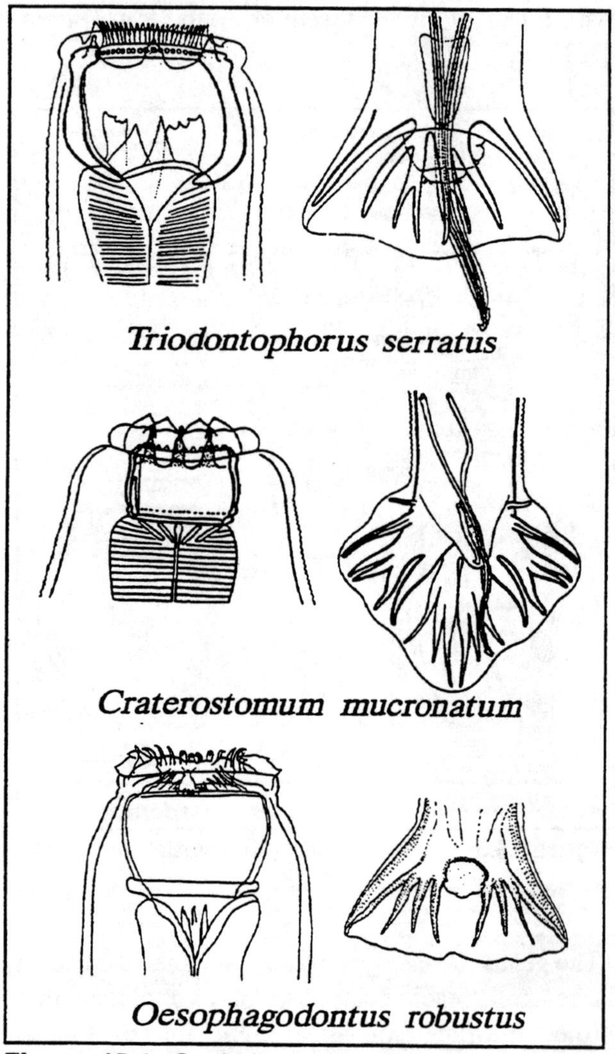


**Figure 15.4.** Cephalic and caudal ends of some Strongylinae of horses.

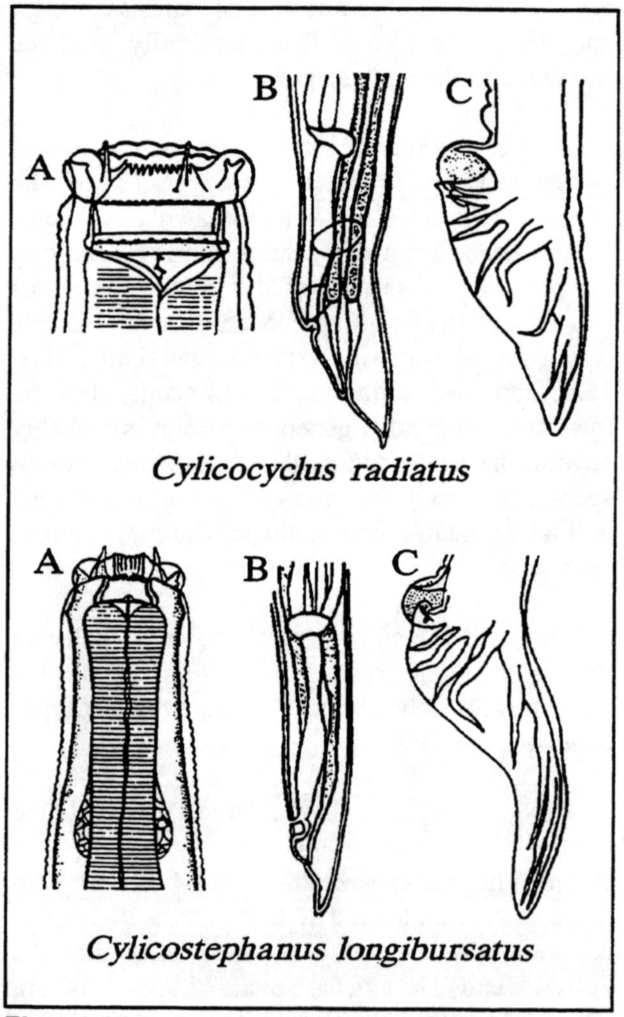


**Figure 15.5.** Cepahlic end (A), caudal end of the female (B) and caudal end of the male (C) of some Cyathostominae of horses.

## 3. Biology

Because *S. vulgaris* is the most dangerous of the horse strongyles, its biology has been studied the most.[2] We will use it as a model for the biology of the strongyles of equines.

### 3.1. Life cycle of *S. vulgaris* outside the host

After mating in the host intestine, the females lay eggs that are passed with the feces of the host containing a few blastomeres. In the presence of adequate temperature, humidity, shade, and oxygen, they will develop successively into free living L1s and L2s, and ensheathed infective L3s.

Development and hatching of eggs occur only between 8 and 38C (46.4 and 100.4F) but the rate of survival is low (< 10%) at both ends of this range. Almost 70% of the eggs develop at the optimal temperature of 20-25C (68-77F), though. The eggs do not hatch below 8C but many may remain alive through the winter and resume development later if they are above the freezing point or protected under the snow. Under more extreme temperatures, a large proportion of eggs dies with time. Free living larvae are more sensitive to low temperature than eggs, but infective larvae are quite resistant.

While in the fecal pad, humidity is normally high enough to assure development but moisture content below 15-20% will inhibit development and the movement of the infective larvae away from the pad. Few larvae migrate more than 15 cm away from the fecal pad or 10 cm from the soil surface even under optimal circumstances. Distribution of infective larvae on the pasture is largely due to moderate rains that disturb the fecal pads. Dryness is much more lethal to eggs and L1s than to L2s and L3s. Infective larvae can survive dehydration for months and resume their activity upon rehydration.

With appropriate humidity, development to infective larvae takes 3-4 days at 30C (86F), 4-5 days at 20-25C, and 16-20 days at 12C (53.6F). Sublethal drying lengthens these periods. Survival of infective larvae on pastures depends mainly on environmental temperature, low temperatures favor survival. About 1% of the larvae survive for 2-3 weeks in the summer but for 7-11 weeks in the winter. Many larvae will survive winters with temperatures near the freezing point but a high proportion will die when the warmth of the spring comes.

### 3.2. Life cycle of *S. vulgaris* inside the host

For many years there was a lively controversy about the path of migration of *S. vulgaris* in the host but the Kikuchi-Enigk model is widely accepted as the true migration nowadays.[3,4]

The infective larvae ingested with the herbage exsheath in the small intestine and burrow into the wall of small intestine, cecum, or ventral colon to reach the submucosa. After a week of infection, the L3s have molted to L4s, penetrate the lumina of small submucosal arteries, and migrate in the intima against the blood flow. By the end of the second week of infection the larvae, which still are only 1-3 mm long, reach the cranial mesenteric artery. Some larvae continue their migration cranially and caudally along the aorta and satellite arteries but most will accumulate in the cranial mesenteric. The larvae remain there, grow to 10-18 mm long, and molt to juveniles. By the 110-120th day of infection they return to the large intestine migrating downstream within the intestinal arteries. Once in the serosal surface, the worms form pea-sized nodules, develop for further 90 or more days, and finally break into the intestinal lumen to become mature adults in six to eight weeks. The first eggs appear in the feces at 6-7 months of infection.

### 3.3. Life cycle of other Strongylinae

Because of the difficulty of identifying the genus of the eggs or early larvae, or establishing infections with a single species of horse strongyle, little work has been done on the life cycles of strongyles other than *S. vulgaris* outside the host. It is believed, however, that the preparasitic phase of the life cycle is comparable in all strongyles of equines.

The infective larvae of *S. edentatus* penetrate the intestinal mucosa of the large intestine, invade the portal veins, and migrate to the liver where they molt to L4s during the second or third week of infection. By the tenth week, the larvae pass through the hepatic ligaments to the abdominal wall of the right flank, under the peritoneum. L4s and juveniles are found at this location during the third month of infection forming hemorrhagic nodules that can reach several centimeters in diameter. Eventually, the juveniles return to the large intestine by the mesentery and form large hemorrhagic nodules in the intestinal wall starting about 4 months after infection. These nodules finally break into the intestine to release the worms that mature in the lumen. It is fairly common to find erratic larvae or juveniles in liver, lungs, other organs, or even the peritoneal cavity. The first eggs are reported to appear in the host feces by the 11th month of infection but patent infections are found in 6 month old foals.

The infective larvae of *S. equinus* penetrate the wall of the cecum and colon and move to the subserosa where the L4's are found in nodules by the 11th day. Subsequently they migrate to the liver by the peritoneal cavity and wander in the organ for 6-7 weeks after which they pass through the hepatic ligament to the pancreas and peritoneal cavity. They molt to juveniles by the end of the fourth month of infection. Shortly thereafter they penetrate the intestinal wall again and emerge in the lumen. The first eggs appear by the 9th month of infection.

Larvae of *Triodontophorus* has been found in the submucosa of cecum and colon, and juveniles and adults in the lumen. There is no evidence that these worms migrate outside the intestine. Apparently, the larval stages develop in the intestinal wall, and the juveniles mature in the lumen of the large intestine. Presumably, the same is true for the other Strongylinae.

### 3.4. Life cycle of the Cyathostominae[5]

The life cycle of the small strongyles outside the host is comparable to that described for *S. vulgaris*. The range of egg development and hatching is from 8 to 30C (46.4-86F) and the infective larvae occurs in 2-4 days at the optimal temperature of 20-25C (68-77F). A minimum water content of 24% in the fecal pad is necessary for development of the infective larvae. Survival in the field is favored by moderate cold: significant numbers of infective larvae last for only 2-3 weeks in hot summers, for 3-8 weeks in spring or autumn, and for 20 or more weeks in cold winters.

Once ingested, the infective larvae exsheath in the small intestine, penetrate the intestinal glands of the cecum and colon, and move to the mucosa or submucosa. Host reaction forms an infiltrate of inflammatory cells and later a fibrous cyst around these larvae. Molting occurs in the cysts in 6-12 days and the L4s remain in them for 1-2 months after which they emerge into the lumen to develop into mature adults. Reports of persistence of L4s in the intestinal wall for several months suggest that they may undergo larval arrest. Most of the adult cyathostominae occur in the colon. The first eggs are found by the 6-14th week of infection in strongyle-naive animals, or by the 12-18th week in previously infected hosts.

## 4. Medical importance

The strongyles are very common parasites of equines. Prevalences of more than 80% for *S. vulgaris* and *S. edentatus*, 50% for *S. equinus*, and 95% for the small strongyles are common in young adult horses. Because the ecology of all horse strongyles is similar, it is the rule that the infected animals harbor a variety of strongyles species. The parasitic load is usually counted in the hundreds for the large strongyles but in the tens or hundreds of thousands for the small strongyles.

Among the horse strongyles, the larval stages are more pathogenic than the adult worms. Also, the pathogenicity increases in the order small strongyles, S. equinus, S. edentatus, and S. vulgaris.

### 4.1. Damage by *S. vulgaris*

Although *S. vulgaris* may constitute no more than 5-10% of all strongyles in an infected horse, its development in the arterial system and the consequent lesions make it the most dangerous of the strongyles. Foals experimentally infected with 800 to 8300 *S. vulgaris* larvae died in 8-19 days

**a. Pathogenesis by the larvae**

The activity of the *S. vulgaris* migrating larvae produces an endoarteritis with thrombus formation of the small intestinal arteries during the first week of infection. The lesions invade the main intestinal arteries and cranial mesenteric artery during the second week. Similar lesions may be found in the aorta and satellite vessels by the third week. Penetration of the larvae in the wall of the cranial mesenteric artery (and other arteries) causes an inflammation that may embrace all three layers of the vessel wall. By the third week of infection, there is thrombus formation, thickening of the intima, and infiltration of plasma cells, lymphocytes, macrophages, and neutrophils. As the lesions evolve, the arterial wall becomes fibrotic and very thick, and large thrombi reduce the blood flow. Although this lesion is commonly called **verminous aneurysm**, true aneurysm formation is rather rare.

The juveniles returning to the intestine cause thrombus formation and endoarteritis during their journey, and an embolus when the lumen turns too narrow. Intestinal nodules containing the parasite surrounded by neutrophils and necrotic tissue are produced at these points. After the worms leave the arteries, organization and resorption of the thrombi and reduction of the fibrosis take place. In the absence of reinfections, the affected artery looks normal again after nine months.

Although estimations that 90% of the colics in horses are caused by *S. vulgaris* are probably exaggerated, infections by this parasite produce important alterations of the intestinal physiology. Arteritis, thrombosis, amd emboli of the small intestinal arteries, at the beginning or end of the migration, cause congestion, hemorrhages, inflammation, ischemia, and necrosis of local tissues. Decreased blood flow by obstruction of the cranial mesenteric artery may produce alterations of the intestinal motility, or intestinal infarction, depending on the severity of the resulting hypoxia. There is also evidence that the enlarged cranial mesenteric artery exerts pressure on, and disturb the funcion of the local nervous plexuses that participate in the motility of the intestine and the dilation-contraction of its vessels.

Infection by *S. vulgaris* larvae is manifested clinically by fever, anorexia, signs of abdominal disconfort, weight loss, depression, and, occasionally, diarrhea. The severity of the symptoms is proportional to the parasitic load. Foals infected with 2500-5000 larvae died in 15-22 days but foals infected with 750 larvae recovered without fatalities. Larvae lodged in aberrant locations (aorta, renal arteries, endocardium, central nervous system, etc.) may give origin to atypical symptoms. Infections of strongyle-naive animals cause more severe symptoms than comparable reinfections which suggests that horses develop some degree of protective immunity against parasitism by preadults.

**b. Pathogenesis by the adults**

Juveniles of *S. vulgaris* cause considerable damage to the intestinal mucosa during their emergency from the parietal nodules. The adults in the lumen bite the intestinal mucosa, withdraw a plug within their buccal capsules, digest the cells, and suck blood. They later move to a new location leaving behind a crater-like ulcer that oozes blood before healing. Little solid information exist on the clinical manifestations of the infection with adults. It is known that they cause an accelerated turn over of the seralbumin and reduce the survival or erythrocytes. Infected animals may show a normocytic anemia, poor weight gain, weakness, and emaciation. Anorexia and diarrhea are uncommon.

## 4.2. Damage by other large strongyles

The migrating stages of *S. edentatus* produce subcapsular hemorrhages and tortuous tracts in the liver. Except in massive infections, the hepatic tissue recovers with little fibrotic reaction after the departure of the parasites. Migration of *S. edentatus* in the peritoneal cavity may cause peritonitis with production of serosanguineous fluid. In experimental infections, this stage has coincided with the occurrence of colic. The subperitoneal nodules containing worms may break open causing hemorrhages or peritonitis. The adults in the intestine behave like those of *S. vulgaris* but the parietal nodules are larger and the damage caused by the emergence of adults into the lumen is consequently more severe. They also suck more blood than *S. vulgaris*. Clinically, the infection is manifested by low-grade fever, moderate anemia, elevated eosinophilia, depression, inapetence, signs of abdominal disconfort, and constipation or diarrhea. Experimental infection with 3000 to 75,000 larvae has resulted in ilness and death in two weeks to two months.

The migrating stages of *S. equinus* cause hemorrhagic tracts in liver and pancreas that heal with fibrosis after the departure of the parasites. The adult stages behave like those of *S. edentatus*. Clinically, the infection is characterized by fever, anorexia, signs of abdominal disconfort, depression, and rapid loss of condition. Experimental infection with 4000 larvae have resulted in serious illness and frequent deaths.

The larvae of *Triodontophorus* spp. penetrate and remain in the submucosa of the large intestine. It is believed that they may cause damage during emergence into the lumen. The adults are blood-suckers and their bites produce profund ulcers, often confluent.

### 4.3. Damage by small strongyles[6]

Invasion of the intestinal mucosa or submucosa by the infective larvae of the small strongyles produces numerous inflammatory nodules of a few millimeters in diameter around the larvae that are replaced by a fibrous cyst later. Emergence of the L4s into the lumen causes inflammation of the tissues overlying the larvae and a small ulcer in the mucosa. When the concentration of larvae is high, a catarrhal or hemorrhagic enteritis occurs at this time. The corresponding clinical manifestations are transient fever and eosinophilia, anorexia, increased intestinal peristalsis, weakness, poor weight gain, and solf fecces or diarrhea. Animals infected with 200,000 to 500,000 larvae started regaining weight only after 5 months. Because symptoms are common in spring but infective larvae on pastures are scarce during winter and spring, it is believed that the larvae that cause these manifestations are those ingested during the previous grazing season. If so, this disease would have a mechanism similar to the ostertagiasis II of cattle.

Adult cyathostomins bite and digest only the superficial cells of the intestinal mucosa. Only a few uncommon species are large enough to reach the vessels and draw blood. It is believed that the adult small strongyles produce little damage under normal circunstances. Massive infections, however, may disrupt the mucosa enough to interfere with the digestive and adsorptive functions and produce a desquamative, catarrhal enteritis.

## 5. Immunity

A number of studies has demostrated that older animals are less affected by *S. vulgaris* infection than younger ones, although all ages remain susceptible to infection. This phenomenon appears to correspond to true age resistance as well as acquired immunity because it occurs in animals of different age raised free of infection, and in animals of comparable age vaccinated by previous exposure.[2] Circulating antibodies have been detected after administration of infective larvae but not after implantation of adult worms. Although larval development appears to be necessary for antibody production, antibody titers did not show a relationship with the severity of the symptoms.

Vaccination with two doses of larvae irradiated with 80-130 kiloroentgens reduced the number of larvae that developed after a challenge and the severity of the symptoms and lesions, but incresed the number of lesions in ectopic sites. These results could not be replicated in other studies.

The only probable manifestations of immunity reported for small strongyles is the arrest of larval development and a prolongation of the prepatent period in previoulsy infected animals.

### 5. Treatment

Numrous treatments againt the migrting larvae of *S. vulgaris* have been attempted. Diethylcarbamazine (110, 220, or 550 mg/kg for 14, 7, or 3 days) or tetramisole (10 mg/kg for 2 days) produce clinical improvement and reduced deaths but did not decrease the number of larvae that were recovered after an infection. Pyrantel (40 mg/kg for 8 days) improved the clinical signs and resulted in no larvae being recovered but caused severe toxic reaction. Thiabendazole (440 mg/kg for 2 days) reduced the symptoms and lesions and killed many larvae.

**Summary:**

1. The Strongylidae are recognized as larged-mouthed bursate nematodes with a leaf-crown (or corona radiata) around their oral opennings.

2. Two subfamilies of the family Strongylidae (Strongylinae and Cyathostominae) encompass the strongyles of equines. The adults live in the large intestine.

3. The Strongylinae (or large-strongyles of equines) are large parasites with a globular buccal cavity and a dorsal gutter (*Strongylus, Triodontophorus,* etc.). The Cyathostominae (or small strongyles of equines) are smaller parasites with a cylindrical buccal cavity and no dorsal gutter (*Cyathostomum, Cylicocyclus, Cylicostephanus,* etc).

4. Infected hosts pass strongyle-type eggs that develop into infective L3 in the pastures and are ingested by new hosts.

5. Preadult stages of *Strongylus* spp. migrate outside the intestine (cranial mesenteric and other arteries for *S. vulgaris*; liver and right abdominal wall for *S. edentatus*, and; liver, pancreas, and abdominal cavity for *S. equinus*) but the other species only invade the intestinal mucosa.

6. Juvenile *Strongylus* spp. mature in nodules in the intestinal wall. They later emerge into the mucosal lumen and develop into adults that bite the mucosa.

7. *Strogylus* spp. cause damage during their migrations, during their maturation in the intestinal wall, during their emergence, and when they bite the mucosa to suck blood. The smaller species also cause some damage on emergence but rarely bite the mucosa.

8. Control of strongyles of equine consists in preventing contamination of pastures and infection of the host. Currently this is done through strategic treatment of the host.

## REFERENCES

1. Lichtenfels JR. 1975. Helminths of domestic equids. Proc. Helm. Soc. Wash. 40 (special issue), 92 pp.

2. Ogbourne CP and Duncan JL. 1985. *Strongylus vulgaris* in the horse: its biology and veterinary importance. 2nd edition. Commonwealth Institute of Parasitology, Farnham Royal, United Kingdom, 68 pp.

3. Enigk K. 1970. The development of the three species of *Strongylus* of the horse during the prepatent period. Proc. II Internat. Conf. on Equine Inf. Dis., Paris, 1969, 2:259-268.

4. Duncan JL and Pirie HM. 1972. The life cycle of *Strongylus vulgaris* in the horse. Res. Vet. Sc. 13:374-379.

5. Reinemeyer CR. 1986. Small strongyles. Recent advances. Vet. Clinics N.A. Equine Practice 2:281-312

6. Ogbourne CP. 1978. Pathogenesis of cyathostome (Trichonema) infections of the horse. A review. Commonwealth Agr. Bureau, Farnham Royal, England, 25 pp.

# The Family Strongylidae. II. The Nodular and Bowel worms

**Preview.** The Nodular (*Oesophagostomum* spp.) and Bowel (*Chabertia* sp.) worms are small parasites of the large intestine of ruminants or pigs. The host is infected by ingestion of L3s with their feed. The preadult parasitic stages develop in the intestinal mucosa and cause considerable damage. The adults graze on the surface of the mucosa and do little harm.

## 1. Morphology

The **Nodular worms** (genus *Oesophagostomum*) and the **Bowel worm** (genus *Chabertia*) are strongyles that belong to the subfamily Oesophagostominae. They are small (10 to 20 cm long by 0.3 to 0.5 mm wide), whitish nematodes of the large intestine of ruminants or pigs. At the anterior end, the cuticule is dilated forming a cephalic vesicle that is separated from the rest of the body by a ventral groove. *Oesophagostomum* (but not *Chabertia*) have two small lateral papillae a short distance behind this groove. Around the mouth, the cuticle forms a circular fold called the mouth collar. Small leaf-crowns are present. The buccal capsule is shallow, narrow, and circular in *Oesophagostomum* but large and globular in *Chabertia* (Figures 15.6 and 15.7) The males have two slender spicules and the females a short tail with the vulva a little anterior to the anus. The eggs are typical strongyle-type eggs.

## 2. Identification and classification

*Chabertia* is easily identified for its large bucal capsule that makes it appear inflated and truncate at the anterior end even with the naked eye. In sheep, *Oesophagostomum* is easily differentiated from *Chabertia* for its small buccal capsule. The position of the cervical papillae and characteristics of the leaf-crowns are important to the identification of species of *Oesophagostomum* but rarely a veterinarian will need identify species. A few simple measurements of the the spicules of the males or the tail and relative position of the vulva of the female will suffice for the most common species.

*Chabertia ovina* is a cosmopolitan parasite of the large intestine of ruminants. The males are 13 to 14 mm long by 0.3 mm wide with spicules 1.3 to 1.7 mm long. The females are 17 to 20 mm long by 0.5 mm wide. Their tails are conical for the most part but form a distinct pointed end (Figure 15.6).

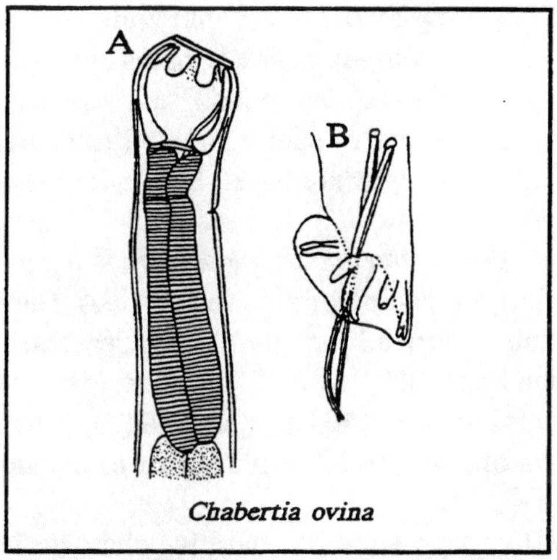


**Figure 15.6.** Anterior (A) and posterior end of the male (B) of *Chabertia ovina*.

*Oesophagostomum radiatum* is a cosmopolitan parasite of the large intestine of large ruminants. The males are 14 to 17 mm long by 0.3 to 0.4 mm wide with spicules 0.7 to 0.8 mm long. The females are 16 to 22 mm long by 0.3 to 0.4 mm wide. Their tails are 0.3 to 0.4 mm long and the vulva is about 1 mm anterior to the anus. The eggs are 70-76 by36-40 µm.

*Oesophagostomum columbianum* is a cosmopolitan parasite of the large intestine of small ruminants. The males are 12 to 16 mm long by 0.2 to 0.4 mm wide with spicules 0.75 to 0.85 mm long. The females are 14 to 18 mm long by 0.3 to 0.4 mm wide. Their tails are 300-600 µm long and the vulva opens 750-800 µm anterior to the anus. The eggs are 74-88 by 45-54 µm.

*Oesophagostomum venulosus* is a cosmopolitan parasite of the large intestine of small ruminants. The males are 11 to 16 mm long by 0.3 to 0.4 mm wide with spicules 1.1 to 1.5 mm long. The females are 13 to 24 mm long by 0.5 to 0.6 mm wide. Their tails are 150-200 µm long and the vulva opens 310 µm anterior to the anus. The eggs are 85-105 by 47-59 µm. In the practice, they are indistinguishable from the eggs of other *Oesophagostomum* species of small ruminants.

*Oesophagostomum dentatum* is a cosmopolitan parasite of the large intestine of pigs.The males are 8 to 10 mm long by 0.2 to 0.3 mm wide with spicules 1.15 to 1.3 mm long. The females are 11 to 14 mm long by 0.4 to 0.5 mm wide. Their tails are 256 µm long and the vulva opens 360-380 µm anterior to the anus. The eggs are 60-80 by 35-45 µm.

*Oesophagostomum quadrispinulatum* is a parasite of the large intestine of pigs in the USA, Europe, and South America.. It resembles O. dentatum but the spicules are 0.91 to 0.95 mm long, the tails of the femals are 400 to 460 µm long and pointed, and the vulva opens 380-460 µm anterior to the anus.

Table 15.I shows the comparative characteristics of thespecies above. Several other species of *Oesophagostomum* of more restricted geographic distribution exist in small ruminants, pigs, and non-human primates.

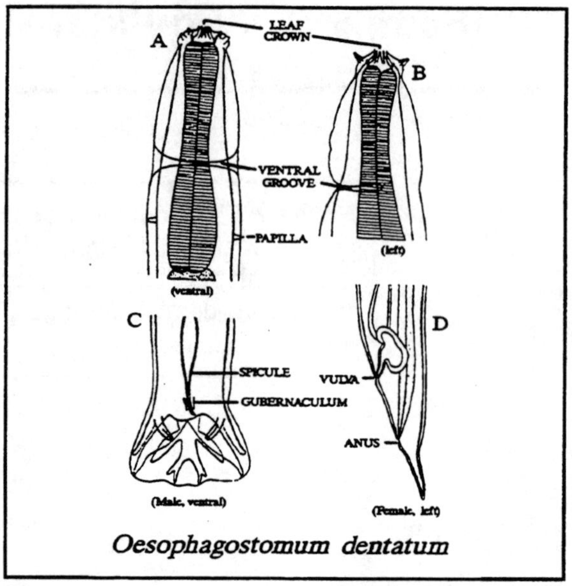


**Figure 15.6.** Views of the anterior end (A and B) and the posterior end of the male (C) and female (D) of *Oesophagostomum dentatum.*

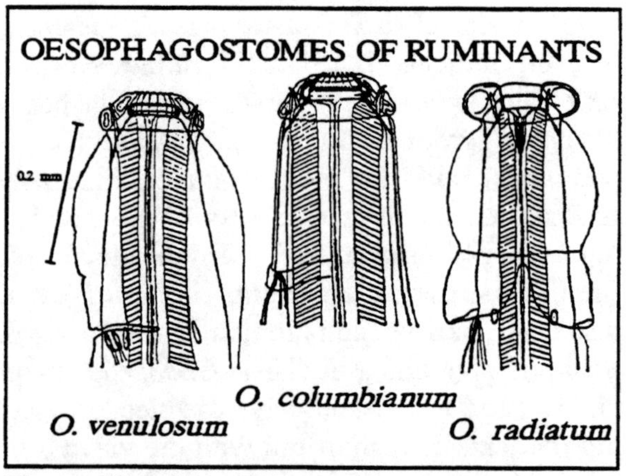


**Figure 15.8.** Morphology af the anterior ends of *Oesophagostomum* of ruminants.

## 3. Biology

At room temperature and in water the eggs hatch within the first day and, provided that the temperature is moderately high and there is plenty of humidity, the L3 stage is reached in 6 to 7 days. After ingestion, the L3s penetrate the mucosa of the small or large intestine, molt to L4s, and grow up to 1.5 to 2.5 mm long. Normally, they return to the intestinal lumen by the 5th to 7th day of infection, accumulate in the large intestine, and molt to the juvenile stage. Adults appear after two or three weeks of infection and the eggs start appearing in the feces by the 4th to 7th week. The prepatent period is 32-42 days for *O. radiatum*, 41 for *O. columbianum*, 28-31 for *O. venulosum*, 49 for *O.dentatum*, and 33 for *O. quadrispiculatum*.

*Oesophagostomum* worms usually reach their peak fertility after a couple of months, keep it high for a few weeks, and then most of the worms are eliminated. A few worms may remain for over a year in their host, however.

The life cycle of *C. ovina* is esentially similar to that of *Oesophagostomun* although its development inside the host is a litlle more prolonged. Prepatency is 47-54 or more days.

**4. Medical importance**

*C. ovina* causes disease particularly at the juvenile stage that develops toward the end of the first month of infection. Like the adults, they suck a plug of mucosa in their large bucca l capsules and digest it. This causes congestion, edema, petechiae, and a lymphocytic-eosinophilic inflammation of the intestinal mucosa. In heavy infections (250 to 300 parasites), the host responds to the damage with diarrhea that may contain abundant blood and mucus. Anemia is often an important component of the disease although it is not clear whether this is caused by the hematophagia or the oozing of blood from the intestinal wounds. The affected animals stop gaining weight or lose weight, and the production and quality of wool is affected in sheep. The first clinical signs commonly appear about a month after infection (before patency) and, without treatment, may persist for one or two months. When death occurs, it is commonly around the 8th week of infection. Larvae and juveniles are often found in the feces during this period. The disease usually becomes less severe by the end of the second month. It is not clear whether the adult parasites are less pathogenic than the juveniles or the expulsion of worms during the preceding period simply diminishes the parasitic load.

*Oesophagostomum* causes disease particularly at the L4 stage. In a first infection, the L4s in the intestinal mucosa cause the production of small nodules of about 1 mm in diameter. These nodules produce little peripheral inflammation but, in about 10 days, become filled with leucocytes and double their size. After the larvae are released, the nodules may become purulent or hemorrhagic and the surrounding mucosa becomes inflammed and edematous. Once the hosts become sensitized to the parasite antigens during a first infection, the nodules are much larger (more than 1 cm in diameter) and the inflammation more intense on subseqeunt infections. Leucocytes, eosinophils, giant cells, and fibroblasts collect around the larva and often delay their release for up to three months, or kill it. Because the most severe clinical signs are associated with the presence of juveniles in the intestinal lumen, probably most of the damage is caused by the larvae abandoning the intestinal nodules and leaving purulent nodules or ulcers that ooze blood and may become infected. The large nodules also intefere with the digestion, absorption, and movement of the intestine. The adults are moderate blood suckers and may produce an intermitten diarrhea that affect weight gain.

Severely affected animals develop an intense, dark green, and foul-smelling diarrhea with abundant mucus and occasionally blood. It begins during the second week of infection (before patency), becomes more severe in the next two to four weeks, and coincides with an intense anorexia. The combined result of inappetence, faulty digestion and absorption, and loss of protein through the intestine has a profound effect on weight gain and the animals emaciate rapidly. An normochromic normocytic anemia attributed mostly to nutritional factors occurs sometimes. The signs commonly subside by the 7th week, in coincidence with the appearance of the adult worms. If the animals survive the acute phase, the diarrhea becomes intermittent but the inappetence persists and emaciation still may occur. In milder infections, less severe signs appear three to fourth weeks after infection and may last for a couple of months.

The acute disease is more common in cattle while the chronic disease is seen more often in sheep. *O. venulosum* is much less pathogenic for sheep than *O. columbianum*, it rarely causes nodule formation. Pigs do not show overt oesophagostomosis as often but their productivity may be affected even by asymptomatic infections.

In 1964, the US Department of Agriculture estimated that oesophagostomosis caused losses of $1.7 million in sheep and $ 7 million in pigs. This does not include the inability to use infected sheep intestines to make catgut or infected pig intestines to make sausage casings.

**5. Diagnosis.**

Because in severely parasitized animals the signs usually appear during prepatency, the search for eggs in the feces during the acute disease is often unsuccessful. Larvae and juveniles, however, can be found in the feces during the acute disease. Otherwise, the presumptive diagnosis is supported by the necropsia of selected animals. The nodules of oesophagostomosis, filled with a caseous, green or yellow material, or even calcified, are quite characteristic. Intestines so affected are often called "pimply guts." The eggs of *Oesophagostomum* cannot be differentiated from the eggs of other strongyles but they can be incubated in the laboratory to examine the larval stages.

**Table 15.I. Characteristics of common *Oesophagostomum* species described in the text**

| Species | Host | Male (mm) | Spicules (µm) | Female (mm) | Female tail (µm) | Vulva* (µm) | Eggs (µm) | Prepatency (days) |
|---|---|---|---|---|---|---|---|---|
| radiatum | cattle | 14-17x 0.3-0.4 | 700-800 | 16-22x 0.3-0.4 | 300-400 | 1000 | 70-76x 36-40 | 32-42 |
| columbianum | sheep, goat | 12-16x 0.2-0.4 | 750-850 | 14-18x 0.3-0.4 | 300-600 | 750-800 | 74-88x 45-54 | 41 |
| venulosus | sheep, goat | 11-16x 0.3-0.4 | 1100-1500 | 13-24x 0.5-0.6 | 150-200 | 310 | 85-105x 47-59 | 28-31 |
| dentatum | pigs | 8-10x 0.2-0.3 | 1150-1300 | 11-14x 0.4-0.5 | 256 | 360-380 | 60-80x 35-45 | 49 |
| quadrispinulatum | pigs | 8-10x 0.2-0.3 | 910-950 | 11-14x 0.4-0.5 | 400-460 | 380-460 | 60-80x 35-45 | 33 |

* Distance from the vulva to the anus.

**Summary:**

1. The Strongylidae are recognized as larged-mouthed bursate nematodes with a leaf-crown (or corona radiata) around their oral openings.

2. The Nodular (*Oesophagostomum* spp.) and Bowel (*Chabertia* sp.) worms are small (10-20 by 0.3-0.5 mm), whitish, strongylidae of the large intestine of ruminants or pigs.

3. The strongyle-type eggs passsed by infected hosts develop into infective L3 in the pastures and are ingested by new hosts.

4. Preadult stages mature in the intestinal mucosa and return to the lumen to develop to adults.

5. Development and emergence of the intramucosal larvae cause considerable damage but the adults mostly graze on the surface of the mucosa.

## REFERENCES

1. Steward TB and Gasbarre LC. 1989. The veterinary importance of nodular worms (*Oesophagostomum* spp). Parasitol. Today 5:209-213.

# Chapter 16

# The Family Ancylostomatidae or Hookworms

**Preview.** The hookworms are small hematophagous nematodes of the small intestine of carnivores, ruminants, pigs, and humans. Their eggs develop into free-living infective larvae that enter the host by mouth or through the skin, migrate to the lungs, and mature to adults in the intestine. A dog species can be transmitted congenitally or with the mother's milk. They may cause cutaneous, respiratory, and intestinal manifestations.

## 1. Morphology

The family **Ancylostomatidae** (from *Ancylostoma*, one of its genera) or **hookworms** is a rather homogeneous group of hematophagous nematodes that parasitize the small intestine of some mammals. They are dull white when starved to dull red when fed, from 5 to 25 mm long and 0.2 to 0.6 mm wide. Their cephalic end is bent dorsally mimicking a hook which explains their common name. The buccal cavity, directed backwards, is large, lacks a leaf-crown, but have teeth or cutting plates on its ventral margin. Most species have additional teeth or lancets in the depth of the buccal cavity. Their strong, club-shaped esophagus can be discerned from the outside. As members of the superfamily strongyloidea, the males have a well developed copulatory bursa.

## 2. Identification and classification

The hookworms of veterinary importance are parasites of ruminants, swine, or domestic carnivores. Their size, location, and characteristic mouth is enough to identify them as ancylostomatidae in these hosts. Identification of species is based on buccal structures, size and shape of the spicules, and characteristics of the copulatory bursa. The rather strict host-specificity of the hookworms makes identification easier because it circumscribes the alternatives to the species existing in a given host. Barriga's[1] review of the hookworms of domestic carnivores and humans includes information for the identification of species. Differentiation of the larvae in the tissues from those of ascarides or *Strongyloides* is difficult and best left to the specialist.[2]

The most important species of hookworms are listed below. Some of their characteristics appear in Table 16.I.

*Bunostomum phlebotomum* of cattle. Cosmopolitan in tropical and temperate regions.

*Bunostomum trigonocephalum* of sheep and goats. Cosmopolitan in tropical and temperate regions.

*Globocephalus* spp. of pigs. In many tropical and temperate regions (Figure 16.1).

*Ancylostoma caninum* of canids. Particularly prevalent in temperate regions. It has three pairs of well evident teeth on the buccal margin.

*Ancylostoma braziliense* of canids and felids. Particularly prevalent in tropical and subtropical regions including the Gulf Coast of the United States. It can be distinguished from *A. caninum* because *A. braziliense* is smaller and has only two pairs of teeth on the buccal margin, the medial ones being very small.

*Ancylostoma ceylanicum* of canids, felids, and humans. Prevalent in tropical and subtropical areas. It can be distinguished from *A. braziliense* because the mediolateral and posterolateral rays of the bursa run close together in *A. ceylanicum* but diverge widely in *A. braziliense*, and the externodorsal rays originate at the same level than the ventral rays in *A. ceylanicum* but much higher than the origin of the ventral rays in *A. braziliense* (Figure 16.2).

*Ancylostoma tubaeforme* of felids. Prevalent in temperate and subtropical regions. It is very similar to *A. caninum* but its esophagus is 0.83 mm long, its spicules 1.1 to 1.5 mm long, and the lateral lobes of the copulatory bursa 0.35 to 0.39 mm wide. The same measurements in *A. caninum* are 1.1, 0.7 to 1.0, and 0.45 to 0.49 mm, respectively.

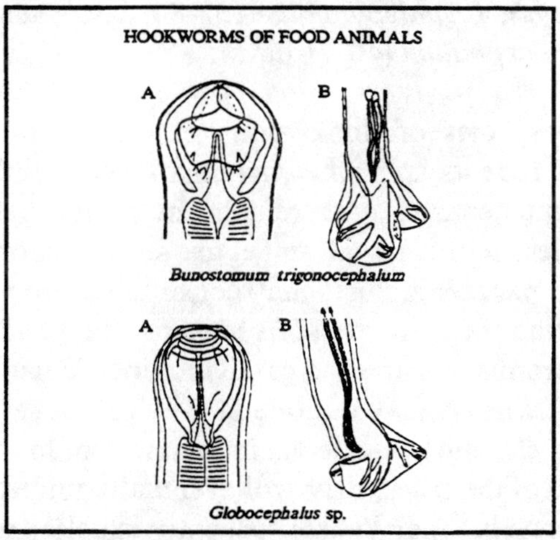


**Figure 16.1.** Ventral view of the head (A) and left view of the bursa copulatrix (B).

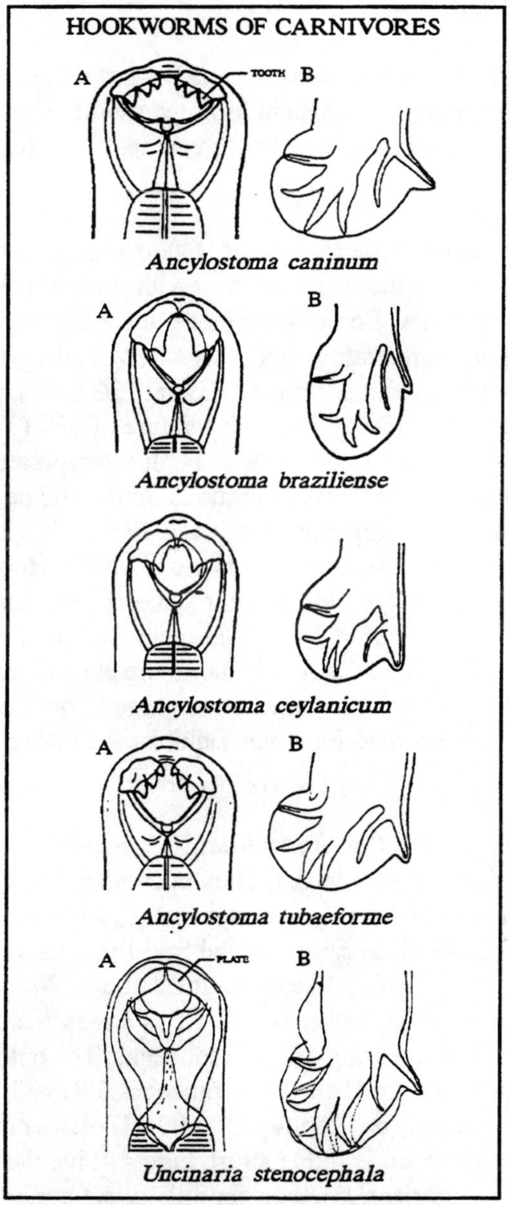


Figure 16.2. Ventral view of the head (A) and left view of the bursa copulatrix (B).

*Uncinaria stenocephala* of canids and felids. Prevalent in the cooler parts of temperate regions including northern United States and Canada. It can be distinguished from Ancylostoma spp. because it has plates rather than teeth on the buccal margin.

*Ancylostoma duodenale* and *Necator americanum* are hookworms of humans that prefer temperate and tropical zones, respectively.[3]

### 3. Biology

Because the hookworms are homogenous not only in morphology but also in biology, the life cycle of *A. caninum* provides a good representation for the group.

A young female lays about 16,000 strongyle-type eggs per day that leave the host with the feces as an early morula. For development, the eggs require adequate temperature, humidity, shade, and oxygen. They produce an L1 in 6-12 days at 12C (54F), in 1 day at the nearly optimal temperature of 23C (73F), and in 9 hours at 37C (99F). Higher temperatures kill the eggs, lower temperatures inhibit the development, and temperatures of 0C (32F) or -5C (23F) kill them in 8 days or 6 hours, respectively. Humidity below 90% inhibits their development and a humidity of about 50% kills them in less than a week. Direct sunlight is lethal to the eggs in a few hours. Lack of oxygen when they are in the center of an undisturbed fecal mass inhibits their development.

The L1s and L2s are free-living organisms with a rhabditiform esophagus. They become infective in 17 days at 15C (59F), 3-4 days at 23C, and 38 hours at 37C. The best range for the free-living larvae is 25-30C (77-86F). Temperatures above 37C are lethal in a couple of days. The L3s are ensheathed larvae with a strongyliform esophagus. The optimal temperature for their development is 30C and few are produced outside the 25-35C (77-95F) range. Their life span is rather short, they survive the fall of the American midwest for only about a month.[4]

The free-living stages of *A. tubaeforme* and *Bunostomum* spp. have temperature requirements similar to those of *A. caninum* but are less resistent to the cold. For this reason, they are less prevalent in the cooler parts of the temperate regions than *A. caninum*. The free-living stages of *A. braziliense* and *A. ceylanicum* need higher temperatures which explains their distribution in the tropical and subtropical regions. *U. stenocephala*, on the other hand, can develop at temperatures as low as 8C (46F), the infective larvae appear in only 4 days at 20C (68F), and most of them survive more than 40 days at 0C.

The infective larvae of *A. caninum* may enter the host by the mouth or through the skin. The larvae that are ingested penetrate the gastric or intestinal mucosa, develop to L4s in 3-4 days, and return to the lumen of the small intestine to mature to adults. The larvae that invade the skin rely on their mechanical activity and a collagenase to open their way through the tissues until reaching the circulation. Taken by the blood or the lymph, they reach the capillaries of the lungs and break into the alveoli where they molt to L4s 44-48 hours after the infection. These larvae crawl up the air passages to reach the pharynx, are swallowed, and molt to early adults in the intestine by the 6th day of infection. Eggs start to appear in the feces during the third week of infection. The adults live for 6-12 months.

In ruminants, a standardized cutaneous infection results in the development of more intestinal parasites than the oral infection. The reverse is true for the species in carnivores. It appears that the ruminant hookworms are particularly adapted to skin invasion whereas the carnivore hookworms are more adapted to oral infection. *U. stenocephala* larvae can penetrate transcutaneously but most remain in the skin and few reach adulthood by this route. The prepatent periods of most hookworms of veterinary importance are similar to that of *A. caninum* with the exception of *A. tubaeforme* (22-25 days), *B. phlebotomum* (52-84 days), and *B. trigonocephalum* (40-71 days).

The species of hookworms of carnivores can infect rodents and other mammals per mouth or transcutaneously, and remain in their skeletal muscles at the larval stage for several months. These **paratenic hosts** may constitute a source of infection for carnivores. In humans, the larvae of hookworms of cattle and carnivores, particularly of *A. braziliense*, may migrate in the skin for several weeks causing a cutaneous inflammation. In about a third of the cases, they will eventually migrate to the lungs but they are subsequently expelled without further development.

A small proportion of the infective larvae of *A. caninum* will become arrested in the skeletal muscles, lung, liver, and other tissues of the dog, particularly in old or resistent animals, during their migration. These hypobiotic parasites become active again during late pregnancy and lactation and may pass to the offspring primarily with the milk and, secondarily, through the uterus.[5] This phenomenon has not been substantiated in other hookworms.

#### 4. Medical importance

The hookworms are particularly prevalent and pathogenic in young hosts. Prolonged or repeated infections stimulate enough immune resistance to eliminate most of the existing intestinal parasites, to reject a large proportion of the newly arrived larvae, and to impair their pathogenic mechanisms. Immunity also kills some of the larvae arrested in the tissues but with less efficiency.[6]

Ancylostomiasis can cause pathology associated with the penetration of the larvae through the skin, their migration through the lungs, or the activities of the adults in the intestine.

Skin penetration by the larvae of *B. phlebotomum* or *U. stenocephala* frequently causes a dermatitis in cattle or dogs. This symptom is rather uncommon with the other hookworms except in the case of hosts that have been exposed to repeated infections before. For this reason, and for the abundance of eosinophils in the inflamed skin, it is widely believed that hookworm **dermatitis** is a manifestation of allergy to products of the parasites. It is also suggestive that, among the hookworms of the carnivores, the most frequent dermatitis is due to *U. stenocephala*, species in which the infective larvae tend to remain in the skin rather than to invade the body.

The cutaneous syndrome usually starts as a pruriginous dermatitis of the interdigital spaces that may extend up the limbs. The affected area shows all the signs of inflammation and develops small vesicles that may become pustules due to secondary pyogenic infection. Occasionally, small areas of necrosis enclosing dead larvae are observed, and sloughing and self-mutilation in dogs may occurs in particularly severe reactions. Most commonly the lesions are transient and subside in less than a week.

Larvae of animal hookworms, particularly *A. braziliense*, can penetrate the human skin and cause a winding track of inflammation that may last for several weeks and is very pruriginous (**cutaneous larva migrans** or **creeping eruption**). Lesions due to scratching and secondary infections are common complications.

Passage of the larvae through the lungs causes points of hemorrhage and some leukocyte infiltration which rarely has a clinical expression. Only in cases of massive infections in very young animals or in previously sensitized hosts, the parasites may cause signs of **pneumonia**. The lesions are traumatic in the first case and allergic in the second.

The activity of the parasites in the intestine is by far the most severe pathogenic mechanism of hookworm disease. The worms bite and digest plugs of intestinal mucosa, at the same time that suck blood with the assistance of an anticoagulant enzyme produced by the esophageal glands. After a few days, they move to a new location leaving an oozing wound behind. Reliable calculations have shown that *A. caninum* and *A. tubaeforme* cause a blood loss of over 0.05 ml per worm per day, and *A. braziliense* and *U. stenocephala* of less than 0.01 ml per worm per day. The blood loss peaks before patency and decreases soon afterward, presumably due to the effect of host's immunity. Consequent with these figures, 50-75 *A. caninum* per lb of body weight approach the $LD^{50}$ in pups younger than 6 months whereas 6,309 *A. braziliense* do not change significantly the hemoglobin values of the host.

Very young hosts are particularly affected by the blood loss due to their low iron reserves, the low content in iron of their milk diet, and their lack of resistance to the infection. The hookworm **anemia** begins as a hemorrhagic type (normocytic and normochromic) but it progresses to the hypoferric type (microcytic and hypochromic) as the iron reserves of the host become exhausted.

The trauma by the bites and the subsequent inflammation of the intestinal mucosa frequently lead to **diarrhea** with feces streaked with blood, frankly bloody, or black due to their digested blood content. Ruminants infected with *Bunostomum* spp., dogs with *A. caninum*, or cats with *A. tubaeforme* may show **anorexia**, and stop gaining weight or lose weight. These signs appear to be more related to the blood loss than to the diarrhea, however, because carnivores with *A. braziliense* or *U. stenocephala* (which take little blood) may develop diarrhea but their general condition is little affected.

Intestinal infection with hookworms also causes atrophy of the intestinal villi, malabsorption, and hypoproteinemia. The **hypoproteinemia**, which may lead to **generalized edema** in severe cases, probably results from an increased turnover of the seralbumin to compensate the losses of plasma proteins into the intestinal lumen. The occasional liver degeneration found in these cases appears to be directly related to the degree of anemia and may be due to tissue anoxia.

**Table 16.I. Characteristics of some common hookworms of domestic animals**

| Species | Male(mm) | Spicules(mm) | Female(mm) | Eggs (um) | Mouth |
|---|---|---|---|---|---|
| *B. phlebotomum* | 10-12x 0.4-0.4 | 3.5-4.0 | 16-19x 0.5-0.6 | 79-117x 47-70 | Plates |
| *B. trigonocephalum* | 12-17x 0.5 | 0.6 | 19-26x 0.7 | 80-102x 35-57 | Plates |
| *Globocephalus* spp. | 5-7x 0.35 | 0.5-0.7 | 6-8x 0.4 | 52-56x 26-35 | Plates |
| *A. caninum* | 11-13x 0.3-0.4 | 0.7-1.0 | 14-20x 0.5-0.6 | 55-72x 34-45 | 3 pairs teeth |
| *A. braziliense* | 5-8x 0.2-0.2 | 0.7-1.0 | 7-9x 0.2 | 55-95x 32-45 | 2 pairs teeth |
| *A. tubaeforme* | 9-11x 0.3 | 1.1-1.5 | 12-15x 0.4 | 5-76x 34-45 | 3 pairs teeth |
| *U. stenocephala* | 5-9x 0.2 | 0.6-0.8 | 7-13x 0.25 | 63-93x 32-55 | Plates |

**Summary:**

1. The Ancylostomatidae or hookworms are recognized as large-mouthed bursate nematodes with teeth or cutting plates (instead of a leaf crown) on the ventral margin of their oral opennings.

2. They infect the small intestine of carnivores, ruminants, pigs, and humans.

3. Infected hosts pass strongyle-type eggs that develop into free-living, infective L3s on the ground.

4. The L3s infest their hosts transcutaneously or orally. The preadult stages migrate by the circulation to the heart and lungs and reach de small intestine to develop to adults.

5. *A. caninum* larvae may arrest in immune hosts and later pass to the offspring congenitally or with the milk.

6. Infective larvae entering transcutaneously may cause skin inflammation in sensitized hosts. Migrating larvae may cause pulmonary manifestations in massive infections or highly sensitized hosts. Hematophagous adults may cause anemia, diarrhea, and malabsorption.

7. Humans may suffer a temporary dermatitis by larvae of animal hookworms.

## REFERENCES

1. Barriga OO. 1982. Ancylostomiasis. In Steele JH (ed.), *CRC Handbook Series in Zoonoses, Section C: Parasitic Zoonoses*, Volume II, CRC Press, Boca Raton, Florida, 3-24.

2. Nichols RL. 1956. The etiology of visceral larva migrans. I. and II. J. Parasit. 42:349-362 and 363-399.

3. Miller TA. 1979. Hookworm infection in man. Adv. Parasit. 17:315-384.

4. Mark DL. 1975. Survival of *Ancylostoma caninum* in blue grass pasture. J. Parasit. 61:484-488.

5. Lee KT, Little MD & Beaver PC. 1975. Intracellular (muscle-fiber) habitat of *Ancylostoma caninum* in some mammalian hosts. J. Parasit. 61:589-598..

6. Miller TA. 1971. Vaccination against the canine hookworm disease. Adv. Parasit. 9:153-183.
- - - 1978. Industrial development and field use of the canine hookworm vaccine. Adv. Parasit. 16:333-342.

# Chapter 17

# THE ORDER STRONGYLIDA OR BURSATE NEMATODES

## THE SUPERFAMILY TRICHOSTRONGYLOIDEA OR SMALL-MOUTHED BURSATE NEMATODES

**Preview.** The Trichostrongyloidea (*Haemonchus, Ostertagia, Trichostrongylus, Cooperia,* and *Nematodirus*) are small bursate nematodes of the stomach and small intestine of ruminants and other livestock. The infective larvae is a free living L3 and the parasitic stages develop without leaving the gut. They are the most pathogenic nematodes of the ruminants.

### 1. Morphology

The superfamily **Trichostrongyloidea** (from Gr *trikho*= hair, and *strongulos*= round, nowadays meaning "round worm") is a rather homogeneous group of small or very small nematodes of the stomach and/or small intestine of a number of mammals, or birds. They are particularly important, however, as parasites of ruminants. The trichostrongylids measure from about 3 to 30 mm long by 0.05 to 0.5 mm wide (Figure 17.1). Different species are whitish, reddish, or brownish. The cuticle of some genera have transverse striations and longitudinal ridges that may be used for identification purposes.[1] The oral opening is small and the buccal cavity very small or non-existing. The males have well developed copulatory bursa and spicules, with an evident gubernaculum in some genera. The females have the vulva located in the posterior half of the body and covered with a flap of cuticle in some genera.

### 2. Identification and classification

The trichostrongyloidea are easily identified by their location in the stomach or small intestine, their small size, the presence of a very small or inapparent buccal cavity, and the well developed bursa of the males. Because of these last two characteristics, they are often referred to as the **small-mouthed bursate nematodes**. The genera most important to veterinary medicine are *Haemonchus, Ostertagia, Trichostrongylus, Cooperia, Nematodirus,* and *Hyostrongylus*. Identification of the genera or species is commonly done by study of the males because the females have fewer identifying fea

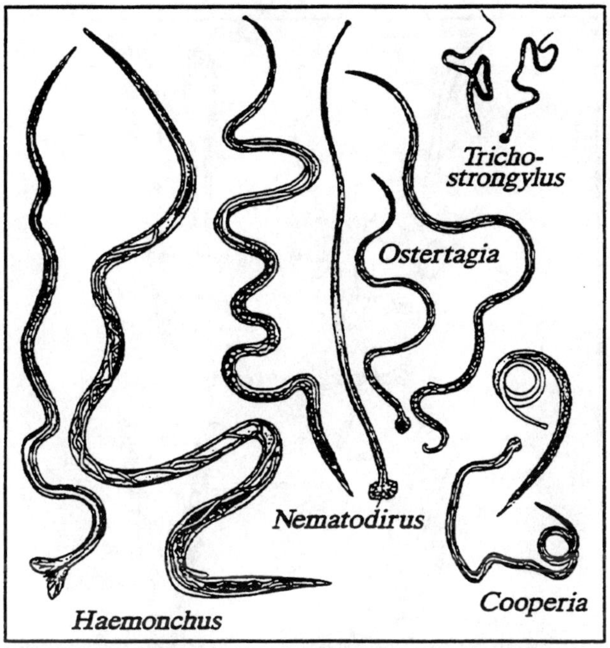


**Figure 17.1**. Some important Trichostrongyloidea drawn at proportional size. Males are recognized by the presence of a capulatory bursa.

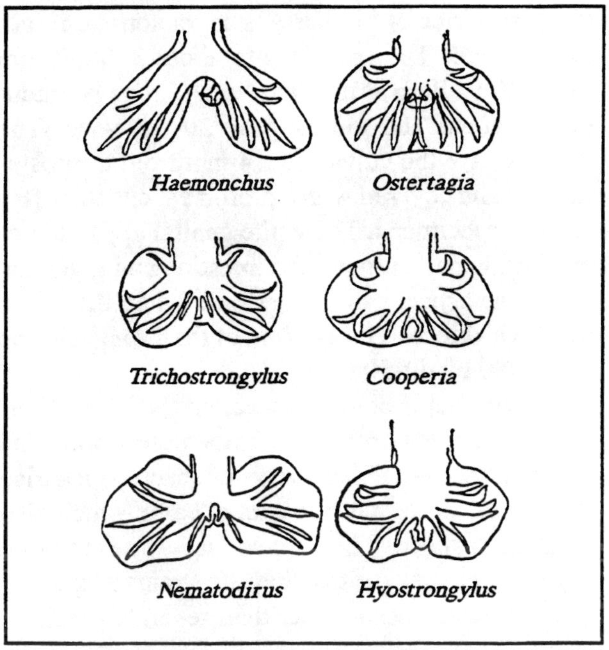


**Figure 17.2.** Copulatory bursa of some important Trichostrongyloidea.

tures. Table 17.I shows the major identifying characteristics of the common genera of trichostrongyloidea of ruminants. Identification of species depends on the observation of subtle characteristics of the bursa or spicules of well prepared specimens (Figure 17.2). This exercise is probably beyond the needs and skills of general practitioners. Levine's[2] and Soulsby's[3,4] books and the Weybridge Manual[5] provide information for the identification of the species of the domestic animals as well as the generic identification of their larvae.

■ *Haemonchus* are parasites of the stomach. They are the largest of the common trichostrongyloidea of ruminants. The males are 10-20 and the females 18-30 mm long, and 0.5 mm wide. They are easily seen at necropsy. Their size and their location in the stomach of ruminants suffice for identification in the field. Microscopically, they have a small buccal cavity with a tooth or lancet that arises from the dorsal wall, and a pair of spine-like cervical papilla a little behind the nerve ring (Figure 17.3). The males have a well developed copulatory bursa with 2 spicules and a gubernaculum. Characteristically,

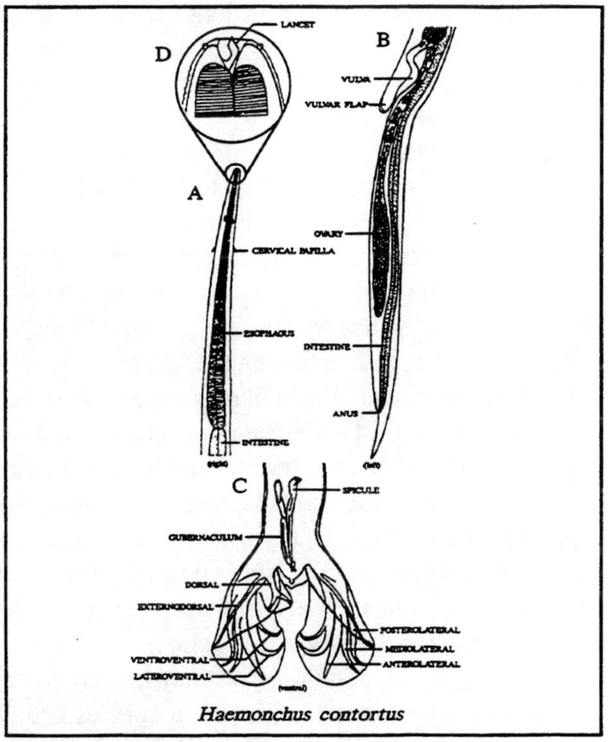


**Figure 17.3.** Anterior end (A), posterior end of the female (B), anterior end of the male (C) and detail of the mouth (D) of *Haemonchus contortus*.

the dorsal lobe of the bursa is asymmetrical rather than medial. The spicules are about 350-450 um long, with a barb at the distal end. The gubernaculum is about 200 um long by 30 um wide. The females have the vulva about 4 mm from the posterior end and covered with a prominent cuticular flap in most specimens. The white genital apparatus of the female coils around the intestine and gives the worm the aspect of a barber pole when the gut is filled with blood. The eggs are of the strongyle-type and 62-90 by 40-50 um.

*Haemonchus* is commonly called the large stomach worm, wireworm, or the barberpole worm. The major species are *H. contortus* of sheep which also parasitizes cattle, and *H. placei* of cattle which also parasitizes sheep. They are so closely related that some authors believe that they are strains adapted to their particular hosts rather than separate species.

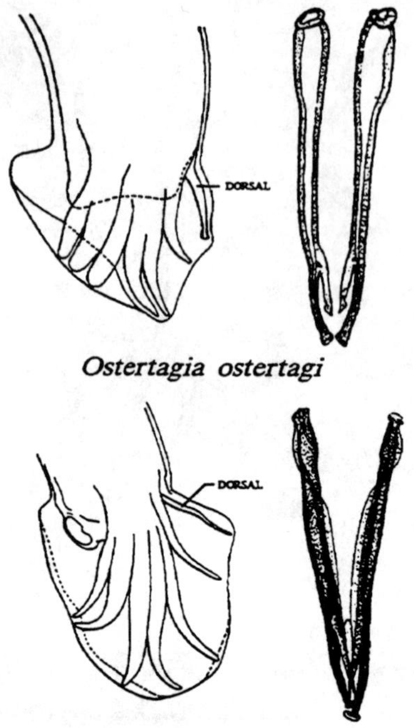


**Figure 17.4.** Copulatory bursae and spicules of two species of *Ostertagia*.

■ *Ostertagia* is also a gastric parasite of ruminants, rarely found in the small intestine. They are reddish-brown and considerably shorter and slender than *Haemonchus*. The males are 7 to 9 mm long and the females 8 to 13 mm long. Both are about 0.1 mm wide. They have cervical papillae en gubernaculum. Their finding during necropsy demands careful observation. The location in the stomach of ruminants and the size smaller than *Haemonchus* is usually enough to identify *Ostertagia* in the field. Differently from *Haemonchus*, the bursa of *Ostertagia* males has a symmetrical dorsal lobe, the gubernaculum is shorter (about 70 to 90 um), and the spicules are smaller (about 200 to 300 um), divided into 2 or 3 branches posteriorly, and the main branch ended in a blunt surface rather than a hook (Figure 17.4). The females may or may not present a flap in front of the vulva which is located 1.3-2.3 mm from the posterior end. The females of *O. circumcincta* and *O. trifurcata* exhibit four annulations around the tail. The eggs are about 75-90 by 35-45 um but they are indistinguishable from those of *Haemonchus* in the practice.

*Ostertagia* are commonly called the brown or medium stomach worm. The main species are *O. ostertagi* and *O. lyrata* of cattle, and *O. circumcincta* and *O. trifurcata* of sheep and goats. The cattle species are occasionally found in sheep and goats, and the sheep and goat species are infrequently found in cattle.

■ *Trichostrongylus* are parasites of the small intestine and occasionally the stomach of ruminants, equines, pigs, rodents, lagomorphs, and rarely, humans. They are pale brown and the smallest of the common trichostrongyloidea of ruminants. The males are about 4-9 mm long by 0.06-0.08 wide and the females about 5-9 mm long by 0.08-0.12 wide. They are virtually invisible to the naked eye during necropsy. *Trichostrongylus* do not have an apparent buccal cavity. The duct of the excretory glands opens ventrally immediately behind the nerve ring forming a distinct notch which is a characteristic feature of the genus. Different from *Haemonchus* or *Ostertagia*, they do not have cervical papillae. The dorsal lobe of the bursa is greatly reduced or absent, the spicules are about 75 to 175 um long and of unequal size in many species, and the gubernaculum is about 55 to 95 um long (Figure 17.5). The females do not have

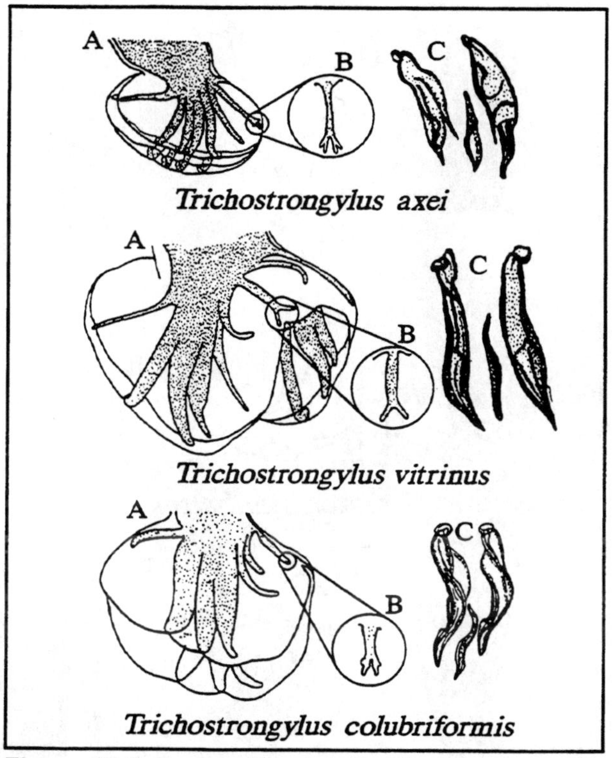


**Figure 17.5.** Bursae (A), detail of thedorsal ray (B), spicules and gubernacula of some *Trichostrongylus*.

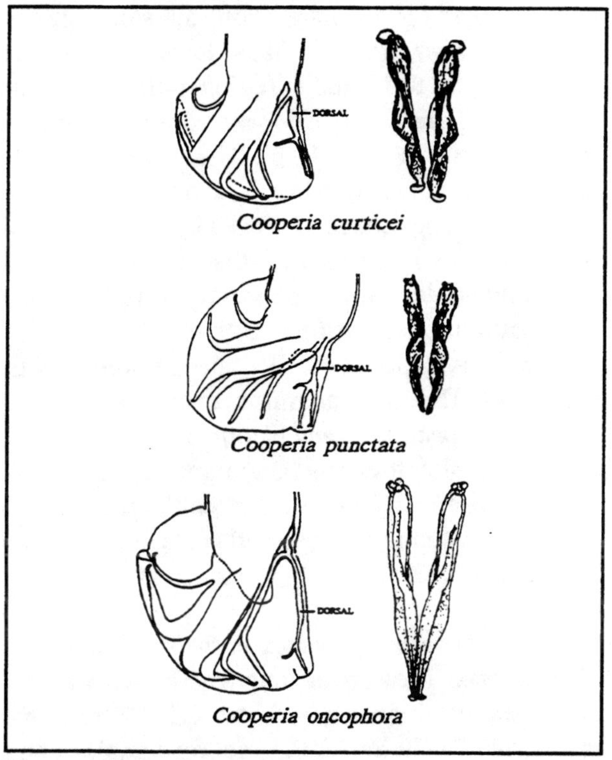


**Figure 17.6.** Copulatory bursae and spicules of some *Cooperia*.

a vulvar flap. The eggs are about 85-125 by 37-50 um and indistinguishable from those of *Haemonchus* or *Ostertagia*. The only common nematodes of comparable size found in the proximal portion of the small intestine are *Strongyloides* (about 3.5-6 mm long and 0.06 mm wide) and *Trichinella* (about 1-3.5 mm long and 0.03-0.07 wide). The most apparent differences with *Strongyloides papillosus* are that there is no parasitic males among *Strongyloides*, the esophagus of the females is 1/3 or more of the body length (versus 1/5 or less in *Trichostrongylus*), and the eggs in the uterus or ovijector are about 40-60 by 20-36 um (versus 85-125 by 37-50 in *Trichostrongylus*). The major differences with *Trichinella* are that the *Trichinella* males end in a pair of tubercules rather than a copulatory bursa, the thin esophagus is embedded in a row of cells in both sexes and it is about half the body length in the males and a fourth in the females, the females contain embryos rather than eggs, and the vulva is located about a fourth of the body length from the mouth. Besides, *Trichinella* in ruminants must be considered an exceptional finding.

*Trichostrongylus* are commonly called the hairworms, bankrupt worms, or black scour worms. The most important species are: *T. axei* of the stomach and occasionally small intestine of cattle but also sheep, goats, equines, and, occasionally, pigs; *T. colubriformis* and *T. vitrinus* of the small intestine and rarely stomach of sheep and goat, and, secondarily, cattle, it also infects other ruminants, primates, lagomorphs, and pigs; and *T. capricola* in the small intestine and stomach of sheep and goats.

■ *Cooperia* are parasites of the small intestine of ruminants, rarely found in the stomach. They are reddish, about the same size as *Ostertagia* (5 to 9 mm long by 0.1 to 0.2 mm wide for males and 6 to 12 mm long by 0.1 to 0.3 mm wide for females), and frequently coiled like a watch spring. They have a small buccal cavity. The cuticle is inflated and presents a number of transverse striation at the anterior end of the body. They do not have cervical papillae. The spicules are about the same size as those of *Ostertagia* but they have a wing-like expansion in the middle region rather than the prongs of *Ostertagia*. *Cooperia* does not have a gubernaculum (Figure 17.6). The females usually have a small vulvar flap but no annulations around the tail. The eggs are about 70-90 by 30-45 um and with the sides more parallel than in the other trichostrongyloidea. However, accurate differentiation is difficult in the practice.

*Cooperia* is sometimes called the medium intestinal worm. The most common species are *C. oncophora*, *C. pectinata*, and *C. punctata* of cattle, *C. surnabada* of cattle, sheep, and goats, and *C. curticei* of sheep and goats. The cattle species are occasionally found in sheep and goats but the sheep and goat species are rarely found in cattle.

■ *Nematodirus* are parasites of the small intestine of ruminants. They are as long as *Haemonchus* but considerably thinner (8-19 by 0.1-0.2 mm for males, and 12-29 by 0.2-0.5 mm for females), and are often found entwined in the intestinal mucus. They have a cephalic inflation and striations like *Cooperia*, and a buccal tooth like *Haemonchus*. The internal surface of the bursal lateral lobes has a number of round circular protuberances (bosses), and the dorsal lobe is greatly reduced or split into two halves, each attached to a lateral lobe. The spicules are long (700 to 1250 um), thin, curved ventrally, and fused to each other at their tips. There is no gubernaculum. The tail of the females ends bluntly and bears a spine at the end (the females of *N. battus* have a needle-sharp tail). The eggs are about 150-230 by 80-110 um, with their sides curve in some species and parallel in others. Their size allows for easy differentiation from the eggs of the other common trichostrongyloidea.

*Nematodirus* are sometimes called the twisted intestinal worms. The common species are *N. helvetianus* of cattle, and *N. spathiger*, *N. abnormalis*, *N. filicollis*, and *N. battus* of sheep and goats. The cattle species is also found in sheep and goats and *N. spathiger* and *N. battus* are occasionally found in cattle.

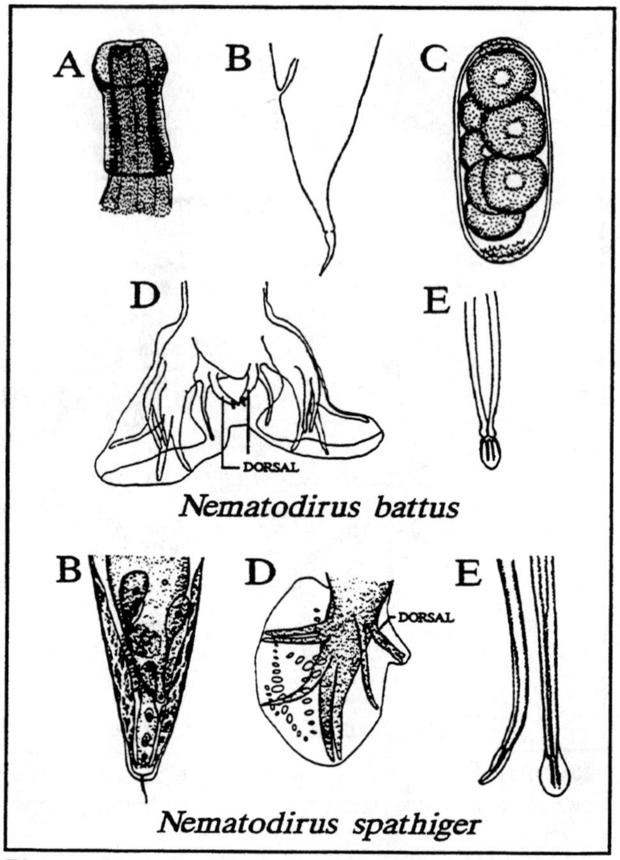


**Figure 17.7.** Anterior end (A), posterior end of the female (B), egg (C), posterior end of the male (D), and spicules (E) of *Nematodirus*.

### 3. Biology

The adult trichostrongylids live in the lumen of the stomach or small intestine, in close association with the mucosa. In heavy infections, they may be found in the glands or crypts, underneath the digestive epithelium, or even inside the mucosa. *Haemonchus* lacerates the mucosa and sucks blood but the other genera appear to feed on mucus and intestinal content. Probably most adult trichostrongyles live for only several weeks to a few months. Their fertility peaks toward the end of the first month of infection and declines markedly in the subsequent weeks. The eggs hatch to free-living L1s, these molt to free-living L2s, and these originate ensheathed, infective L3s.

Under laboratory conditions, at constant 20-25C and with appropriate humidity, the eggs hatch in 1-2 days and the L3s appear in 6-9 days. With the fluctuations of temperature, humidity, and available oxygen bound to occur in nature, formation of L3s in the field probably takes 2 or more weeks. The range of temperature for development is 9-41C for *Haemonchus*, 4-34C for *Ostertagia*, and somewhere in between for the other genera. In each genera there are parasites adapted to colder or warmer environments. An *Haemonchus* strain from England, for example, developed between 9 and 36C whereas an *Haemonchus* strain from New York developed between 15 and 40C.

The survival of the larvae in the environment is limited by the intrinsic longevity of the parasites and the effect of the climate. In pastures, over 80% of *Haemonchus* die within 2 months and few live for 3-4 months under optimal conditions for survival (4-18C and 2-3 inches of rainfall). The larvae of the other genera probably have comparable life spans. Virtually no *Haemonchus* survives the drought of the summer or the cold of the winter in temperate regions. *Ostertagia* is more tolerant of the cold; enough larvae to cause new infections may survive the winter. *Trichostrongylus* larvae survive winter better than *Haemonchus* but not as well as *Ostertagia*, and die rapidly in summer. *Cooperia* larvae do not withstand winters or summers. *Nematodirus* survives the winter quite well (the eggs of *N. battus* need exposure to low temperature to hatch) but withstands the summer poorly.

The infective larvae are ingested by a new host with its forage, exsheath in the rumen or stomach, and molt to L4s by day 3-7 of infection, and to young adults by day 10-15 (but see Arrested Development, below). Passage of eggs begins by day 11-23 of infection in most genera, but after the third week in *Nematodirus*. With the exception of *Haemonchus* and *Ostertagia*, the larvae (and adults) of the trichostrongylids develop among the intestinal crypts without entering the mucosa. The L3s of *Haemonchus* develop inside the gastric mucosa but the L4s return to the lumen to lacerate the mucosa and absorb blood. The L3s of *Ostertagia* invade the gastric glands, develop in this location during the 4th larval stage, and return to the lumen as young adults.

**Arrested development**

Not all nematode larvae ingested by a host develop immediately to the adult stage. It has been observed in many nematode species that a variable proportion of the pre-adult parasites acquired by the host remains hypobiotic for several weeks to a few months before reaching adulthood. This phenomenon, comparable to the diapause of the insects, has been called **larval arrest**, arrested development, inhibition of larval development, or hypobiosis.[6,7] Larval arrest occurs at the L4 stage in most nematodes, at the L3 stage in the ascarides, ancylostomids, and *Trichostrongylus*, and at the early adult stage in *Dictyocaulus*.

The exact causes of larval arrest have not been determined. Some research done mainly with *Haemonchus* indicated that hypobiosis is a parasite response to specific host immunity. Work with *Ostertagia*, on the other hand, revealed that the cold of late autumn acts on the infective larvae on the ground to trigger the larval arrest once the parasites are in the host. Other investigations suggest that the ability to arrest is a genetic property of some subpopulations of parasites. Arrested development is so important to the survival of the parasitic species, however, that is its likely that parasites use host immunity, environmental signals, or genetic characteristics as alternatives or in combination to achieve their goals.

It seems clear that larval arrest is an adaptation to parasite survival. It occurs only in geographic areas with seasons unfavorable to parasite development (cold winters, dry summers), and takes place during these periods. Hypobiosis not only permits the parasite to elude the adverse weather in the comparatively milder host environment, but, since it occurs at an immature stage, it allows the parasites to avoid senility and preserve their fleeting fecundity. Larval arrest is viewed nowadays as an efficient mechanism that the nematodes developed to coordinate their peak fertility with the most suitable seasons for free-living development and infection of a new generation of hosts (see Epidemiology, below).

Two other consequences of larval hypobiosis are worth mentioning. On one hand, parasites with a reduced metabolism are less pathogenic and produce less antigen. As a consequence, larval arrest lessens the host-parasite confrontation and favors the survival of the parasitic species. On the other hand, most anthelmintics act by competition with biochemical pathways so a reduced metabolism affects severely their efficacy. This comparative insusceptibility of arrested larvae to anthelmintics is a major obstacle to the control of nematode infections.

## 4. Medical importance

The trichostrongylids are the most harmful parasites of small ruminants, and second only to the arthropods in large ruminants. It has been calculated that internal parasitism, largely by trichostrongyle nematodes, causes losses equivalent to 19% of the sheep industry or 1.6% of the cattle industry. *Ostertagia* and *Trichostrongylus* are particularly important in large ruminants, and *Haemonchus* and *Trichostrongylus* in small ruminants

**4.1. Haemonchosis.** The major pathogenic mechanism of *Haemonchus* is its hematophagia. It has been estimated in sheep that 2,000 worms increase 5 times the physiologic losses of erythrocytes, and 1600 worms increase 3-7 times the physiological losses of plasma. Evidence of blood in the feces of the host is found during the second week of infection. A sudden decrease of erythrocytes (that causes a normocytic hypochromic anemia) commonly occurs during prepatency. In the early patency, the erythrocyte drainage is compensated by a faster turnover of body iron and the anemia remains stable. Severe and prolonged infections may lead to a subsequent iron depletion and bone marrow exhaustion with intense microcytic hypochromic **anemia** and death.[8] The loss of plasma proteins increases the protein turnover in the body with the subsequent **loss of weight**. The hypovolemia and low colloid osmotic pressure that result from the loss of plasma and plasma proteins cause the production of **edema** that is first seen in the intermandibular space (**bottle jaw**) but may extend to the entire body later. Although the buffering effect of the plasma proteins in the stomach raises the gastric pH in the chronic infection (from 2.5 to 5.0-6.5 in massive infections) and presumably interferes with digestion, diarrhea does not occur and the appetite is commonly preserved.

Haemonchosis may be an hyperacute, acute, or chronic disease depending on the previous physiologic condition of the host and the severity and duration of the infection. The hyperacute condition generally occurs only in very young or debilitated hosts that ingest a massive dose of parasites; it is infrequent in sheep, and rare in cattle. The affected animals may die within a week with little or no other manifestation of disease. The acute disease is characterized by severe anemia and generalized edema. In the chronic disease the anemia is less severe, the edema is commonly localized, but the animals stop gaining weight or lose weight.

**4.2. Ostertagiasis**. Most of the damage produced by *Ostertagia* is due to the growth of the L4s in the gastric mucosa and the emergence of the young adults into the lumen. The larvae in the mucosa stimulate an inflammatory response and the accelerated growth of the enterocytes of the surrounding tissue, and the emergence of the worms ruptures the epithelium. These actions disrupt the normal differentiation of the zymogen, parietal, and mucous cells, and the architecture of the gastric mucosa. As a result, pepsinogen and HCl production become depressed, mucus production is enhanced, and pepsinogen leaks into the blood, and plasma into the stomach. The shortage of HCl and the buffering action of the plasma proteins causes the gastric pH to increase (from 2.5-3.0 to 6.0-7.0 in severe infections). The loss of gastric acidity, in turn, promotes bacterial growth and inhibits the conversion of pepsinogen to pepsin. The combination of extra fluid leaked into the stomach, the action of bacterial products, and the presence of undigested gastric content in the duodenum is the responsible for the characteristic **diarrhea** of ostertagiasis. The diarrhea, in turn, interferes with normal digestion and adsorption, and results in malnutrition and loss of weight.

The increased permeability of the digestive epithelium to plasma proteins is a characteristic of a number of digestive diseases that are gathered under the common name of **protein-losing enteropathies**. The loss of proteins to the gastric lumen reduces the half life of plasma albumin and immunoglobulins up to 50%, and accelerates their catabolism up to 2-3 times.[9] Since the infected animals eat little and utilize food poorly, these proteins (and those of the gastric mucus and epithelium) are re-synthesized at the expense of skeletal muscle, wool production, bone formation, and milk secretion. As a consequence, the animals experience poor growth or weight loss, and nurse poorly. The hypovolemia and loss of plasma proteins could lead to edema formation but the diarrhea commonly causes enough dehydration to avoid it. **Anorexia** is a characteristic sign of trichostrongyle infections (with the exception of haemonchosis). It used to be blamed by most of the weight loss but nowadays it appears that poor utilization of the food contributes more to the pathogenesis of these infections than anorexia.[10] The **anemia** sometimes reported in ostertagiasis, particularly ostertagiasis type II (see below), is probably of nutritional origin.

*Ostertagia* is more pathogenic in cattle than in sheep or goats. Two clinical entities occur in cattle: ostertagiasis type 1 and ostertagiasis type 2. **Ostertagiasis type 1** results from the ingestion of a large number of infective larvae that develop to adults in about 3 weeks. It occurs at the peak of the season most favorable for transmission, when large number of infective larvae are available in the pastures (late summer and early autumn in temperate regions, and late winter and early spring in semi-tropical regions). It is more common in animals during their first year of life, and often affects a large proportion of the animals that were exposed to the infection. Because all the parasites in an animal mature at about the same time, treatment is usually successful. **Ostertagiasis type 2** results from the maturation of hypobiotic larvae that accumulated in the host during the unfavorable seasons. It occurs at the end of the season unfavorable for transmission (late winter and early spring in temperate regions, and late summer to autumn in semi-tropical regions). It is more common in animals during their second year of life, and affects only those few animals that accumulated a large number of hypobiotic larvae. Because the hypobiotic parasites often mature in successive waves, treatment is not very effective.

**4.3. Trichostrongylosis.** The gastric *Trichostrongylus* (*T. axei*) produces erosion of the cells of the gastric epithelium which triggers phenomena comparable to those discussed for *Ostertagia*. The *Trichostrongylus* of the small intestine lie just underneath the epithelial layer causing separation of the epithelium, inflammation, and acceleration of the epithelial cell turnover. This last phenomenon causes the villi to become atrophic and distorted and permit leakage of plasma into the lumen. The increase of fluid in the intestine is compounded by the catarrhal secretions contributed by the inflamed tissues. Because digestion and absorption of food is often compromised, the excess of fluid is eliminated as **diarrhea**. Although hypoproteinemia often occurs in trichostrongylosis, edemas are rare because they are compensated by the dehydration resulting from the intense diarrhea. The loss of proteins into the intestine (due to plasma leakage, production of inflammatory secretions, and increased cell turnover), the **anorexia** typical of the disease, and the deficient digestion and absorption of food are major factors causing **malnutrition**. It has been reported that infected sheep retain the ingested food in the rumen and stomach, and some studies have shown that food is underutilized in infected animals. Malnutrition, in turn, is the responsible for the weight loss, the slow wool growth typical of the infection, and the anemia occasionally reported in trichostrongylosis. It has been found experimentally that infected sheep show an increased rate of protein synthesis in the liver and intestine (presumably to offset the losses of plasma proteins and intestinal cells) and a decreased rate in muscle and wool (presumably because the available amino acids are diverted to liver and intestine).[11] This phenomenon appears to be common in protein-losing enteropathies. In the case of trichostrongylosis, it has been found that infected animals have depressed levels of insulin and thyroxine, and elevated levels of corticosteroids. The known effects of these hormones could explain the changes in the rates of protein synthesis.[12] The increase in corticosteroids with its known action as immunodepressants may explain the greater susceptibility of animals with trichostrongylosis to concurrent infections.

**4.4. Cooperiasis.** The pathogenesis of pure *Cooperia* infections has been less studied than that of the other trichostrongyles. Heavy *Cooperia* infection in cattle produces inflammation of the jejunal mucosa with fragmentation of the epithelium and a catarrhal exudate. The portions more parasitized may show degeneration and necrosis of the epithelium with a fibrino-necrotic exudate and destruction of the villous tips. In massive infections the animals reduce their food and water intake by the 3rd week of infection, develop an intense **diarrhea**, show a large increase in packed cell volume (hemoconcentration), lose body weight, and may die.

Like in the other trichostrongylid infections, the mechanism of **anorexia** is unknown. The diarrhea is probably due to a combination of defective absorption, poor digestion, and increased volume of the jejunal content due to the exudates and transudate (see below). The hemoconcentration is only partially explained by the reduced water intake, or the loss of water and sodium with the diarrhea. Actually, the infected animals retain water as compared to uninfected cattle subjected to the same food and water intake. The weight loss may have a mechanism similar to other protein-losing enteropathies (v. g., trichostrongylosis) because important losses of plasma to the intestinal lumen have been reported in infected cattle.[13] Death appears to be due to vascular shock.

**4.5. Nematodiriasis.** Most of the pathology of *Nematodirus* is caused by the L4s and young adults. Signs of disease are observed only with heavy infections and they usually subside by the time that egg production reaches a peak. Sick animals develop anorexia, diarrhea, dehydration, weakness, and poor growth. Depending on the number of parasites, the jejunal mucosa may show from a catarrhal inflammation with superficial erosion to intense inflammation with distortion and necrosis of the villi. The pathogenesis of the infection has not been studied but the lesions suggest that it may be similar to that of trichostrongylosis.

**4.6. Parasitic gastro-enteritis.** Because the trichostrongylids have similar ecologic requirements, they usually coexist in a same geographic area and are acquired together by the exposed animals. As a result, infections with a single species are rare and most animals carry mixed infections. This syndrome is commonly called parasitic gastro-enteritis of the ruminants. The clinical signs of the disease depend on the species that predominates. For example, anemia and edemas will be important when *Haemonchus* is abundant, anorexia and diarrhea will be prominent when *Ostertagia* or *Trichostrongylus* are the major genera, and instances of disease may occur in late winter or early spring when *Ostertagia* is predominant. Unfortunately, the pathogenesis of each parasite is independent from, or even synergistic with, that of the other genera. Parasitic gastro-enteritis is often more severe than the single individual infections.

**TABLE 17.I. CHARACTERISTICS OF THE COMMON TRICHOSTRONGYLOIDEA GENERA OF RUMINANTS (*)**

| | Size | Cephalic end | Bursa | Eggs | Special features |
|---|---|---|---|---|---|
| *Haemonchus* | M: 10-20x 0.4mm F: 18-30x 0.5mm | Attenuated; buccal lancet; spine-like papillae | Asymmetrical dorsal lobe; 425um, barbed spicules; gubernaculum | 62-90x 40-50um | Barber pole effect and vulvar flap in females; in stomach |
| *Ostertagia* | M: 7-10x 0.1mm F: 8-13x 0.1mm | Attenuated; small buccal cavity | 200-300um trifurcated spicules with terminal knob; gubernaculum | 75-90x 35-45um | Vulvar flap and caudal annulations in females; in stomach |
| *Trichostrongylus* | M: 4-9x 0.07mm F: 5-9x 0.1mm | Attenuated; no buccal cavity; excretory notch | Reduced dorsal lobe; 75-175um, pointed, unequal spicules; gubernaculum | 85-125x 37-50um | In stomach or small intestine |
| *Cooperia* | M: 5-9x 0.1mm F: 6-12x 0.2mm | Inflated, with transverse striations | 160-300um spicules, with wing-like expansions; no gubernaculum | 70-70x 30-45um; parallel sides | Often coiled; small vulvar flap in females; in small intestine |
| *Nematodirus* | M: 8-19x 0.2mm F: 12-29x 0.3mm | Inflated, with transverse striations; buccal tooth | Bosses on lateral lobes; dorsal lobe split or reduced; 700-1250um spicules fused at tip; no gubernaculum | 150-230x 80-110um | Often entwined; spine on blunt female tail; in small intestine |

**Summary:**

1. The Trichostrongyloidea are small bursate nematodes with a well developed copulatory bursa but a small or non-existent buccal cavity.

2. The most important genera are *Haemonchus, Ostertagia, Trichostrongylus, Cooperia,* and *Nematodirus.*

3. They are mostly parasites of the stomach or small intestine, particularly of ruminants.

4. The females lay strongyle-type eggs that developed into free living L3s.

5. The infective larvae are acquired by a new host with the herbage and develop into adults without leaving the gut.

6. They may arrest at a larval stage and resume development when the conditions for transmission are appropriate.

7. They are the most common and pathogenic nematodes of ruminants, often affecting them as mixed infections.

## REFERENCES

1. Lichtenfels, JR. 1977. Proc. Helm. Soc. Wash. 44:111-119.

2. Levine, N.D. 1980. *Nematode Parasites of Domestic Animals and of Man.* 2nd ed. Burgess, Minneapolis, 477 pp.

3. Soulsby, E.J. L. 1965. *Textbook of Veterinary Clinical Parasitology.* Blackwell, Oxford, 1120 pp.

4. Soulsby, E.J.L. 1982. *Helminths, Arthropods and Protozoa of Domesticated Animals.* 7th ed. Lea & Febiger, Philadelphia, 809 pp.

5. Ministry of Agriculture, Fisheries and Food. 1987. *Manual of Veterinary Parasitological Laboratory Techniques,* Her Majesty's Stationary Office, London, 159 pp.

6. Michel, J.F. 1974. Arrested development of nematodes and some related phenomena. Adv. Parasit. 12:279-366.

7. Gibbs, H.C. 1986. Hypobiosis in parasitic nematodes - An update. Adv. Parasit. 129-174.

8. Jennings, F.W. 1976. The anemias of parasitic infections. In Soulsby, E.J. L. (ed.), *Pathophysiology of Parasitic Infection*, Academic Press, New York, 41-67.

9. Nielsen, K. 1976. Plasma protein metabolism, In Soulsby, E.J.L. (ed.), *Pathophysiology of Parasitic Infection*, Academic Press, New York, 23-40.

10. Symons, L.E.A. 1985. Anorexia: occurrence, pathophysiology, and possible causes in parasitic infections. Adv. Parasit. 24:103-133.

11. Steel, J.W. and Symons, L.E.A. 1982. Nitrogen metabolism in nematodosis of sheep in relation to productivity. In Symons, L.E.a., Donald, A.D. and Dineen, J.K. (eds.), *Biology and Control of Endoparasites*, Academic Press, Sidney, 235-256.

12. Prichard, R.K., Hennessy, D.R. and Griffiths, D.A. 1974. Endocrine responses of sheep to infection with *Trichostrongylus colubriformis*. Res. Vet. Sci. 17:182-187.

13. Bremner, K.C. 1982. The pathophysiology of parasite gastro-enteritis of cattle. In Symons, L.E.A., Donald, A.D. and Dineen, J.K. (eds.), *Biology and Control of Endoparasites*, Academic Press, Sidney, 277-289.

# Chapter 18

# THE ORDER STRONGYLIDA OR BURSATE NEMATODES

## THE SUPERFAMILY METASTRONGYLOIDEA OR LUNGWORMS

**Preview.** The Metastrongyolidea are parasites of the respirtory system of ruminants, pigs, horses, and domestic carnivores. Most require an intermediate host but the most patogenic species (*Dictyocaulus*) produce free livng infective larvae. *Dictyocaulus* may cause severe bronchitis and bronchopneumonia. The other species are little pathogenic.

### 1. Morphology

The superfamily **Mestastrongyloidea** (Gr *meta*= beyond) is a heterogenous group of nematodes. The only characteristics most species of veterinary importance have in common are that they are slender and mostly small worms, with very small or nonexistant buccal cavities and poorly developed bursas. All live in the respiratory apparatus of their hosts. Most species are whitish. Some are less than 1 cm long but others may reach up to 11 cm. Their thin bodies make them appear as small parasites, nevertheless. Except *Metastrongylus* of pigs and *Filaroides osleri* of dogs, all pass L1s rather than eggs in the host's feces. Except in *Dictyocaulus* of sheep or equines, where they are larger, the L1s are 300 to 350 µm long and their tails may be conic, pointed, or undulated. Some species bear a dorsal spine on the tail. In all species, the L1s have coarse brown granules of food reserve in their intestines.

### 2. Identification and classification

The Metastrongyles are commonly identified simply because they are thin worms located in the lungs. The host species, the specific location of the worms in the lungs, and their size are important considerations for the presumptive identification of genera. Rarely a veterinarian will need identify species of adult specimens. The species of the larvae found in the host's feces are diagnosed by the species of host, size of the larvae, and characteristics of their tails. *Dictyocaulus* of sheep has a typical cephalic button (see below).

☛ *Dictyocaulus viviparus* is a cosmopolitan parasite of the trachea, bronchi, and bronchioles of cattle and other large ruminants. The males are 17-50 mm long by 0.5 mm wide, with a small, unlobed bursa. The dorsal ray ends in three lobes and the mediolateral and posterolateral rays are fused . The spicules are brown, short, and thick (195-215 µm long and 48 µm wide). The females are 23-80 mm long and have a short, pointed tail. The eggs are 82-88 by 33-38 µm and are embryonated when laid. The stage regularly found in the host's feces is an L1 with a pointed tail that measures 310-360 µm long by 16-19 µm wide.

☛ *Dictyocaulus filaria* is a cosmopolitan parasite of the bronchioles of sheep, goats, and other ruminants. It infects cattle only rarely. The males are 25-80 mm long , have a short bursa similar to that of *D. viviparus* but the mediolateral and posterolateral rays are separated at the tip and their brown spicules are 400-550 µm long by 48-96 µm wide (Figure 18.1). The females are 43-112 mm long with a conic tail. The eggs are 112-135 by 52-67 µm and contain an embryo when laid. The L1 commonly found in the host's feces has a conic tail, is 500-585 µm long by 25 µm wide, and has a dome-like cuticular knob at the anterior end ("cephalic button," Figure 18.2).

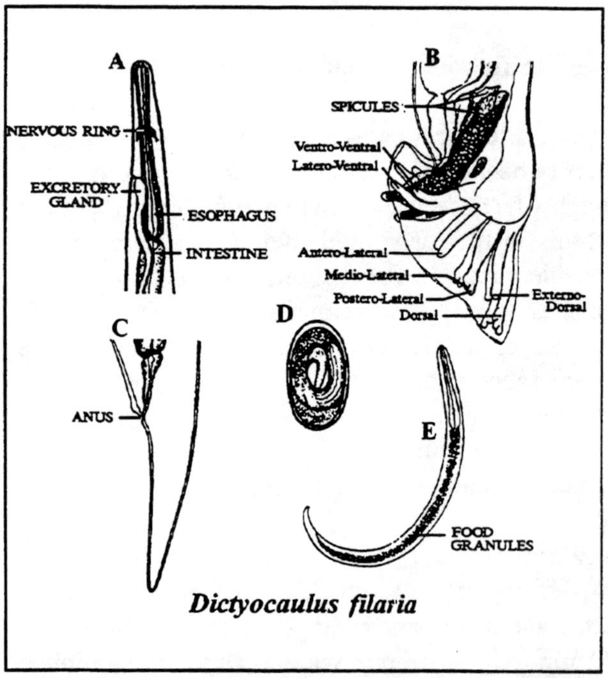


**Figure 18.1.** Anterior end (A), posterior ends of male (B) and female (C), egg (D), and L1 (E) of *Dictyocaulus filaria.*

☛ *Dictyocaulus arnfieldi* is a cosmopolitan parasite of the bronchi and bronchioles of equines. The males are 25-43 mm long by 0.13-0.26 mm wide, have a short bursa with the ventral rays side by side but with the ventroventral ray much shorter than the lateroventral ray. The spicules are 199-250 µm long. The females are 43-68 mm long by 0.4-0.5 mm wide with a short, blunt tail. The eggs are 80-100 by 50-60 µm and embryonated when laid.. The L1s found in the host's feces along with eggs is 420-480 µm long and has a sharp pointed tail.

☛ *Muellerius capillaris* is a cosmopolitan brown and very thin nematode of the lung parenchyma of sheep and goats. The males are 11-14 mm long, with a posterior end coiled in about a dozen turns, and a tiny bursa. The spicules are 140-160 µ long and each is divided into two branches caudally. The females are 19-23 mm long by 40-50 µm wide. The eggs are 100 by 20 µm. They contain a zygote when laid but develop and hatch an L1 before leaving the host. The L1 is 300-320 µm long, lacks a cephalic button, and has an undulated tail that bears a small dorsal spine (Figure 18.2).

☛ *Protostrongylus rufescens* is a virtually cosmopolitan, thin, reddish nematode of the bronchioles of sheep and goats. The males are 16-46 mm long by 0.1-0.2 mm wide and have a short bursa with bow-shaped plates at its base (Figure 18.3). The dorsal ray is very thick and bears 6 ventral papillae, the posterolateral and mediolateral rays are fused for their proximal half. The spicules are 230-340 µm long and have membranous expansions at their tips. The females are 25-65 mm long by 0.15-0.3 mm wide. The egg are 75-120 by 40-85 µm and unsegmented when laid. The larvae in the host's feces (250-320 µm long) lack a cephalic buton and their tails are undulated but lack a dorsal spine (Figure 18.2).

☛ *Metastrongylus apri, M. salmi,* and *M. pudendotectus* are cosmopolitan thin nematodes of the small bronchi and bronchioles of pigs. The males are about 10-25 mm long and 0.2-0.3 mm wide, with a fairly well-developed bursa (Figure 18.3). These species can be distinguished by the size of

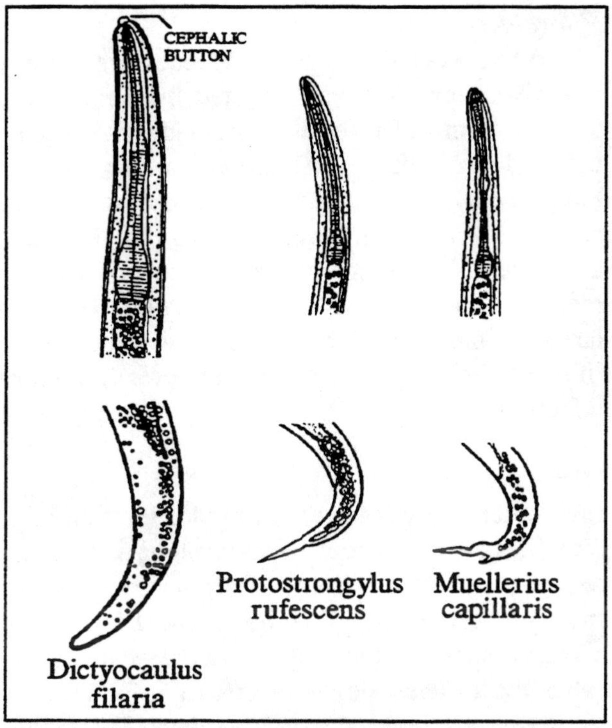


Figure 18.2. Anterior and posterior ends of L1s of Metrastrongyloidea of sheep.

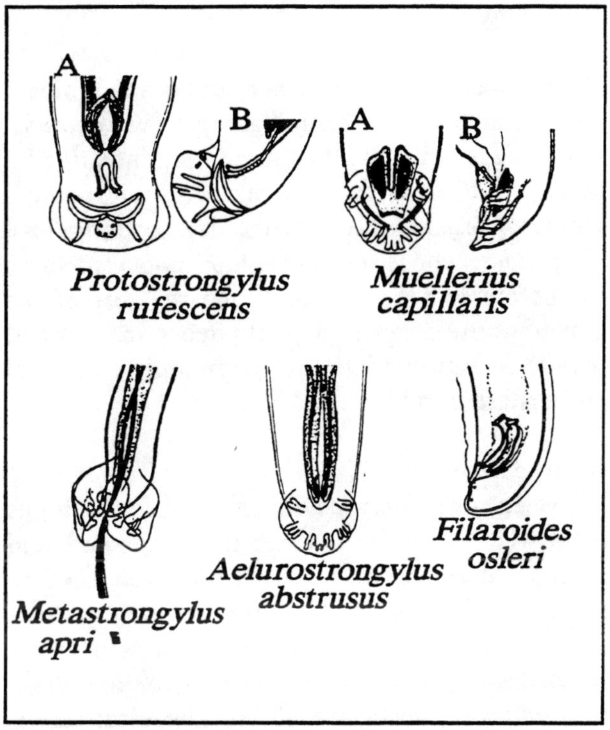


**Figure 18.3.** Bursae of some Metastrongyles, ventral (A) and left (B) views.

the long spicules on the males: 3.9-5.5 mm for *M. apri*, 2.1-2.4 mm for *M. salmi*, and 1.3-1.9 mm for *M. pudendotectus*. The spicules of the first two species have a hook at the distal end but the spicules of *M. pudendotectus* bear a double hook. The females are about 20-50 mm long by 0.3-0.4 mm wide. The vulva opens near the anus and is covered by a swelling of the cuticle ("prevulvar swelling"). The eggs are about 45-60 by 38-42 µm and embryonated when laid. They rarely hatch before being voided.

☛ *Filaroides* (syn. *Oslerus*) *osleri* is a parasite of the trachea or bronchi, and *F. milksi* and *F. hirthi* of the lung parenchyma, of dogs. The males are 4-7, 3-4, and 2-3 mm long, respectively, and about 0.1 mm wide. Their bursas are so small that only short papilla-like rays are visible (Figue 18.3). The spicules are 99-113, 31-60, and 45-48 µm long in the respective species. The females are about 7-15 mm long by 0.1-0.2 mm wide, with the vulva opening near the anus. The eggs of *F. osleri* are 80 by 50 µm and contain a larvae when laid. *F. milksi* and *F. hirthi* are ovoviviparous..The larvae found in the feces are about 320-400 µm long. The tail of the larvae of *F. osleri* is undulated but that of *F. hirthi* is straight.

☛ *Aelurostrongylus abstrusus* is a wide-spead parasite of the lung parenchyma and lung vessels of cats. The males are 4-6 mm long by 0.5 mm wide, with a small but distinct bursa (Figure 18.3). The females are 9-10 mm long by 0.8 mm wide. The eggs are 60-85 by 55-80 µm and are laid unsegmented but they hatch before leaving the lungs. The larva in the feces of the host is about 360 µm long and has an undulating tail with a dorsal spine.

☛ *Parelaphostrongylus* (syn. *Odocoileostrongylus*, *Pneumostrongylus*, *Elaphostrongylus*) *tenuis* is a parasite of the venous sinuses of the cranium and subdural spaces of deer in the United States and Canada. The larvae may infect and cause neurological disease in moose, sheep, goats, and other ruminants that eat the slug or snail intermediate host.

## 3. Biology

The Metastrongyles are heterogeneous in biology. They constitute three natural groups: *Dictyocaulus*, whose eggs develop into a free-living infective L3 outside the host (for this reason, some authors include *Dictyocaulus* with the Trichostrongyles), *Filaroides*, whose eggs develop into an infective L1 before leaving the host, and the rest of the bunch, whose eggs develop into free living L1s that invade an intermediate host (commonly a molusc) and mature into infective L3s in it.

### *Dictyocaulus*

The eggs of *Dictyocaulus* are laid in the lungs from where they are coughed up, swallowed, and reach the digestive tract. Usually they hatch before leaving the intestine and L1s (rather than eggs) are found in the host's feces. The L1s passed in the feces develop in the fecal pad into L2s and these into infective, ensheated L3s. Under ideal conditions the infective stage appears in 4-7 days. None of the larval stages is very migratory and most of the infective larvae are found still in the feces. Rains, growing grass, wind, the activity of coprophagous insects, and even the burst of the sporangia of *Pilobolus* fungi (which grow in the bovine fecal pads) help the spreading of the infective larvae. The longevity of the infective larvae is not very long so they must be ingested by a new host with the herbage within a few weeks or months.

The gastric pepsin and HCl stimulate the exsheathment of the larvae that proceed to the small intestine and penetrate the intestinal wall. They first reach the mesenteric lymph nodes in 24 hours, and continue by the lymph and blood toward the lungs where they start appearing by the 3rd day. In the lungs they break the capillaries, fall into the alveoli, and molt to juveniles. Molting to L4 occurs in the mesenteric lymph nodes in *D. viviparus* but in the alveoli in *D. filaria*. Adults appear by the 22nd (*D. viviparus*) to 28th (*D. filaria*) day of infection and the first larvae in the feces are observed at 3-4 (*D. viviparus*) or 5-8 (*D. filaria*) weeks of infection. The longevity of the adults is also limited:, the larvae disappear from the feces after 30-72 days of patency.

### *Filaroides*

The L1s voided in the host's feces are already infective. New dogs get infected by eating fresh feces or vomit of infected dogs, and, enventually, infected lung tissue. Autoinfection may occur. Puppies may be infected from their mother's saliva when she licks them. Ingested L1s go by the blood or lymph to the lungs where they are present already within the first day of infection. The first larvae in the host's feces are observed during the fifth (*F. hirthi*) or after the tenth (*F. osleri*) week of infection.

### Other genera

All other genera of metastrongyles have an indirect life cycle. Except *Metastrongylus* spp., all requiere any of a variety of moluscs (slugs or snails) as an intermediate host. The L1s usually invade the foot of the molusc but they can also be eaten by it. They develop into an infective, ensheated larvae in 30, 45, or more days. The definitive hosts get infected when they eat the mollusc. In the case of *Aelurostrongylus*, a number of transport hosts (frogs, lizards, birds, rodents) may facilitate the infection of cats. The prepatent period in most species is 30 to 40 days.

*Metastrongylus* spp. pass embryonated eggs (rather than larvae) in the host's feces. The L1s, hatched or still in the eggshell, are ingested by any of a variety of earthworms. The larvae accumulate in its heart and reach the ensheated, infective stage in 10 to 30 days. When the earthworm is eaten by a pig, the L3s reach the lungs by the blood and lymph system and develop into fertile adults in 24 or more days.

## 4. Medical importance

In **cattle**, dictyocaulosis is an disease mostly of calves and only when many worms are present. Experimentally, infection with 70,000 larvae caused acute, fatal disease but 5,000 larvae produced mild disease.

Migration to the lungs does not cause clinical manifestations. The presence of predult parasites in the alveoli and bronchioles during the second and third week of infection, however, triggers an intense inflammation with neutrophils, eosinophils, macrophages, and giant cells. The infiltrates block the fine air passages and cause collapse of the distal alveoli. Epithelialization of the open alveoli occurs and emphisema, edema, and formation of hyaline membranes appear rapidly. These changes produce respiratory stress with coughing, tachypnea, and hyperpnea. Death may occur already during the third week in heavily infected animals.

The presence of adult parasites after the third week provokes a copious exudate. The exudate, eggs, and L1s that are aspirated cause an hyperplasia of the alveolar epithelium and an eosinophil and neutrophil inflitrate of the lamina propria. Macrophages and giant cells are seen around the eggs and larvae. Consolidation of lung lobules and intertitial emphysema may occur. The clinical manifestations at this time are a respiratory rate that may be faster than the cardiac rate. frequent cough, loss of appetite, and failure to gain weight. The animals that survive start recovering by the beginning of the third month. A few animals may develop bronchiestiasis or pulmonary fibrosis and continue with a chronic cough.[1]

A first infection usually leaves strong protection against reinfections. Animals that undergo a heavy reinfection, however, may develop a brief, nonlethal disease with severe coughing and tachypnea. In these cases the larvae cause a strong immune reaction that results in the formation of pea-size nodules on the surfice of the lung. The nodules contains remnants of the parasites surrounded by macrophages, giant cells, eosinophils, plasma cells, and lymphocytes.

An irradiated vaccine against *D. viviparus* was designed in England in the early 1960's (Dictol, Glaxovet, Greenford, Midlesex, England) and it is still being used in Europe.[2] (Urquart et al., 1981)..

In **sheep**, dictyocaulosis may affect lambs but it is mostly a chronic infection of the adults. The tissue changes are similar to those observed in cattle dictyocaulosis but the tachypnea and coughing are considerably milder than in cattle.

The other lungworms of sheep cause even less clinical manifestations and are regarded as minor problems that rarely cause overt disease. Clinical manifestations are occasionally seen in older animals. *Muellerius* larvae are rapidly enclosed by eosinophils in the lungs and form nodules that grow with the parasite. The nodules reach up to a couple of millimeters and feel like lead shot under the lung surface. *Protostrongylus* causes obtruction of bronchioles with formation of conic areas of infarction in the lung. The smaller bronchioles in these areas are filled with adult parasites, eggs, macrophages, eosinophils, and lymphocytes.

In **swine**, metastrongyle infections may cause bronchitis with considerable coughing and failure to gain weight. They are less severe than dictyocaulosis of ruminants, however.

In **horses**, dictyocaulosis is not very severe and afects mostly the upper respiratory tract. Donkeys are very resistant to the disease.

In **carnivores**, F. *osleri* causes the formation of mucosal nodules near the tracheobronchial junction, particularly in young dogs, which may result in persistant cough and, infrequently, loss of condition. *F. milksi* infection does not produce overt clinical manifestations normally but very heavy infections, particularly in dogs with immune suppressive treatments, may produce extensive and fatal lung granulomas. *A. abstrusus* of cats is commonly an asymptomatic infection but some cats, probably with heavy inections, develop coughing and annorexia, and even respiratory distress.

**TABLE 18.I. SOME CHARACTERISTICS OF COMMON METASTRONGYLOIDEA SPECIES**

| Species | Host | Location | Male size (mm) | Spicules length (µm) | Female size (mm) | Larvae (µm) |
|---|---|---|---|---|---|---|
| *Dictyocaulus viviparus* | Cattle | Trachea to bronchioles | 17-50 x 0.5 | 195 x 215 | 23-28, pointed tail | 310-360, pointed tail |
| *D. filaria* | Sheep, goats | Bronchioles | 25-80 x 0.4-0.6 | 400-550 | 43-112, conic tail | 500 x 585, conic tail, cephalic button |
| *D. arnfieldi* | Horses | Bronchi and bronchioles | 25-43 x 0.1-0.3 | 199-250 | 43-68, blunt tail | 420-480, pointed tail |
| *Muellerius capillaris* | Sheep, goats | Parenchyma | 11-14 x 0.2 | 140-160 | 19-23 | 300-320, undulated tail with spine |
| *Protostrong. rufescens* | Sheep, goats | Bronchioles | 16-46 x 0.1-0.2 | 230-340 | 25-65 | 250-320, undulated tail |
| *Metastrong.* species | Pigs | Brobchi and bronchioles | 10-25 x 0.2-0.3 | *390-550<br>*210-240<br>*130-190 | 20-50 | 45-60x38-42 larvated eggs |
| *Filaroides* species | Dogs | *Trachea & bronchi<br>*Parenchyma | *4-7x0.1<br>*3-4x0.1 | *990-1130<br>*310-600<br>*450-480 | 7-15 | *80-50 larvated eggs<br>*320-400 undulated tail<br>*320-400? straight tail |
| *Aelurostrong. abstrusus* | Cats | Parenchyma | 4-6 x0.5 | 75-130 | 9-10 | 360, undulated tail with spine |

(*) Different species, see text.

**Summary:**

1. The Metastrongyloidea are bursate nematodes generally with a reduced bursa that live in the respiratory system..

2. The most important genera are *Dictyocaulus, Muellerius, Protostrongylus*, *Metastrongylus, Filaroides*, and *Aelurostrongylus*..

3. In most species the eggs hatch into an L1 before leaving the host.

4. With the exception of *Dictyocaulus* which have a direct life cycle, all other species need an intermediate host, usually a mollusc, to develop into an infective L3.

5. The infective larvae (free living for *Dictyocaulus* or in an intermediate host for the other species) are ingested by the final host with its food or water.

6. The preadults migrate to the mesenteric lymph nodes and then by the lymph and blood to the lungs.

7. The adults live in the respiratory passages (*Dictyocaulus, Protostrongylus, Metastrongylus, Filaroides osleri*) or in the lung parenchyma (*Muellerius, Filaroides milksi, F. hirthi, Aelurostrongylus*).

8. The most pathogenic species belong to the genus *Dictyocaulus* that cause bronchitis and bronchopneumonia.

## REFERENCES

1. Urquart, G. M., Jarret, W. F. H., and McIntyre, W. I M. 1973. Bovine dictyocauliasis: Pathology, clinical signs, epidemiology, trreatment and control. In Urquart, G. M. and Armour, J. (eds), *Helminth Diseases of Cattle, Sheep, and Horses in Europe,* Maclehose, Glasgow, 23-30.

2.Urquart, G. M., Jarret, W. F. H., Bairden, K. and Bonazzi, E. F. 1981. Control of parasitic bronchitis in cattle: vaccination or treatment. Vet. Rec. 108:180-182.

## Chapter 19

# THE ORDER ASCARIDIDA OR ASCARIDES

**Preview.** The ascarides are large nematodes of the small intestine, particularly prevalent in piglets, colts, pups, kittens, and poultry. The larvae develop in the intestinal mucosa in some species, migrate through liver and lungs to the intestine in others, or remain in the tissues for long periods in still others.

All can be transmitted by ingestion of embryonated eggs, but milk or transplacental transmission is more efficient for some species. Infection by consumption of infected paratenic hosts is common among carnivores.

They cause digestive and, occasionally, respiratory disturbances. Losses in production occur even in asymptomatic cases. Toxocara canis of dogs is a Public Health concern.

### 1. Morphology

The **Ascaroidea** (from *Ascaris*, the oldest genus) are medium to large nematodes of the small intestine. Most species are 8 to 25 cm (3 to 10 inches) long and 0.2 to 0.8 cm wide.

The most characteristic feature of the morphology of the ascarides is the scarcity of noticeable external structures such as prominent buccal capsules or copulatory bursas. Their body is smooth and pointed at both ends. Some species have delicate cephalic alae. The mouth is a simple orifice surrounded by three small lips (Figure 19.1) that leads to a club-shaped esophagus. The presence of the three lips and the shape of the esophagus are characteristic of the group. The caudal end, coiled in the males and straight in the females, ends in a cone and the anus opens near its tip. The males have two equal spicules and a number of small papillae in front and behind the cloaca. The females produce thick-shelled eggs that are discharge through a vulva located in the anterior half of the body.

The transverse section of the larvae reveals few but large muscle cells that fill the body cavity, and lateral expansions of the cuticle that look like spines in the section.

### 2. Identification and Classification

The ascarides are easy to identify by their large size, the lack of prominent external features, and their location in the small intestine. Examination of the typical lips will confirm the diagnosis. Preliminary identification of the larvae in sections of host's tissues can be attempted by the characteristics explained under Morphology but the definitive diagnosis is best left to the specialist.[1]

The Ascaroidea contains five genera of great veterinary importance (*Ascaris, Parascaris, Toxocara, Toxascaris,* and *Ascaridia*) and a few genera of minor importance that belong to the subfamily Anisakinae. The measurements of the adults and eggs of the major species are presented in Table 19.I.

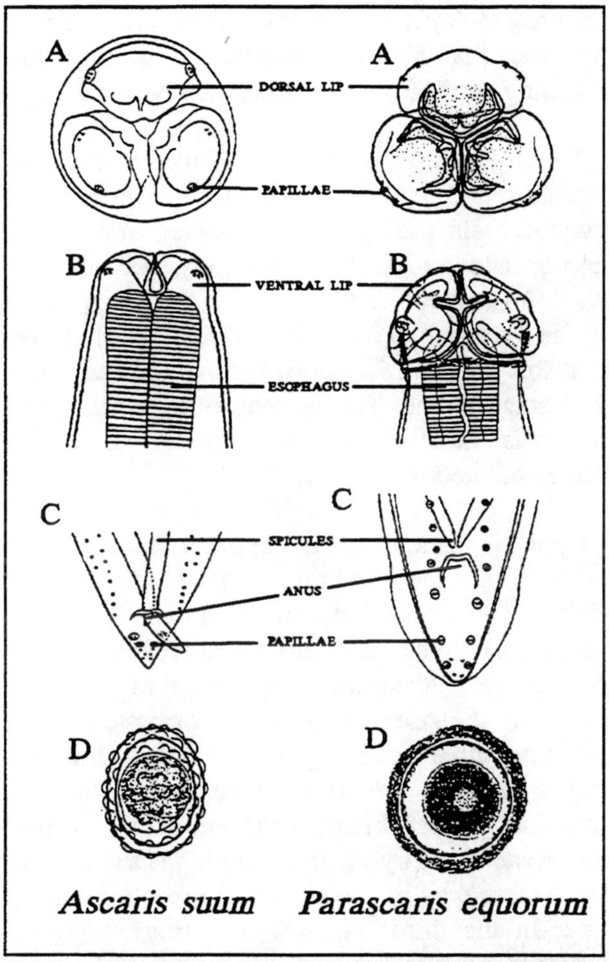


**Figure 19.1.** Face view of the lips (A), ventral view of the anterior (B) and posterior (C) ends of the male, and eggs (D) of representative Ascaridida.

☛ *Ascaris suum* is the pig ascarid (Figure 19.1). They are large worms the females of which lay oval eggs covered by a mamillated outer layer.

☛ *Ascaris lumbricoides* is the human ascarid. The only known morphologic difference with the pig ascarid is in the shape of the denticles of the lips.[2]

☛ *Parascaris equorum* (syn. *A. megalocephala*) is the ascarid of the equines. They are very large worms. The females lay eggs that are dark, subspherical, and with a finely pitted outer layer.

☛ *Toxocara vitulorum* (syn. *Neoascaris vitulorum*) is the ascarid of cattle and, rarely, sheep. They are also very large worms. The eggs are subspherical, and with a finely pitted outer layer.

☛ *Toxocara canis* is one of the two common ascarides of canids. Its larval stages can infect many other vertebrates including ruminants, rodents, lagomorpha, and humans, but without reaching the adult stage in them. They are rather large worms with eggs that are dark, subspherical, and with a finely pitted outer shell (Figure 19.2).

In the dog, *T. canis* can be distinguished from *Toxascaris leonina* by several criteria (Table 19.II). The transverse striations of the cuticle near the cephalic end are more widely separated in *T. canis* than in *T. leonina*, and the cephalic end is commonly bent ventrally in *T. canis* (which gives the worm the shape of a letter C) whereas it is bent dorsally in *T. leonina* (which gives the parasite the shape of a letter S). This latter criterium is not totally reliable, however. The tail of the males of *Toxocara* spp. ends in a digitiform appendix that is lacking in the males of *T. leonina* (Figure 19.2). Their eggs are also different (Figure 19.2).

☛ *Toxocara cati* (syn. *T. mystax*) is one of the two common ascarides of felines. Their size and eggs are very similar to those of *T. canis*. If necessary, both species can be separated by the criteria shown in Table 19.II. The eggs of *T. cati* are somewhat smaller than those of *T. canis* but they are indistinguishable in the practice.

☛ *Toxascaris leonina* is one of the common ascarides of felines and canines. The worms are very similar to *T. canis* and *T. cati* but their eggs are light yellow, ovoid, and covered by a smooth outer layer (Figure 19.2). *T. leonina* can be distinguished from *T. canis* and *T. cati* by the criteria shown in Table 19.II.

☛ *Ascaridia* are the ascarides of birds. *A. galli* is the most common ascarid of chickens but also infects other gallinaceous birds. *A. dissimilis* is the most common ascarid of turkeys. These species are somewhat smaller than the ascarides of carnivores and their eggs are light yellow, ovoid, and have a smooth outer layer.

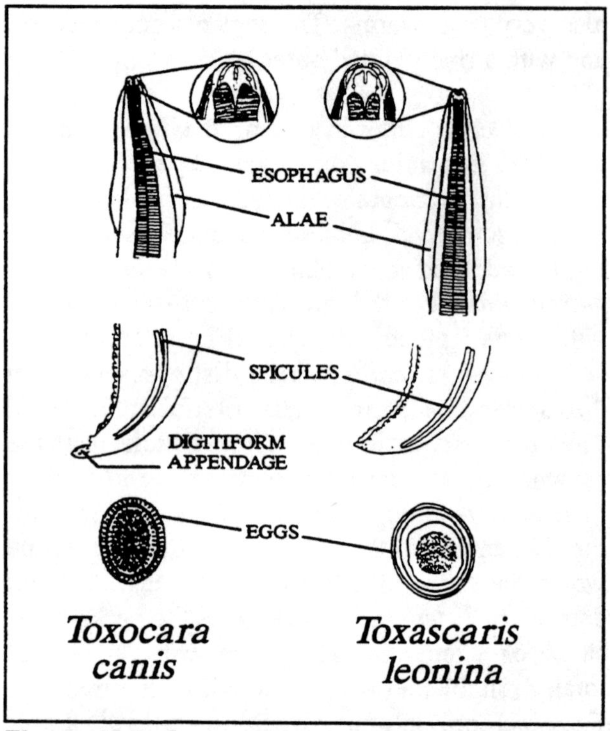


**Figure 19.2.** Comparative features of *T. canis* and *T. leonina*.

The subfamily Anisakinae contains several genera (*Anisakis, Contracaecum, Phocanema*) that are parasites of marine mammals when adults, and of fish when larvae. The larvae are occasionally found as gastric or intestinal parasites of humans, pigs, or domestic carnivores that eat uncooked infected fish.[3]

Because the ascarides very rarely develop to the adult stage in abnormal hosts, the host from whom the adult parasites were collected constitutes an important criterium for the identification of the species.

### 3. Biology

Although rather homogenous in morphology, the ascarides are heterogeneous in biology. Some authorities have speculated that they originated from worms with intermediate hosts and are evolving toward a direct life cycle. Others are of the contrary opinion. Whatever the situation may be, the present-day ascarides of domestic animals need a period of larval development in the tissues before reaching adulthood in the intestinal lumen.

The eggs are deposited by the female in the host's intestine and leave with the feces. The fertilized eggs contain a zygote when passed and require appropriate temperature, humidity, oxygen, and shade to develop to the infective 3rd stage larvae inside the eggshell. For a long time it was believed that the infective larvae of the Ascaroidea was a 2nd stage larvae. The current evidence indicates that it is actually a 3rd stage larvae like in most other nematodes.[4]

Upon ingestion by an appropriate host, the physico-chemical conditions of the host's digestive tract stimulate the larva to hatch. The new larva needs a stay in the host's tissues to proceed with its development. According to the extent of this tissue invasion, the Ascaroidea of the domestic animals fall into three natural groups. In one (**mucosal migration**) the infective larvae invade only the intestinal mucosa. In another (**tracheal migration**) the larvae travel by the liver and lungs to the pharynx where they are swallowed to reach the intestine. In the third one (**somatic migration**) the larvae migrate to the systemic tissues and remain dormant there until passing to the new generation congenitally.

*Toxascaris* and *Ascaridia* belong to the mucosal migration group. Upon hatching, their larvae penetrate the mucosa of the small intestine for about two weeks and then return to the lumen to complete their development to adults. The first egg-laying females appear after the tenth week of infection in *Toxascaris* and after the fifth in *Ascaridia*. When the infection with *Toxascaris* occurs by ingestion of paratenic hosts rather than eggs (see below), the larvae already underwent some development in this host and patency occurs in only eight weeks.

*Ascaris* and *Parascaris* belong to the tracheal migration group. The hatched larvae penetrate the blood vessels of the small intestine and go by the portal system to the liver where they reach their

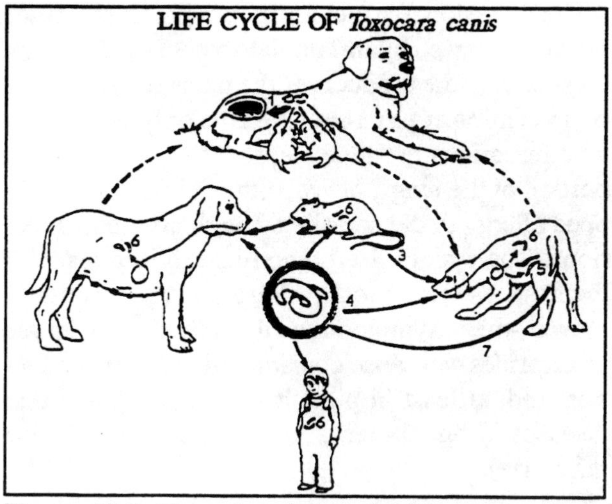


**Figure 19.3**. *T. canis* is transmitted in uterus (1), in the milk (2), by paratenic hosts (3), and by larvated eggs (4). Only young dogs develop adult parasites (5). Young dogs and other hosts accumulate tissue larvae (6).

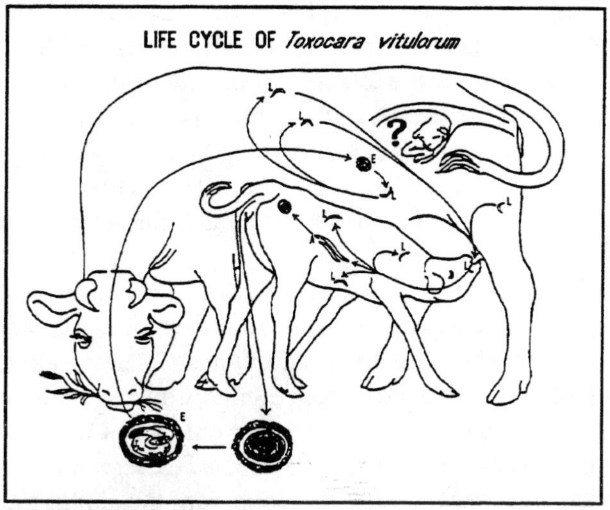


**Figure 19.4.** *T. vitulorum* acquired by larvate eggs accumulate tissue larvae in the adult hosts that pass to the calves with the milk. In uterus tranmission is suspected but unproven.

peak concentration about the fourth day of infection. From there they continue by the circulation to the heart and lungs where they accumulate about the ninth day. The parasites break the vessels and alveoli, crawl up the air passages and reach the pharynx from where they are swallowed to start reaching the intestine about the fourteenth day of infection. The first egg-laying adults appear at 40 days of infection in *Ascaris* and at 80 in *Parascaris*.

*Toxocara* belongs to the somatic migration group. The larvae initiate their journey as in the tracheal migration but some are retained in the liver, others in the lungs, and others bypass the lungs and become distributed in the muscles and different organs (e.g., kidney). These larvae grow somewhat but do not develop any further and remain dormant for months or years. When the host reproduces and starts lactation, part of the dormant parasites resumes their migration and passes to the new generation through the placenta or with the colostrum and milk. Resumption of migration appears to be related to a relaxation of host's immunity caused by advanced pregnancy and lactation.[5] In the new host the larvae develop to adults in the intestine without further tissue migration. Patency may begin about day 15 in *T. vitulorum*, 23 in *T. canis*, and 31 in *T. cati*. New waves of dormant parasites become reactivated in succeeding lactations.

In addition to the colonization of somatic tissues, ingestion of embryonated eggs of *Toxocara* spp. may also result in patent infections in some cases. Administration of infective eggs of *T. vitulorum* will result in patent infection (by day 30) in new born calves but not in animals older than 1-2 days. Infective eggs of *T. canis* can produce patent infections (by day 28) in dogs up to 1-3 months old but infrequently in older animals. *T. canis* favors tracheal migration in very young animals but switches rapidly toward somatic migration as the host grows older. Infective eggs of *T. cati* appear to cause patent infection (by day 55) as well as colonization the tissues in cats of any age.

Different from *T. vitulorum* and *T. cati*, the dormant larvae of *T. canis* become reactivated as early as day 40 of pregnancy and go through the placenta to infect the offspring in uterus (Figure 19.3). Speculations that the same occurs with *T. vitulorum* have not been supported experimentally (Figure 19.4). The pups are usually born with larvae in their lungs and become patent after the 23th day of life. Although lactogenic infection also occurs with *T. canis*, transuterine transmission is more important. Some of the reactivated larvae may also reach the intestine of the bitch and develop to adults. Patency in the bitch may begin 14 days after whelping and persist for a few weeks to a couple of months.

With the exception of *Ascaridia*, all the ascarides mentioned above are able to infect mammalian species other than their natural hosts. They do not develop beyond the infective stage, however, and in most cases they remain alive for only a few days in the tissues of the incidental host. The larvae of *T. canis, T. cati* and *T. leonina*, on the contrary, remain alive for months in rodents or other mammals and constitute an effective source of infection for the definitive host. This is probably an adaptation of the parasite to the carnivorous habit of its host because it protects the parasite from the vicissitudes of the external environment and facilitates its contact with the definitive host. The larvae of *T. canis* is of particular importance because this species is the major agent of visceral larva migrans in humans (see below).

**4. Medical importance**

The ascarides are very common parasites, particularly prevalent in young hosts. The prevalence and magnitude of the infections diminish markedly toward puberty and the parasites are rather rare in adult animals.

Ascarides can cause systemic tissue pathology at the larval stages, or intestinal pathology at the adult stage.

The passage of the larvae through the liver produces small foci of trauma and inflammation that rarely have clinical manifestations. These foci heal with formation of fibrous tissue, particularly after repeated infections that produced immune reactions against the parasite. The fibrotic lesions are especially frequent in the pig's liver where they are called **milky spots** and often require condemnation of the organ at the slaughter house.

The invasion of the lungs produces traumatic lesions followed by inflammatory foci, and allergic responses to the products of the parasite. Symptoms of a **verminous pneumonia** ensue only when massive infections produce damage to a significantly portion of the lungs, or when the animal has developed allergy to the parasite through previous infections. The lesions are predominantly traumatic in the first case, and mostly allergic in the second.

Even when asymptomatic, the infection by larvae of ascarides can cause considerable loss of production and, at least in pigs, it may exacerbate other diseases (hog cholera, viral pneumonia, swine influenza).

Larvae are occasionally found in other organs (skeletal muscle, kidney, brain, eye) but they rarely have a clinical expression in domestic animals. In humans, the larvae of *T. canis* (and, possibly, of *T. cati*) that invade the internal organs cause **visceral larva migrans**. This infection is more frequent in children (because they are more often in contact with contaminated soil) and produces low fever, malacia, hepatomegaly, eosinophilia, hyperglobulinemia, and other symptoms that commonly last for 6-24 months. The location in the eye (**ocular larva migrans**) affects visual acuity and may require enucleation of the organ. Studies in healthy people suggest that 4-7% of the apparently healthy population has been infected with the parasite sometime in their lives.[6]

Although there is no evidence that the adult ascarides feed on the host's mucosa, heavy infections commonly cause a **catarrhal enteritis** with all the attendant symptoms. Some authors believe that the intestinal pathology is a manifestation of an allergic response to the parasite or its products. Upon necropsy, the mucosa looks edematous, congestive, and often inflamed and with small ulcers.

Large numbers of parasites may cause **intestinal obstruction**. On occasions, they migrate inside the common duct and occlude the passage of bile. In a few cases, they can perforate the intestinal wall and produce peritonitis. Even in cases with little or no symptoms, the intestinal parasites may reduce the weight gain of food animals.

In studies with pigs, four parasitized animals gained 48 lb of body weight in the same period that four unparasitized controls gained 100. Levine[7] calculated that infected pigs need 150-200 lb more grain than unparasitized pigs to reach market weight. The extra feed and the condemnations at the slaughter house were estimated in $ 385 million per year in the United States in the late 1970's.

Normal hosts do not react very effectively against the larvae of the ascarides that undergo somatic migration. The larvae of *T. canis* survive for at least a year in bitches[8] and the same must occurs with *T. vitulorum* and *T. cati*. Lack of immune resistance is attributed to the facts that dormant larvae produce little antigen, and they cause depression and deviation of host's protective immunity.

Most of the intestinal worms are eliminated by the host by 4-6 months of age. Because previously infected animals are more resistance to reinfection than parasite-naive animals, the elimination is generally attributed to an immunologic response. It is widely believed that older animals are more resistent to the infection than younger ones, but there is no solid evidence that it is so.

## 5. Diagnosis

Ascaridiasis is suspected by the symptoms, the age of the host, and the known presence of the infection in the area. In addition to the symptoms from the affected organ (hepatitis, pneumonia, or enteritis), heavily infected animals look unthrifty, have a dull coat, eat poorly, may present a potbelly, and the carnivores may vomit.

The larval infection with *T. canis* is diagnosed by serology in humans[9] but no practical methods for the diagnosis of other species in domestic animals have been developed. An elevated peripheral eosinophilia may add to the clinical suspicion though.

The intestinal infection is diagnosed by the finding of the typical eggs in the feces. Because the ascarides are very prolific (*T.canis* may lay 20,000 eggs/female/day and *A. suum* one million), a simple smear often shows the presence of eggs. Enrichment methods are rarely necessary for the diagnosis of ascarid infections heavy enough as to be of veterinary importance. The eggs appear in the feces, however, only after a month or more of infection (see above), when symptoms may have already ensued in heavy or repeated infections. On occasions, juvenile or adult parasites are passed with the feces or, in the carnivores, with the vomit. In cases of recent, prepatent infections, or of infections with males only (females are eliminated earlier in the infection), carnivores with a negative fecal exam may pass one or a few worms in the vomit.

## 6. Treatment

There is no satisfactory treatment for the infection with larvae of ascarides which is unfortunate because the tissue infection causes more losses than the intestinal infection. Levamisole or ivermectin appear to be the most effective drugs against tissue ascarides but their administration to mice for 13 days at doses twice as high as the therapeutic recommendations kills only 64% and 43% of the *T. canis* larvae, respectively.[10] Prolonged treatment of pregnant bitches with fenbendazole may prevent lactogenic infection of the pups (see below).

A number of drugs is effective against the intestinal parasites. Possibly the mildest and cheapest is piperazine but the benzimidazoles (with the exception of thiabendazole), the imidazothiazoles (with the exception of butamisole), the organophosphorus compounds, pyrantel, morantel, ivermectin, dithiazanine iodide, diethylcarbamazine, n-butyl chloride, and toluene are also effective and most have a broader spectrum of activity. Sodium fluoride and cadmium compounds are still used occasionally for pigs but they may cause intoxication. The antibiotic, hygromycin B, is effective when given in the feed for 3 or more weeks.

Phenothiazine, thenium closylate, disophenol, phthalofyne, and glycobiarsol, although effective against other nematodes, have little activity against ascarides (see Therapeutic notes).

In animals living in a heavily contaminated environment, the treatment should be repeated periodically, either by permanent administration with the feed (as for pigs and poultry) or repeated dosage (as for dogs or horses). This schedule eliminates the intestinal parasites with one dosage, and kills those that were in migration at the time with the next dosage.

**7. Epidemiology**

The ascarides are very common parasites. With the exception of *T. vitulorum*, they are universal in distribution and affect a very large proportion of the young hosts unless special precautions to prevent infection are taken. As the host approaches puberty, the frequency and magnitude of the infections diminish. The infection is infrequent in adult animals that experienced infections when young.

*T. vitulorum* is very prevalent in the northern part of Africa and in the southern part of Asia. It is less prevalent elsewhere and uncommon in the United States. The human infection by *A. lumbricoides* is also common in countries where contamination of the ground or waters with human feces is prevalent.

As a rule, infections with ascarides are acquired by ingestion of eggs passed with the feces of infected hosts that contaminate pastures, feed, or water. *Toxocara* spp., however, are transmitted mainly with the mother's milk, and *T. canis* is mostly transmitted transplacentally. The ascarides of the carnivores are also acquired by ingestion of paratenic hosts.

The eggs are quite resistant to environmental factors including chemicals (2% formalin, copper sulfate, sodium hypochlorite, lye). The shortest longevity corresponds to the eggs of *Ascaridia* that survive in the external environment for up to 10 months. Eggs of *Ascaris suum* survive outside for up to 5-6 years. The eggs of the other species are believed to have an intermediate longevity, possibly closer to that of *Ascaris*. In order to develop an infective larva, the eggs need temperature, humidity, oxygen and shade. They survive best in loose soil with a thick vegetable cover that retains humidity and protects them from direct sun light. At the ideal temperature of about 30C (86F), the infective larva develops in about a week. At 19C (66F), it takes about three weeks. The eggs die rapidly above 35C (95F) or below -20C (-4F). They do not develop below 12 to 15C (54 to 59F) but moderately low temperatures favor their survival. Under common environmental conditions, probably few eggs become infective in less than two to four weeks. The ideal humidity for development is above 85%. Direct sunlight kills the eggs rapidly due to heat, desiccation, and ultraviolet rays.

Domestic carnivores can be infected with *T. canis, T. cati,* or *T. leonina* by ingestion of rodents infected with the larval stages of the corresponding parasites. The existence of these paratenic hosts presumably protects the larvae against the vicissitudes of the external environment and favors the survival of the parasite species. The larvae remain alive in the rodents only for a few months, however.

The most important mechanism of transmission of *T. vitulorum* and *T. cati* is with the milk (Figure 19.4). The most important for *T. canis* is transplacentally (Figure 19.3). A number of surveys has demonstrated that virtually all pups are born infected with *T. canis*: examination of more than 600 newly born pups in five studies showed that 99.4% were infected.

**8. Control**

The control of most ascarides consists in avoiding that the susceptible hosts ingest viable eggs with their food or water. In order to achieve this, one must:

a) Prevent the passage of eggs from infected

animals and the consequent contamination of the environment,

b) Remove the eggs from the environment before they embryonate, and/or

c) Make the environment unsuitable for egg embryonation.

Because *Toxocara* spp. are transmitted with the mother's milk, *T. canis* in uterus, and all the ascarides of carnivores by ingestion of transport hosts, these parasites pose particular problems of control.

Passage of eggs in the feces can be prevented by the permanent administration of an effective anthelmintic in the food or water (as in the case of pigs and poultry), or by the repeated administration of individual treatments (as in the case of dogs and horses). In areas of high prevalence, it is convenient to assume that infection takes place shortly after birth (before birth in the case of *T. canis*). Because the available drugs are ineffective against the tissue larvae, prevention of environmental contamination requires that the first treatment be administered when the parasites are already in the intestine but before the first eggs appear in the feces. Subsequent treatments should be repeated before the new larvae that arrived in the intestine had the opportunity to develop into egg-laying parasites.

With **pigs**, permanent or periodic administration of anthelmintics in the feed will keep the infection at a low level if contamination is not very severe. In heavily infected herds, the McLean County System of Swine Sanitation may provide a new start. A few days before farrowing, the pregnant sow is treated against *Ascaris*, scrubbed to eliminate eggs that may be adhered to her body, and moved to a clean farrowing pen. During the second week after farrowing, the sow and her litter are moved to an *Ascaris*-free pasture, and the sow is removed after weaning. At about 4 month of age, when the piglets are believed to be comparatively resistant to the infection, they can be moved into the herd.

With **cattle**, treatment of the calves must be initiated at 2 weeks of age, since prepatent periods as short as 15 days are reported. Another treatment after 2-3 weeks would kill the parasites that might have been migrating at the time of the first treatment. Further treatments may not be necessary because calves older than 1-2 days do not develop patent infections on ingestion of infective eggs. Infection of the calves can be prevented by withholding or boiling the colostrum and milk of infected cows. Unfortunately, there is not a practical method yet to identify infected cows.

With **horses**, satisfactory control is achieved with a first treatment at 8 weeks of age, and repeated treatments every 6-8 weeks for the first year of life. If the infection is not very prevalent, regular and thorough cleansing of the premises may suffice.

With **dogs**, the major concern is to avoid contamination of the environment with eggs of *T. canis* because of the danger of visceral larva migrans in humans. The first treatment should be given to the pups and the bitch when the pups are 2 weeks old. At this time, some larvae have already reached the intestine of the pups and the new worms that may have developed in the bitch are about to start to lay eggs. Since it takes a little over 2 weeks for the larvae arrived in the intestine to develop into egg-laying adults, further treatment should be repeated every 2 weeks to kill the migrating larvae that escaped the prior treatment before they become adults. By two months of age, most pups will not develop patent infections so the treatments may be suspended after this age. This results in four treatments, at 2, 4, 6, and 8 weeks of age. Because of this insusceptibility of the grown dogs to patent infections and the fact that many dogs spontaneously eliminate their intestinal parasites at 6-8 months of age, treatment of adult dogs is regarded as unnecessary. Most studies, however, have found 10-40% patent *T. canis* infection in general dog populations.[6] This figure certainly recommends regular deworming of dogs, whatever their age is. Daily treatment of the bitch with 50 mg of fenbendazole/kg from day 40 of pregnancy to day 14 after whelping is reported to prevent infection of the pups.[11]

With **cats**, the first treatment of the kittens should be administered before day 31 of life (when patency of transmammary infections begins) and repeated every 10 days until 3 weeks after the end of nursing. Because grown cats are still susceptible to patent infections from eggs or paratenic host, periodic treatments are indicated.

Because ascarid eggs need at least two weeks to embryonate under natural conditions, removal and burning of feces every two weeks should keep environmental contamination at a low level. The eggs are sticky, however, so scrubbing of the floors, walls, and animals, or at least washing with a strong jet of water, may be necessary. Flaming, steam, hot lye solution (1 kg/167 l or 1 lb/20 gall), 4% cresol for 5 minutes, 1% sodium pentachlorophenate (at 30-35 g per $m^2$), or dibromomethane fumigation (50 ml per $m^2$) are reported to kill the eggs.

Keeping the environment unsuitable for development of the larvae means to keep the premises free of feces and other materials that protect the eggs, a low humidity on the ground, and plenty of direct sunlight. The effect of direct sunlight and dryness on clean surfaces cannot be stressed enough: clean eggs of *A. suum* exposed to sunlight die in less than 5 hours when dry, and in less than 9 when in water. When possibly, concrete floors are recommended.

In the case of *T. canis, T. mystax,* and *T. leonina*, it is also necessary to prevent the host from ingesting infected rodents.

Prevention of human visceral larva migrans is rightfully a veterinary concern. The current recommendations are:

a) To prevent the infection of dogs (see above),

b) To discourage dog defecation in public places (streets, parks, playgrounds),

c) To reduce the number of stray dogs, and,

d) To educate the public about visceral larva migrans.[12]

Unfortunately, nowhere have these goals been achieved and there are some questions whether it is realistic to expect better compliance. As a result, the conventional control of human toxocariasis is little effective at present.

**TABLE 19.I. MEASUREMENTS AND PREPATENCY OF THE MAJOR SPECIES OF ASCARIDES**

| Species | Male (cm) | Female (cm) | Eggs (µm) | Prepatency(days) |
|---|---|---|---|---|
| *Ascaris suum* and *A. lumbricoides* | 15-25x0.3-0.4 | 20-40x0.5-0.6 | 50-80x40-60 | 40 |
| *Parascaris equorum* | 15-28x0.3-0.6 | 15-50x0.5-0.8 | 90-100 | 80 |
| *Toxocara vitulorum* | 15-26x0.3-0.5 | 22-30x0.5-0.6 | 68-102x60-86 | 15-30 |
| *Toxocara canis* | 4-10x0.2 | 5-18x0.2-0.3 | 85-90x75 | 23 or 30 |
| *Toxocara cati* | 3-7x0.15 | 4-12x0.2 | 65-75 | 31 or 56 |
| *Toxascaris leonina* | 2-7x0.15-0.2 | 2-10x0.2-0.25 | 75-85x60-75 | 56 or 70 |
| *Ascaridia galli* | 3-7x0.1 | 5-11x0.1-0.2 | 75-85x45-55 | 35 |

**TABLE 19.II. DIFFERENTIATION AMONG ASCARIDES OF DOMESTIC CARNIVORES**

| Species | Body shape | Cephalic alae end | Cuticular striations | Spicules length | Digitiform appendix | Eggs |
|---|---|---|---|---|---|---|
| *T. canis* | Bent in a C | Caudally smooth | 16-22 um apart | 0.75-1.3 mm | Present | Round, dark, pitted shell |
| *T. cati* | Bent in a C | Caudally abrupt | 12-16 um apart | 1.6-2.1 mm | Present | Round, dark, pitted shell |
| *T. leonina* | Bent in an S | Caudally smooth | 6-12 um apart | 0.7-15 mm | Absent | Oval, clear, smooth shell |

**Summary:**

1. Ascarides are common parasites of the small intestine of pigs (*Ascaris suum*), equines (*Parascaris equorum*), domestic carnivores (*Toxocara canis, T. cati,* and *Toxascaris leonina*), and poultry (*Ascaridia* spp.).

2. The larvae of *Toxascaris* and *Ascaridia* develop in the intestinal mucosa, those of *Ascaris* and *Parascaris* migrate through the liver and lungs to the intestine, and those of *Toxocara* remain in the tissues until the end of the host's next pregnancy and beyond.

3. They affect young hosts causing digestive disturbances and losses in production. In heavy or repeated infections they may also produce respiratory symptoms.

4. The diagnosis is made by observation of the typical eggs in the feces, or of worms in the feces or vomit.

5. There is no satisfactory treatment for the tissue larvae but many anthelmintics are effective against the intestinal forms.

6. Except for *Toxocara*, transmission depends on the ingestion of eggs from a fecally contaminated environment. *Toxocara* spp. are transmitted with the mothers' milk and *T. canis* is also transmitted transplacentally. All ascarides of carnivores can be transmitted by ingestion of infected paratenic hosts.

7. Control consists in treating the animals passing eggs to prevent the environmental contamination, eliminating the eggs in the environment, and making the environment unsuitable for egg embryonation.

8. *Toxocara canis* causes visceral larva migrans in humans.

## REFERENCES

1. Nichols RL. 1956. The etiology of visceral larva migrans. I and II. J. Parasit. 42:349-399.

2. Ansel M & Thibaut M. 1973. Value of the specific distinction between *Ascaris lumbricoides* Linne 1758 and *Ascaris suum* Goeze 1782. Internat. J. Parasit. 3:317-319.

3. Smith JW & Wootten R. 1978. Anisakis and anisakiasis. Adv. Parasit. 16:93-163.

4. Maung M. 1978. The occurrence of the second moult of *Ascaris lumbricoides* and *Ascaris suum*. Internat. J. Parasit. 8:371-378.

5. Lloyd S, Amerasinghe PH & Soulsby EJL. 1983. Periparturient immunosuppression in the bitch and its influence on infection with *Toxocara canis*. J. small Anim. Pract. 24:237-247.

6. Barriga O.O. 1988. A critical look at the importance, prevalence, control, and possibilities of immunological control of toxocariasis. Vet. Parasit. 29:195-234.

7.Levine ND. 1980. *Nematode parasites of domestic animals and of man.* 2nd ed., Burgess, Minneapolis, 269.

8. Douglas JR & Baker NR. 1959. The chronology of experimental intrauterine infection with Toxocara canis (Werner, 1782) in the dog. J. Parasit. (suppl.) 47:15.

9. Glickman L, Schantz P, Dombroske R & Cypess R. 1978. Evaluation of serodiagnostic tests for visceral larva migrans. Am. J. Trop. Med. Hyg. 27:492-498.

10. Carrillo M & Barriga OO. 1987. Effect of levamisole chlorhydrate or ivermectin on tissue toxocariasis of the mouse. Am. J. Vet. Res. 48:281-283.

11. Duwel vD & Strassar H. 1978. Versuche zur Geburt helminthen-freier Hundewelpen durch Fenbendazol-Behandlung. Dtsch. Tierarztl. Wschr. 85:239-241.

12. Schantz PM & Glickman LT. 1979. Canine and human toxocariasis: the public health problem and the veterinarian's role in prevention. J.A.V.M.A. 175:1270-1273.

# Chapter 20

# THE ORDER OXYURIDA OR PINWORMS

**Preview.** The oxyurids are parasites of the large intestine characterized by an esophagus with a well developed posterior bulb. They are acquired by ingestion of embryonated eggs. The oxyurids are little pathogenic but *O. equi* of horses produces anal pruritus which annoys the animals and causes tail rubbing.

## 1. Morphology

The **Oxyurida** (from *Oxyuris*, one of its genera, from Gr *oxus*= sharp, and Lat *uro*= tail, see below) are small, whitish nematodes of the large intestine. Their most characteristic feature is the presence of an esophagus with a well developed bulb, often preceded by a narrow isthmus and a well marked corpus (Figure 20.1). They may have 3, 6, or no lips. The males of most species have a truncated posterior end, small caudal alae, and a single spicule. The females commonly end in a long, pointed tail. Because the females of the human oxyurid occasionally passed with the feces have the size and shape of a white pin, the name **pinworms** is commonly applied to this group. The eggs are usually thin-shelled, flattened on one side, and may contain a tadpole stage when laid.

## 2. Identification and classification

The identity of the oxyurids is suspected by their size, color, location in the large intestine, and the sharp tail of the females. It is confirmed by observation of their characteristic esophagus. No other parasitic nematodes of domestic animals have a comparable structure. Recent authors classify the oxyurids as a subgroup of the ascaridida. We will continue considering them as an independent order[1] because this allows us to discuss together several nematodes that have comparable morphology and biology.

The oxyurids that may be of the concern of a practicing veterinarian are:

☛ *Oxyuris equi* of the equines, a cosmopolitan and common parasite. The males are 9-12 mm long, with small caudal alae, one spicule, and no gubernaculum. The females are 40-150 mm long (the tail alone may be a half to three-quarters of it in some females). There are females with long or short tails. The eggs are 85-95x40-45 µm, operculated, with a side flattened, and contain a tadpole when laid (Figure 20.2)

☛ *Probstmayria vivipara* of the equines, an uncommon but potentially impressive finding. They are small oxyurids, about 2-3 mm long. Both sexes have a long tail. The males have 2 spicules but no gubernaculum or caudal alae. The females have eggs or embryos inside the uteri.

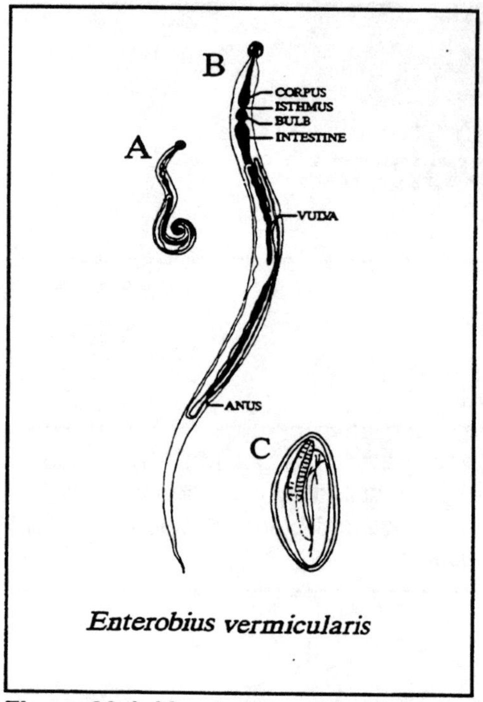


**Figure 20.1.** Morphology of the male (A), female (B) and egg (C) of the pinworm of humans.

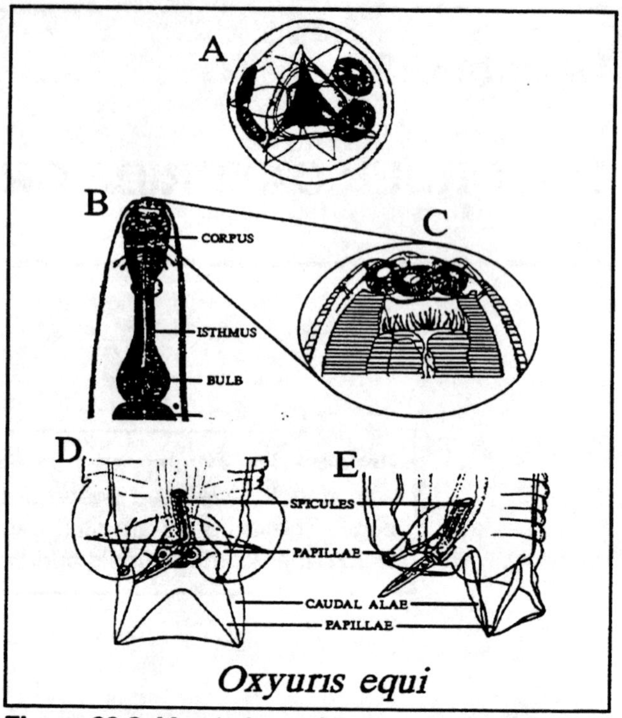


**Figure 20.2.** Morphology of the lips (A), anterior end (B and C), and posterior end (D ventral, E left) of the pinworm of horses.

☛ *Skrjabinema ovis* of sheep and goats, widely spread but not very common. The males are 2-4 mm long by 0.1-0.2 mm wide, the females 5-10 by 0.3-0.6 mm, and the eggs 47-67x27-36 μm, with a flattened side, and contain an infective larva when laid.

☛ *Passalurus ambiguus* of rabbits and hares. The males are 3-5 mm long by 0.2 0.3 mm wide and with a long tail. The females are 8-12 mm long by 0.5-0.6 mm wide. The eggs, 95-103x43 μm, have a side flattened and contain a blastula when laid.

☛ *Syphacia* spp. of mice, rats, and other rodents. The males (1.1-1.5 mm long) have 2 or 3 circular mamelons ("bosses") on its ventral surface, a spicule, and a gubernaculum. The females are 3-6 mm long and lay eggs with a flattened side that contain an infective larva.

☛ *Aspiculuris* spp. of mouse and other rodents. The males (2-4 mm long) lack bosses, spicules, or gubernaculum. The females are 3-4 mm long and lay 70-98x29-50 μm, symmetrical, unembryonated eggs.

☛ *Heterakis gallinarum*, the cecal worm of the chicken and other birds. The males are 4-13 mm long, with a prominent circular sucker before the cloaca, 2 spicules of unequal size, and caudal alae. The females are 7-15 mm long and lay symmetrical, unembryonated, thick-shelled, 63-75x36-48 μm eggs. Several other species of *Heterakis* exist. They are distinguished by the structure of the spicules and lips.

☛ *Enterobius vermicularis* of humans and, occasionally, apes. The males are 2-5 mm long by 0.1-0.2 mm wide, the females 8-13 mm long by 0.3-0.5 mm wide. The eggs are 50-60x20-32 μm, with a flattened side, and contain a tadpole when laid (Figure 20.1).

The domestic carnivores do not have oxyurids and, although often blamed for them, they are not the responsible for human infections.

### 3. Biology

The adults pinworms live in the lumen of the large intestine, probably feeding on intestinal content. The gravid females of *O. equi, S. ovis,* and *E. vermicularis* migrate to the anus and lay their eggs on the perianal area, gluing them on the host skin with a yellowish gelatinous material. The eggs of *S. ovis* are already infective when laid but the eggs of *O. equi* need 3-5 days, and those of *E. vermicularis* 1-2 days, to reach the infective stage.
Among the domestic animals, the eggs usually fall to the ground and infect other hosts when they are ingested with food or water. The infective larvae hatch in the small intestine, rapidly move to the large intestine, and penetrate the crypts where they develop to the 4th stage by day 8-10 of infection. The L4s return to the lumen and feed attached to the mucosa. Because the L4s of *O. equi* are brownish, they are believed to ingest blood. The first eggs are detected by the 5th month of infection with *O. equi*, the end of the 1st month with *S. ovis*, and during the 2nd month with *E. vermicularis*.

The life cycles of *Passalurus, Syphacia,* and *Aspiculurus* is comparable to that discussed above but they lay their eggs inside the intestine.

*P. vivipara* is the only nematode of domestic animals that multiplies inside its host. The female lays larvae that grow to adult without leaving the host intestine. Immense populations of these worms may develop in infected horses. Infection is believed to occur by ingestion of feces containing larvae.

*H. gallinae* lays thick-shelled eggs that resemble those of *A. galli*. They become infective in 14 days at 27C (80.6F) or in 9-11 days at 33C (91.4F), and may survive 4 months in water at room temperature or almost 8 months in humid soil. Prepatency is 24-36 days. In the remaining, its life cycle is as discussed above.

The survival of the thin-shelled oxyurid eggs has been studied only for *E. vermicularis*. Mature eggs kept in an humid environment died in 6 weeks at 3-7C (37-45F), 4-5 days at 12-19C (54-66F), 2-3 days at 20-24C (68-75F), or 6 hours at 45-48C (113-118F). Humidity is important for survival: 55% of the eggs survived for 2 days at 20-25C and 54-91% of relative humidity, but only 10% survived at 30-54% of relative humidity.

### 4. Medical importance

The oxyurids appear to be parasites well adapted to their hosts. Millions of *P. vivipara* have been recovered from apparently healthy horses, thousands of *P. ambiguus* from clinically normal rabbits, and no differences in weight gains were found between healthy chickens and chickens infected with *H. gallinae*. No pathology has been found in association with *S. ovis* or the rodent oxyurids either.

It is speculated that large numbers of *O. equi* L4s might cause intestinal inflammation with digestive discomfort, but there is no solid evidence for it. The main pathology of *O. equi* (or *E. vermicularis*) is related to the pruritus produced by the gluing of the eggs to the perianal area. Infected animals rub their tails against posts or fences so the rump may become inflamed and hairless. Secondary infections may occur. Presumably, the intense and constant pruritus makes the animals nervous and restless. *H. gallinarum* is important as the vector of *Histomonas meleagridis* (see respective chapter)

### 5. Diagnosis

Equine oxyuriasis is suspected for the signs of tail rubbing, and confirmed by observation of the characteristic eggs. Because *O. equi, E. vermicularis,* and *S. ovis* glue their eggs to the perianal region, eggs are rarely found in the feces. For example, only 5% of infected humans are positive to the conventional coprologic exam. In these cases, eggs for microscopic examination can be recovered by touching the perianal area with a transparent Scotch tape, rubbing with a swab moistened with glycerin, or removing the flakes of gluing material.

The tape can be attached to a microscope slide and the eggs observed through it. With some frequency, pinworms are passed with the feces, or found attached to the arm during rectal palpation. *P. vivipara* infection is confirmed by examination of feces for adults or larvae. Eggs of the other oxyurids can be found by conventional coprologic exams for nematodes.

**Summary:**

1. The oxyurids are parasites of the large intestine of equines, sheep and goats, lagomorphs, rodents, fowl, and humans.

2. They are recognized by the presence of an esophagus with a well developed posterior bulb, often preceded by a narrow isthmus and a well marked corpus.

3. The females of some species (*Oxyuris equi, Skrjabinema ovis,* and *Enterobius vermicularis*) glue their eggs on the peri-anal area. The others oviposit in the intestine. *Probstmayria vivipara* can produce new generations without leaving the intestine.

4. New infections are acquired by ingestion of embryonated eggs that survive in the external environment for only a few days.

5. The oxyurids are little pathogenic but *O. equi* produces anal pruritus which makes the horses nervous and induces them to rub their tails against nearby objects.

6. The eggs of the species that glue their eggs on the peri-anal area are rarely found in the feces.

## REFERENCES

1. Hyman, L.H. 1951. The Invertebrates: Acanthocephala, Aschelminthes, and Entoprocta. Mc-Graw-Hill, New York, 572 pp.

# Chapter 21

# ORDER SPIRURIDA:

# SUPERFAMILIES FILAROIDEA AND SPIRUROIDEA

**Preview**. The Spirurida are nematodes of the circulation, connective tissue, body cavities, or stomach of a variety of hosts. All require an intermediate host that, sometimes, acts as a biologic vector. The Spirurida of veterinary importance are divided into two major superfamilies: the Filaroidea or filarial worms and the Spiruroidea. The canine heartworm belongs to the first group whereas the agent of stomach or cutaneous habronemiasis belongs to the second group.

The **Spirurida** are nematodes that parasitize the anterior part of the gut (stomach or esophagus) or extradigestive spaces (blood or lymph, body cavities, or connective tissue) of humans or domestic animals. The mouth is simple and without lips, or have two or four paired lips. A distinctive characteristic is their cylindrical esophagus that is divided into an anterior, short and slender portion that is muscular, and a posterior, longer and wider part that is glandular. The division is not evident in all species, however. The males usually have two unequal and dissimilar spicules, variable caudal alae, and papillae on a tail that is coiled in spiral. All need intermediate hosts.

The spirurids important to veterinary medicine belong to either of two superfamilies: the Filaroidea or the Spiruroidea. We will discuss each group separately.

# The superfamily Filaroidea or Filarial Worms

**Preview.** The Filaroidea or filarial worms are parasites of the circulation, connective tissue, or body cavities of a number of species. The females are viviparous and lay larvae called microfilariae. All need a hematophagous insect as a biological vector. The most important to veterinary medicine is probably the canine heartworm, *Dirofilaria immitis*.

## 1 Morphology

The **Filaroidea** are small to large, whitish and thin worms of the body fluids, connective tissue, or body cavities. They commonly lack lips and a buccal cavity but have cephalic papillae, small caudal alae, and caudal papillae. The males have two spicules that are very unequal in length and dissimilar in shape. The vagina is tubular and long and opens in a vulva that often is very close to the anterior end. Characteristically, the Filaroidea lay larvae rather than eggs. The larvae are called **microfilariae.** In some species, the microfilariae keep the eggshell as a thin sheath around them but, in others, they leave the eggshell promptly. The presence or absence of a sheath is a further criteria for species identification. Not having easy access to the external environment, the filarial worms require the assistance of a hematophagous biological vector to be transferred to a new host.

## 2. Identification and clarification

The filarial nematodes are rather easy to identify as very thin and whitish nematodes of the connective tissue, cavities, or body fluids. Adult specimens may be identified preliminarily by their size, location, and host. Accurate identification is a task for the specialist. Species identification of microfilariae requires careful observation of internal structures, task that is better left to the specialist. Because of its significance in the veterinary practice, we will discuss the identification of the microfilariae of *Dirofilaria immitis* below. There is a large number of genera and species but the most important species to veterinary medicine belong to the genera *Dirofilaria, Dipetalonema, Setaria, Onchocerca* and *Stephanofilaria*. The most important species are described below and in Table 21.I.

☛ *Dirofilaria immitis* is a white, long, and thin nematode (about 10-30 cm x 1.0 mm) that lives in the heart and associated large vessels of dogs, other canids, and occasionally, felids and other carnivores. Its mouth is a single opening and the esophagus is clearly divided into a muscular and a glandular part. The caudal end of the males is coiled, has small caudal alae, and bears five pairs of preanal and six pairs of postanal papillae. The spicules are unequal and dissimilar, about 300-400 µm the left one and 200-300 µm the right one. The caudal end of the female is rounded and with a very short tail. The vulva is at the junction of the esophagus with the intestine, about 3 mm from the anterior end. The microfilariae are not sheathed and 308x7 µm on average. The infective L3s are 1.3 mm long. *D. immitis* can be distinguished from other *Dirofilaria* because it has a smooth cuticle

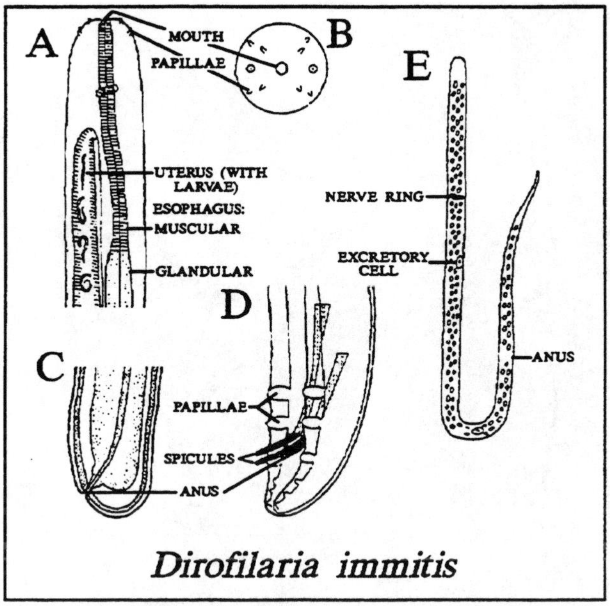


**Figure 21.1.** Morphology of the anterior end (A, lateral view; B, face view), posterior end of the female (C)and the male (D),microfilaria (E).

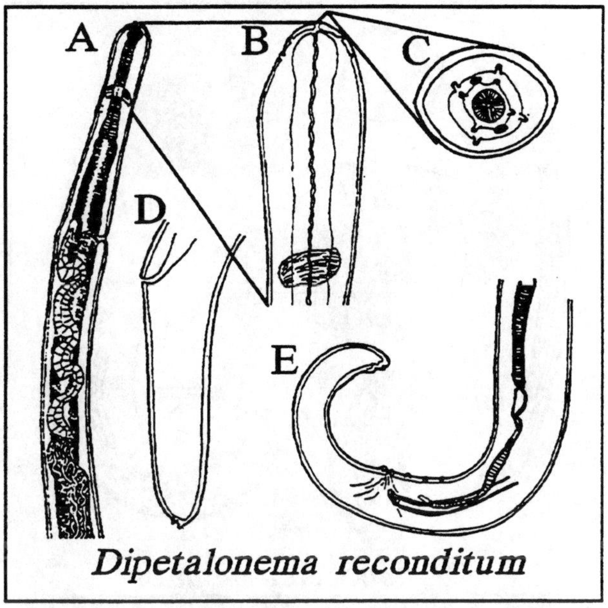


**Figure 21.2.** Morphology of the anterior end (A; B, detail of lateral view; C, face view), posterior end of the female (D) and the male (E).

whereas most other species show conspicuous longitudinal ridges. Morphological details to differentiate *D. immitis* from *Dipetalonema reconditum* microfilariae are given under Diagnosis and in Table 21.II.

☛ *Dirofilaria repens* (about 5-17 cm x 0.5 mm) is a parasite of the subcutaneous tissue of dogs, cats, and, rarely, humans, in southern Europe, southeast Asia, and Africa.

☛ *Dipetalonema* (syn. *Acanthocheilonema*) *reconditum* is smaller than *D. immitis* (about 1-3 cm x 0.1 mm) and lives in the subcutaneous tissue of canids. The morphology of the microfilaria is commented on under Diagnosis and in Table 21.II.

☛ *Onchocerca* are medium size filariae of the subcutaneous or dense connective tissue of large mammals. Most species are cosmopolitan. *Onchocerca cervicalis* (about 6-50 cm x 0.3 mm) and *O. reticulata* (about 27-75 cm x 0.3 mm) infect the ligamentum nuchae and the suspensory ligament of the fetlock of horses, respectively. The microfilariae are in the skin, near the location of the adults. *O. gutturosa* (about 3-55 cm x 0.2 mm) and *O. lienalis* (about 3-55 cm x 0.3) infect the ligamentum nuchae and the femuro-tibial ligaments, and the aponeuroses of the gastrosplenic region of cattle, respectively. The microfilariae of *O. gutturosa* occur in the skin of the neck and back and those of *O. lienalis* in the skin of the belly, particularly near the umbilicus.

☛ *Setaria* are filarias of the abdominal cavity of large hervivores that lay sheathed microfilariae: *S. equina* (about 5-13 cm x 0.8 mm) of equines and *S. labiatopapillosa* (about 4-12 cm x 0.6 mm) of cattle and other ruminants occur in most of the world.

☛ *Stephanofilaria stilesi* (about 0.3-8.0 cm x 0.1 mm) are small filaroids of cattle that live in the dermis, only 1-2 mm below the epidermis, of the midventral line, between the brisket and the navel. The sheathed microfilariae occurs in the dermal papillae in the same location.

☛ *Brugia malayi* (about 1-5 cm x 0.1 mm) infects the lymphatic nodes and vessels of primates (including humans) and domestic carnivores and *B. pahangi* (about 1-4 cm x 0.1 mm) infects the lymphatic nodes and vessels of domestic carnivores

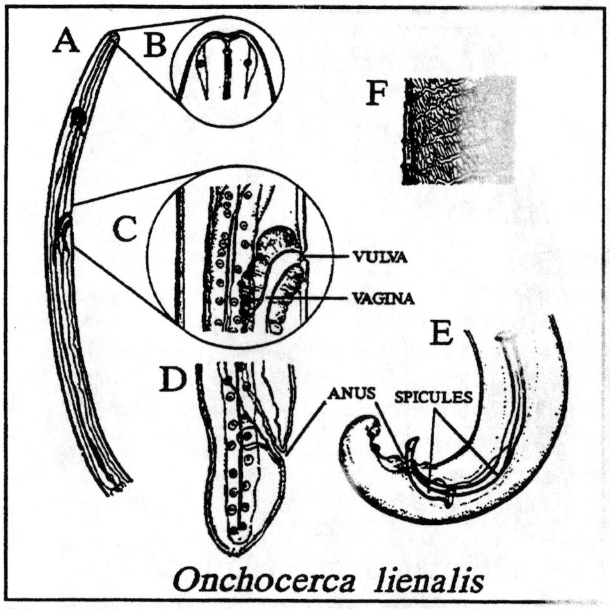


**Figure 21.3.** Morphology of the anterior end (A, B detail; C, detail of the vulva), posterior end of the female (D) and the male (E), cuticle (F).

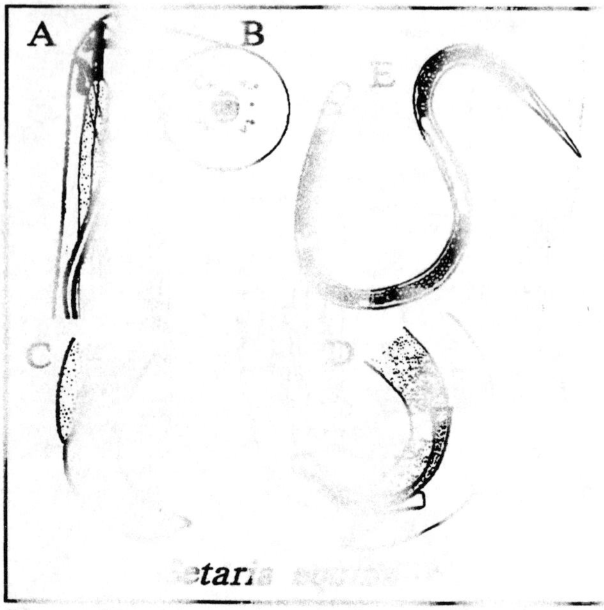


Figure [illegible]. Morphology of the anterior [illegible] lateral [illegible] face view), posterior end [illegible] female [illegible] and male (D), microfilaria (E).

and, occasionally, humans. Both are common laboratory models for the study of filariases.

### 3. Biology

*D. immitis* is possibly the most important parasite in this group and, consequently, much has been written about it.[1,2,3] More than 60 species of mosquitoes are able to transmit *D. immitis* biologically. *Aedes* (particularly *A. vexans*), *Culex* (particularly *C. quinquefasciatus*), *Anopheles*, *Mansonia*, and other genera are appropriate vectors. The non sheathed microfilariae are taken by a susceptible mosquito during its blood meal and invade the cells of the malpighian tubes in 48 hours where they develop into a "sausage" stage. By the end of the week, they move to the lumen of the tubes and molt to L2s by day 10 and to L3s by day 13. The infective larvae (about 1.3 mm long) migrate to the spaces inside the head or the proboscis. Invasion of malpighian cells or head spaces causes considerable mosquito mortality. Larval development does not proceed below about 15C but, if the mosquito hibernates, the larvae hibernate with it and resume development when the temperature rises to about 26C [illegible]

During a later mosquito meal, the L3s escape to the host skin with a drop of hemolymph. They use the puncture left by the mosquito to enter the new host. The L3s remain in the subcutaneous tissue nearby and molt to L4s by the third day. L4s (about [illegible] mm long) start then a migration through the intermuscular connective tissue to the abdomen, thorax, and head. They molt to juveniles between the 50th and [illegible] day, when they are 12 to 15 mm long. By day 70, all L4s have molted to juveniles and are able to penetrate the vein walls. The first juveniles appear in the heart between days 70 and 85. Ovum-bearing females are seen at 100 days and inseminated females at 120 days. The size of the worms is 50-60 mm at this time. The first microfilariae appear in the blood by 7 to 9 months post-infection. The adults live up to 5 years and the microfilariae up to 2.5 years.

The greatest concentration of microfilariae occurs from late afternoon to late evening (when most vectors are out biting) but it may fall to something between 1/5 and 1/20 at other times. Reports of different periodicities have been reported by other workers, however.

There are occasions in which infected dogs do not

exhibit microfilaremia (because of prepatent or unisexual infections, sterilizing treatments, or strong protective immunity). These are called "occult" infections.

*D. reconditum* has a life cycle comparable to *D. immitis* outside the host but the biological vectors are fleas and, occasionally, lice. The infective larvae develop in 7 or more days. The non sheathed microfilariae occur in the blood.

The vectors of *Onchocerca* are simuliids (black flies) and ceratopogonids (biting midgets). The infective L3 develop in 7-10 days. The sheathed microfilariae occur in the skin.

The vectors of *Setaria equina* and *S. labiatopapillosa* are *Aedes* mosquitoes. The infective larvae develop in 15 or 10 days, respectively. The sheathed microfilariae occur in the blood.

The vector of *Stephanofilaria stilesi* is the fly *Haematobia irritans*. The infective L3s develop in about 20 days.

The vectors of *B. malayi* and *B. pahangi* are mosquitoes of the genera *Mansonia*, *Anopheles*, and others.

**4. Medical importance**

As a rule, infections with filarial worms are chronic affairs of reduced pathogenicity. In some cases, however, they may cause very serious disease. The infamous elephantiasis of humans, for example, is caused by two filarial worms (*Wuchereria bancrofti* and *Brugia malayi*) that infect more than 250 million people in the world. The most dangerous of the Filaroidea of veterinary importance is probably *D. immitis*.

*D. immitis* is fundamentally a parasite of the pulmonary arteries. Only when the number of worms exceed about 25 in a medium size dog the parasites invade the right ventricle. Only when they exceed about 50, they are found in the right atrium and venae cavae. The basis of its pathogenesis is also morphophysiologic changes in the pulmonary arteries. The contact of the parasites with the arteria causes a **villose proliferation** of the intima which may begin as early as 3 months after infection and may develop severe lesions in only two months. The early lesions produce an intense inflammation that includes the media, may lead to an important arteritis with secondary fibrosis, and certainly favor the formation of thrombi. Dead parasites, on the other hand, form **emboli** in the distal arterial branches that obstruct the vessel and trigger granulomatous reactions of the vessel wall and the surrounding parenchyma. **Hemorrhages** by rupture of vessels are common at this stage. The remnants of parasites are disposed of first by neutrophils (**suppuration**) and later by mononuclear cells (**fibrosis**). In a week or so, most of the lumen of the vessel has been occluded by fibrous tissue, its wall has lost its elasticity, and the vessel is surrounded by an area of **interstitial pneumonia**.

As an effect of the living and dead worms, the lumen and the elasticity of the pulmonary arteries diminish and foci of pneumonia develop. Elimination of the adult worms results in recovery of the intima proliferation in as early as a month and resolution of the whole process in about a year. Persistence of the worms, however, keeps adding to the problem.

The partial occlusion and loss of elasticity of the pulmonary arteries elevate the pulmonary arterial pressure and makes more difficult for the right ventricle to propel blood through the lung arteries. With time, the ventricle responds with **dilation**, **hypertrophy**, and **failure**. Large number of worms in the ventricle may also interfere mechanically with its function causing **valvular insufficiency**. In turn, the failing ventricle triggers an increase in the pressures of the atrium, venae cavae, and so forth. The blood stasis in the venous side causes **congestion** of the tissues with the consequent increase of capillary filtration and formation of **edemas**. Long standing liver congestion eventually leads to liver fibrosis (**cirrhosis**) and the associated **ascites**.

During exercise, the arterial side dilates to accept more blood from the increased cardiac output but the damaged pulmonary vessels impede to supply it at the correct rate. The blood pressure drops, oxygenation of the muscles diminishes so **exercise tolerance decreases** and, in severe cases, cerebral ischemia may develop and cause **syncope**. The foci of pneumonia and the congestion (that eventually reaches the lung) conspire against the correct gas exchange, contribute to the exercise intolerance, and may cause **dyspnea** and **cough**.

Occasionally, dogs with heartworm develop **glomerulonephritis**. The major cause seems to be the kidney deposition of antigen-antibody complexes but other etiologies may exist. On occasions, dogs without prior signs develop an acute episode of weakness, anorexia, depression, and intense dyspnea. Hemoglobinuria and bilirubinuria are common. Often this represents a massive accumulation of parasites in the right atrium and vena cava which has been called **vena cava syndrome**. This syndrome is believed to correspond to an acute liver failure due to the venous stasis and hemolysis. The hemolysis, in turn, is believed to result from blood turbulence around the parasites. No evidence of immune hemolysis has been found.

*D. reconditum* and *Brugia* spp. are not known to cause disease in domestic carnivores.

*Onchocerca* spp. are infrequent cause of disease but the invasion of the ligaments by the adults may cause an inflammation that subsides in 3 or 4 weeks. The ligaments may remain swollen for some time and, eventually may develop nodules and even calcify. Larva of Onchocerca have been associated with dermatitis but it is likely that the skin lesions are due to the bites of the vector more than to the worms.

*Setaria* does not cause disease in its peritoneal location but the larvae has been found occasionally in the eye causing a verminous ophthalmia.

*Stephanofilaria* may cause a circumscribed dermatitis along the midventral line of cattle that begins in 8-10 month old calves and may last for 2-3 years if not treated. The skin may look raw and bloody, or covered with a serous exudate.

## 5. Diagnosis

The diagnosis of filarial infections is generally suspected by the signs of the disease and confirmed by observation of the microfilariae in the blood, lymph, or skin, or the finding of adult specimens. Here we will discuss the diagnosis of canine dirofilariasis.

Dirofilariasis is a disease of adult or old dogs that did not follow appropriate preventive treatment and had access to infected mosquitoes. Mild cases (commonly with fewer than 25 worms) have few and slight clinical signs and are usually diagnosed by elective testing. Moderate cases (usually with about 50 worms) may have a history of loss of condition, a dry hair coat, and chronic cough. Severe cases (with 100 or more worms) commonly exhibit clear signs of exercise intolerance, with severe tachypnea and tachycardia, and even syncope, with exercise. The mucosae are pale (rather than cyanotic) due to the anemia and deficient peripheral perfusion. Manifestations of right-sided congestive heart failure and ascites are common. Vena cava syndrome cases (about 60 worms in the right atrium and cava vein) are acute episodes of weakness, anorexia, depression, and intense dyspnea.

Clinical suspicion of the infection justifies attempts to diagnose it by demonstrating the presence of microfilariae. Wet smears of blood with anticoagulant reveal moving larvae when they are abundant enough. Enrichment methods, like the modified Knott tests, are more sensitive. One ml of blood with EDTA are mixed with 9 ml of 2% formalin to lyse the cells and centrifuged at 400-600 x *G* (1000-1500 rpm on a clinical centrifuge) for 5 minutes. All but 1 ml of supernate is decanted and 1 ml of stain (1/500 methyl green or 1/2000 methylene blue) is added. The fixed, stained microfilaria may be observed on microscope slides and quantified in counting chambers if desired. Kits for filtration of hemolyzed blood and recovery and staining of the microfilariae are available. Although the recommendations of the manufacturer must be followed, they usually consist of lysing the cells of a fresh blood sample, passing the lysate through a filter with a syringe, washing the filter, and staining the microfilariae. For observing morphology, the Knott tests is generally better. There are also kits similar to the filter kits that permit to stain the larvae for acid phosphatase. *D. immitis* microfilariae are suppose to stain at the excretory and anal pores and *D. reconditum* uniformly, but conflicting results have been reported.

Specific antibody-detecting serological test kits are available in the commerce but they often cross react with *D. reconditum*. They may be useful in cases of occult dirofilariasis. Several specific antigen-detecting serological test kits have appeared lately. They seem to be less cross reactive than the antibody-detecting tests and permit a rough estimation of the parasitic load in the patient. Because parasitic load is somewhat related to the potential for thromboembolic problems during treatment for adult worms, this information may tell the practitioner how aggressive the treatment can be. It can also inform about the effectiveness of the treatment by comparing antigen titters before and after adulticide treatment.

Other tests (radiography, arteriography, electrocardiography, echocardiography, etc.) will assist in the clinical evaluation of the patient or the treatment.

A common problem in the diagnosis of canine heartworm disease is the differentiation between microfilariae of *D. immitis* (which requires treatment) and those of *D. reconditum* (which doesn't). Examined by the Knott technique, the microfilariae of *D. immitis* are usually longer than 290 µm and wider than 5.5 µm. The cephalic end is slightly tapered and the caudal end is commonly straight (Table 21.II). The microfilariae of *D. reconditum*, on the contrary, is usually shorter than 290 µm and narrower than 5.5 µm. The cephalic end has parallel sides and the caudal end is commonly curve. When observed in wet smears, *D. immitis* microfilariae commonly wiggle in a same place whereas those of *D. reconditum* progress to the point that they move out of the microscope field.

These differences should be enough for diagnosis but, because they demand careful observation and measurements, a number of other supposedly diagnostic characteristics have been reported. *D. reconditum* ends caudally in a buttonhook but this is observed only in about half the microfilariae fixed with formalin. It also has a hook in its mouth but it is of difficult visualization. Some workers measure the cephalic or caudal "empty" spaces (zones at either end that do not take the stain well) or observe annular striations in hematoxylin stained specimens. The size of the empty spaces is overlapping (7.5-14.0 and 22.5-33.5 µm for *D. immitis* versus 8.5-10 and 21.0-26.0 µm for *D. reconditum*), however, and the striations of *D. immitis* are too subjective to be of great diagnostic value. Finally, histochemical staining for acid phosphatase shows the enzyme concentrated at the level of the excretory pore and, secondarily, the anal pore in *D. immitis* microfilariae. Similar staining of *D. reconditum* microfilaria is supposed to show the enzyme distributed uniformly over the entire body but there are reports of staining patterns similar to *D. immitis*.

## 6. Treatment

A treatment strategy has been recommended by the American Heartworm Society[4] and periodic updates are published in its Bulletin or Symposia.

Because killing the adult parasites reproduces the embolus pathology explained above and killing the microfilariae may exacerbate the deposition of antigen-antibody complexes, apart from the toxic potential of the drugs themselves, it is very important that the patient is in good health before any attempt at treatment. This means that any preexisting condition, or clinical signs of heartworm disease, must be investigated and dealt with before initiating treatment.

It is common to perform at least thoracic radiology and a complete blood count before treatment. Other exams (complete blood count, urine analysis, serum chemistry, etc.) may be ordered according to the findings and the age of the dog.

Normally, infected dogs are treated with an adulticide drug followed by a microflaricide after 6-8 weeks, if the dog had microfilariae in its circulation.

**Table 21.I. Characteristics of some common species of Filaroidea**

| Species | Host | Location | Male size (mm) | Spicule size (µm)* | Female size (mm) | Tail length (µm) | Vulva (mm) ** | Microfilariae Sheath | Size (µm) |
|---|---|---|---|---|---|---|---|---|---|
| *Dirofilaria immitis* | Dogs, occ. cats | Heart, vessels | 120-200 x0.7-0.9 | R 175-299 L 300-375 | 250-310 x1.0-1.3 | Very short | 2.7 | No | 295-325x5-7.5 |
| *Dirofilaria repens* | Carnivores | Subcut-aneous | 50-70 x0.4 | R 180-210 L 460-590 | 100-170 x0.6 | Very short | 1.1-1.6 | No | 268-360x5-8 |
| *Dipetalonema reconditum* | Canids | Subcut-aneous | 9-17 x0.1 | R 92-104 L 220-300 | 30-32 x0.16 | 180-300 | 0.68-0.92 | No | 250-288x4.5-5.5 |
| *Onchocerca lienalis* | Cattle | Liga-ments | 28-55 x0.09 | R 64-92 L 168-295 | 40-55 x0.2-0.4 | 95-181 | 0.40-0.65 | No | 170-265x4.2-4.5 |
| *Onchocerca gutturosa* | Cattle | Ligaments | 28-33 x0.09-0.1 | R 75-88 L 225-295 | 550 x0.3 | | 0.55 | No | 170-195x4 |
| *Onchocerca cervicalis* | Horses | Ligaments | 60-70 x0.07-0.1 | R 100-120 L 320-360 | <500 x0.4 | 115-130 | 0.63-0.67 | No | 207-240x4-5 |
| *Onchocerca reticulata* | Horses | Ligaments | < 27 x0.02 | R 116-121 L 248-295 | 400-750 x0.3-0.4 | 270-290 | 0.36-0.40 | No | 330-360x6-7 |
| *Setaria equina* | Horses | Perito-neum | 50-80 x0.4-0.6 | R 140-290 L 610-660 | 70-130 x0.7-1.2 | 340-550 | 0.41-0.82 | Yes | 240-260x7-8 |
| *Seraria labia-topapillosa* | Cattle, other ruminants | Perito-neum | 40-60 x0.4 | R 100-120 L 260-270 | 60-120 x0.8 | 430-650 | 0.46-0.86 | Yes | 140-230 |
| *Stephanofilaria stilesi* | Cattle | Skin | 3-3.5 x0.08 | R 45 L 228 | 56-85 x0.1 | Very short | 0.48-0.57 | Yes | 45-60x2-4 |
| *Brugia malayi* | Primates, cats | Lymph-atics | 13-20 x0.08 | R 100-120 L 290-365 | 43-52 x0.1-0.2 | 135-230 | 0.63-0.73 | Yes | 177-260x5-6 |
| *Brugia pahangi* | Carnivores, occ. humans | Lymphatics | 13-17 x0.08 | R 75-90 L 200-215 | 40 x0.1 | 140-155 | 0.45-0.49 | Yes | 250-300x5-6 |

* R = right spicule, L = left spicule, ** Distance from vulva to cephalic end

**Table 21.II. Differentiation between *D. immitis* and *D. reconditum* microfilariae**

| **Characteristic and test** | ***D. immitis*** | ***D. reconditum*** |
|---|---|---|
| **Number in blood** | Few to many | Usually few |
| **Size;** | | |
| **Wet smear** | > 310 μm | < 310 μm |
| **Straight Knott** | 295-325x5.0-7.5 μm | 250-288x4.5-5.5 μm |
| **Stained Knott** | 285-315x4.0-5.0 μm | 260-274x4.0-5.0 μm |
| **Filter tecnique** | > 240 μm | < 240 μm |
| **Shape (Knott)** | Usually straight | Usually curve |
| **Movement (Wet smear)** | Stationary | Progressive |
| **Head (Knott, Filter)** | Slightly tapered | Parallel sides, with hook |
| **Tail (Knott)** | Mostly straight | Curved |
| **Acid phophatase** | At excretory and anal pores | Uniform |

**Summary:**

1. The Filaroidea are thin nematodes of the circulation, body cavities, or connective tissue.

2. The are viviparous and lay L1s that are called microfilariae.

3. Some microfilariae are enclosed in a sheath which is actually the stretched eggshell.

4. All Filaroidea need a hematophagous biological vector to pass from one host to the next.

5. Most filarial infections are chronic and little pathogenic.

6. A few (*Wuchereria* and *Brugia* in humans, *Dirofilaria* in dogs) may cause important disease.

7. *Dirofilaria immitis* of dogs causes occlusion, inflammation, and stiffness of the pulmonary arteries.

8. This provokes circulatory and pulmonary alterations that endanger the life of the host.

9. Because adulticide treatment of *D. immitis* reproduces the pulmonary pathology, it must be performed carefully and on animals clinically sound.

## REFERENCES

1. Boreham, PFL and Atwell RB (eds). 1988. *Dirofilariasis*, CRC Press, Boca Raton, Florida, 249 pp.

2. Rawlings CA. 1986. *Heartworm Disease in Dogs and Cats*. Saunders, Philadephia, 329 pp.

3.Soll MD and Coleman MW (eds). 1992. *Heartworm Symposium 1992*. Proc. Hrtwm. Symp. 92, Austin, Texas, Amer. Hrtwm. Assoc., Batavia, Illinois, 319 pp.

4. American Heartworm Society, Executive Offices, P.O. Box 667, Batavia, Illinois 69510-0667.

# Chapter 22

# THE ORDER TRICHINELLIDA: *Trichinella, Trichuris,* AND *Capillaria*

**Preview.** The orders Trichinellida and Dioctophymatida constitute the subclass Adenophorea (formerly, Aphasmidia), characterized by the lack of phasmids and lateral excretory canals and the presence of a ventral excretory gland. The order Trichinellida, in turn, is characterized by a thin esophagus surrounded by a single row of esophageal glands called stichocytes. Three genera of veterinary importance are found in this order: *Trichinella, Trichuris,* and *Capillaria.*

The **Trichinellida**, with the Dioctophymatida, constitute the subclass **Adenophorea** (from Gr *adenos* = gland, and *phoros* = to bear), formerly called Aphasmidia (from Gr *a* = without, and phasmid, a pair of caudal chemoreceptors). The nematodes in this group lack phasmids and lateral excretory canals but have a large excretory cell underneath the esophagus that opens ventrally on the midline, near the nerve ring. Recent evidence suggests that this cell has more to do with the neurohormonal regulation of molting than with osmoregulation. Observation of these features is often difficult for untrained people. Fortunately, the genera of adenophorea nematodes are characteristic enough to be easily identified by their generic features so determination of subclass, or even order, is rarely necessary. The Trichinellida (from *Trichinella*, one of its genera), also called Trichurida (from *Trichuris*, one of its genera), are very small to medium size parasites characterized by a narrow esophagus surrounded by numerous esophageal glands disposed in a single longitudinal row of cells. The individual cells are called **stichocytes** and the body they form, **stichosome** (Figure 22.1). The order Trichinellida contains three genera of veterinary importance: *Trichinella, Trichuris,* and *Capillaria.* They share the morphologic characteristics of the order but differ so much in biology and host-parasite relationships that it is best to discuss them separately.

# Genus *Trichinella*: the trichina worms

**Preview.** Trichinella are tiny nematodes that infect the small intestine and skeletal muscles of a variety of species, particularly humans, pigs, domestic carnivores, and wildlife. They rarely cause disease in domestic animals but veterinarians play a critical role in the prevention of the human infection.

## 1.Morphology

*Trichinella* are very small, translucent-white worms. The female is 2.5-4.0 mm in length by 0.05-0.06 mm in width, the male is 1.0-1.6 mm by 0.03-0.04 mm, and both are found in the small intestine of their hosts. The first stage larva is 1.0 mm by 0.03 mm. It is found in the circulation of their hosts for a few hours after birth, and then inside the skeletal muscle fibers for months or years. The stichosome is a clearly visible single row of about 40 to 50 cells surrounding the esophagus. Details of their morphology are presented in Figure 22.1.

## 2. Identification and classification

Female *Trichinella* are distinguished from males by their larger size, lack of caudal appendages, a birth pore behind the stichosome, and the presence of embryos inside when they are fertilized. The males are distinguished by their smaller size, and the presence of a pair of large tubercles (but not spicules or spicular sheath) at the caudal end. The larvae are distinguished from the larvae of other nematodes by their presence inside skeletal muscle fibers, and a long stichosome that occupies 2/3 of the length of their body.

The only other common nematodes of comparable size that can be found as adults in the intestine of the hosts of *Trichinella* are *Strongyloides* spp. and *Trichostrongylus* spp. but neither has a stichosome. *Capillaria* spp. of rodents, also with a stichosome, should not be a source of confusion because they are considerable larger than *Trichinella*, the females show eggs in their interior, and the males have a spicule and/or a spicular sheath.

Until the early 1970's the only *Trichinella* species known was *T. spiralis*. In 1972, Soviet workers described a number of differences among *Trichinella* worms recovered from various hosts or geographic locations.[1,2] Because morphologic differences (still the main criterium of practical taxonomists) among these isolates are subtle, many parasitologists refuse to accept them as species and restrict them to the status of varieties, strains, sibling species, or subspecies. Although these isolates seem to be in the early stages of speciation, they generally do not interbreed, or do so with production of sterile progeny, so their status as species appears justified.

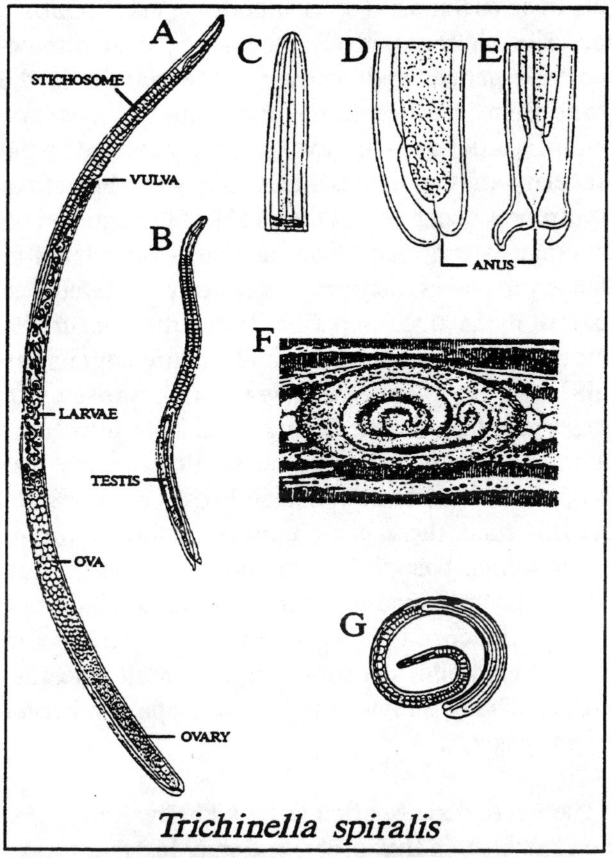


Figure 22.1. Morphology of the female (A), male (B), anterior end (C), posterior end of the female (D) and male (E), larva in muscle (F) and released larva (G).

The new species and their major characteristics are as follows:

♦ *T. spiralis*: known to exist in areas of pig raising; length in mm, 1.1-2.2 for males, 1.5-3.3 for females, and 1.0-1.1 or larvae; highly infective for mouse, rat, guinea pig, rabbit, or pig, moderately infective for hamster, does not infect birds; highly pathogenic for mouse or rat; moderate pathogenicity for humans; form index of the cyst (length to width ratio), 1.7-2.3; larvae in muscle dies in 10-20 days at -15C;

♦ *T. nativa*: known to exist in the circumpolar regions (above the 40th parallel) of Asia, Europe, and North America; length in mm, 1.0-1.2 for males, 1.5-2.1 for females, and 0.8-1.1 for larvae; highly infective for mouse, little infective for rat, hamster, guinea pig, rabbit, or pig, does not infect birds; highly pathogenic for mouse, more pathogenic than *T. spiralis* for humans; form index of the cyst, 1.2-1.5; larvae in muscle survives -15C for 12 or more months;

♦ *T. nelsoni*: known to exist in Africa, southern Europe, southern Soviet Union, and middle Asia; length in mm, 1.1 for males and 2.2 for females; little infective for mouse, rat, hamster, or pig, does not infect birds; moderately pathogenic for mouse, little pathogenic for rats, less pathogenic than *T spiralis* for humans; form index of the cyst, 1.8-2.2; larvae in muscle survives -12 to -17C for 6 or more months and is particularly resistance to high temperatures;

♦ *T. pseudospiralis*: known to exist in the Soviet Union, India, and North America; length in mm, 0.6-1.0 for males, 1.3-2.0 for females, and 0.6-0.8 for larvae; highly infective for hamster, little infective for rats, infects birds, less pathogenic than *T. spiralis* for Macaca monkeys (and presumably for humans); the larvae does not form cysts; larvae in muscle dies in 3 days at -12 to -17C;

These species appear to be just rising as a result of ecological isolation: *T. spiralis* in temperate zones, *T. nativa* in Arctic environments, *T. nelsoni* in a tropical setup, and *T. pseudospiralis* in connection with prey birds. Their definitive identification and significance to public health still require further study. Almost all our present knowledge of the biology and significance of *Trichinella* is the result of studies with the classic species, *T. spiralis*.

### 3. Biology

*Trichinella* infection begins with the ingestion of flesh containing infective larvae of the parasite. The host digests the flesh and releases the larvae which penetrate a row of columnar cells of the epithelium of the small intestine villi in a matter of minutes. The infective larvae rapidly molt 4 times to become adults and mate by the second day of infection. The females start laying living L1's on the 5th day of infection with peak production during the 9th day. A female may produce 200 to 1700 larvae during its lifespan which is limited by the immune response of the host. During primary infections, the parasites remain in the intestine for about 6 weeks in humans, and for 10-20 days in mice or rats.

The larvae leave the small intestine mostly by the lymphatic vessels, and spread throughout the body with the circulation. Within a few hours, they penetrate skeletal muscle fibers. A few larvae may invade other tissues but they do not develop further in them. Once within the myocyte, the larva grows and develops (but does not molt) for the next 20 days. The infective stage for a new host is reached in 16 days. During this period, the larva induces a number of chemical, metabolic, and structural changes of the host myocyte which becomes a **nurse cell** adapted to protect and nurture the parasite.[3] A capsule of collagen starts being deposited by the myocyte around the larva by day 10 of muscle invasion, it becomes well visible about 20 days later, and fully constituted in about 3 months. The nurse cell with the infective L1, both surrounded by the capsule, is known as a **cyst**. Some cysts may begin to calcify 6-9 months after infection but in many of them, calcified or otherwise, some larvae may remain alive for several years.

## 4. Host-parasite relationship

*Trichinella* is particularly important as a parasite of humans, pigs, domestic carnivores, and rats. Only in humans the parasite produces a discernible clinical entity. Human trichinosis may go from an inapparent infection to a lethal disease. The severity of the illness relates closely to the number of parasites in the muscles of the patient: less than 10 larvae per gram often correspond to asymptomatic infections or mild disease whereas more than 100 larvae per gram commonly produce overt symptoms. Other factors like pathogenicy of the particular strain of *Trichinella* or the reactivity of the host also influence the severity of the disease.

Human trichinosis (or trichinelliases) is commonly described in four periods: incubation, acute disease, convalescence, and recovery. **Incubation** is the time from infection to the appearance of systemic manifestations (5-30 days, inversely related to the severity of the illness). Because gastrointestinal symptoms occur in less than 15% of the patients on average, are non-specific, and may be related to dietary excesses, they are customarily considered as part of the incubation period. When they occur, the most common gastrointestinal manifestations are **abdominal pain**, **diarrhea**, and **nausea**. In experimental animals, the intestinal infection causes a mild inflammation of the small intestine that begins on day 4 of infection and peaks on day 8-10. At this time, there is a panmucosal infiltration of eosinophils, basophils, lymphocytes, and plasma cells. The inflammation starts to subside on day 14 and the mucosa is again normal by day 38. As in other nematode infections of the small intestine with, trichinosis may cause villus atrophy and crypt hyperplasia.

The **acute disease** often starts with fever, myalgia, and malaise, in that order, and may last 1-8 weeks depending on the severity of the illness. Because **fever** may appear very soon after systemic infection, before evidence of muscle inflammation or synthesis of specific antibodies, production of endogenous pyrogen is probably induced by proteins of parasites in the circulation. Its production may be sustained later by products generated during muscle inflammation and by antigen-antibody complexes. **Myalgia** is the clinical expression of the myositis caused by penetration of parasites into the muscle fibers. In moderate to severe cases, **vascularities** (of mechanical and allergic origin) appear shortly afterwards. The vascularities is expressed as **edemas**, particularly of the eyelids and sometimes of the whole face, and hemorrhages that are evident in the conjunctiva and under the fingernails. Myocardial, encephalic, or pulmonary complications may appear later in 5-20% of the patients with severe illness. They are attributed to transient invasion of the corresponding organs by larvae, or to manifestations of allergy caused by deposition of antigen-antibody complexes. Myocarditis, encephalitis, and pneumonitis are actually the major causes of death of trichinosis patients. Bacterial pneumonia is often the cause of death in cases of prolonged course (3-7 weeks)

**Eosinophils** (often over 1000 cells/ul) is one of the most consistent laboratory findings in trichinosis. It is usually first detected by the 2nd or 3rd week of infection. Leukocytosis, hypoalbuminemia (which contributes to the edema), and an increase in circulating creatine phosphokinase (an expression of damage to muscle tissue) are also common findings in this period.

The **convalescence** period is heralded by the recovery of the symptoms of the acute disease and is characterized by vague muscle pain and feeling of weakness that may persist for a few months. The period of **recovery** is marked by the absence of all symptoms although living parasites may persist in the patients for several years.

Experimental infection of domestic or laboratory animals with massive doses of *Trichinella* produces evidence manifestations of disease and may cause death. Natural infections are normally undetected, however, probably for the inability of the patient to communicate its discomfort.

Work with laboratory animals has produced evidence that primary infections with *Trichinella* results in immunological responses in the intestine that inhibit the growth and fecundity of the females, and expel the parasites from the intestine in 10-20 days. Abrogation of fertility is mediated by B cells but expulsion requires T cells. In secondary infections, 80% or more of the administered worms are expelled during the first day, and the remaining are disposed of more rapidly than in the primary infection. The presence of migrating larvae in the host of a primary infection awakes a systemic immunity that kills 85% or better of the migrating larvae of a later infection. The killing is effected by neutrophils and monocytes assisted by specific antibodies and complement factors. Recent research has demonstrated that eosinophils are lethal only to 20-hour old larvae which may not be effective in actual infections.

There is also evidence that *Trichinella* infections may affect the capacity of the host to mount immune reactions to unrelated antigens. For example, the intestinal worms do not affect the host's macrophage function but the migratory parasites stimulate phagocytosis and the muscle worms inhibits it.[4] These effects on host immunity may facilitate the bacterial pneumonitis characteristic of protracted severe cases.

## 5. Diagnosis

Diagnosis of the infection in animals will be discussed under Control. Here we will consider only the diagnosis of human trichinosis. Trichinosis is clinically suspected when a human patient has been exposed to an infected meat, has typical symptoms, has an unexplained eosinophilia, or by any combination of these. Presence of symptoms in several people that partook of the infective meal is an important additional consideration. The definitive diagnosis is established by serology or demonstration of the parasite.

The intradermic reaction (of Bachman) with extracts of the parasite is an old and simple test. Unfortunately, it is little sensitive (it detects only about 60% of the cases) and becomes positive only during the second month of infection. There is some evidence that the use of purified antigens could produce better results.

**Summary:**

1. *Trichinella* are tiny nematodes of the small intestine and skeletal muscle.

2. They infect a number of host species but are important agent of disease only in humans.

3. Pigs, rats, domestic carnivores, and wildlife ate important in its epidemiology.

4. The infection is acquired by eating poorly cooked, infected meats, particularly pork.

5. The viviparous adults live for a few weeks in the small intestine but the larvae invade, and may live for several years in, the skeletal muscles.

6. Although clinical disease is exceptional in domestic animals, veterinarians play a critical role in the prevention of the human infection.

## REFERENCES

1. Boev, S.N., Britov, V.A., and Orlov, I.V. 1979. Species composition of *Trichinellae*. Wiad. Parazytol. 25:495-503.

2. Dick, T.A. 1983. Species, and infraspecific variation. Chapter 2 in Campbell, W.C. (ed), *Trichinella and Trichinosis*, Plenum Press, New York, 31-73.

3. Steward, G.L. 1983. Pathophysiology of the muscle phase. Chapter 7 in Campbell, W.C. (ed.), *Trichinella and Trichinosis*, Plenum Press, New York, 241-264.

4. Barriga, O.O. 1980. Modulation of particle uptake in *Trichinella spiralis* infected mice. Inf. Immun. 30:832-834.

# Genus *Trichuris*: the Whipworms

**Preview**. *Trichuris* are medium size nematodes that infect the large intestine of a variety of host species. Because of their shape, they are commonly called whipworms. They are acquired by ingestion and do not migrate outside the intestine. They may cause important disease when numerous.

## 1. Morphology

The **trichurids** are whitish to pinkish nematodes from about 30 to 70 mm in length and about 0.5 to 1 mm in width. The anterior 2/3 to 3/4 of the body encloses the esophagus and is much narrower (0.15 to 0.2 mm in width) than the posterior part (Figure 22.2). This gives the worms the shape of a whip and accounts for their common name of **whipworms**. The esophagus is filiform and surrounded by a row of cells called **stichocytes**.

The posterior part of the males is coiled dorsally in a spiral and bears a single spicule in an evaginable sheath (Figure 22.3). The external surface of the sheath is smooth in some species and spiny in others. The posterior half of the females is bent in a wide arch with the vulva close to the junction between the thin and thick parts. The eggs have a thick, brown shell with a plug at each end. Their shape reminds one of a lemon (Figure 22.2).

## 2. Identification and classification

Along with *Trichinella* and *Capillaria*, the trichurids belong to the order Trichinellida or Trichurida which is characterized by the presence of stichocytes around a very narrow esophagus. All the trichurids belong to the genus *Trichuris* which is easily identified by the clear division between a narrow anterior part and a tick posterior part, and by the presence of the worms in the large intestine of the host. The name *Trichuris* (from Gr *trikho* = hair, and *oura* = tail) commemorates a mistake since the thinner part corresponds to the mouth end. The more correct name *Trichocephalus* (from Gr *trikho*, and *kephalo* = head) has been proposed for this genus but it cannot be accepted by the rules of Zoological Nomenclature.

The most important species of trichurids are the following:

♦ *T. ovis*, a cosmopolitan species in sheep, goats, cattle, and many wild ruminants. The male is 50-80 mm long by 0.5 mm wide with a pointed spicule 4.8-6.9 mm long Figure 22.3). The female is 37-70 mm long by 1 mm wide with eggs of 70-80x30-42 µm. It has been reported in up to 25% of cattle in Illinois.

♦ *T. discolor*, a widespread species in cattle, sheep and goats. The male is 45-59 mm long and 0.45 mm wide with a blunt spicule 1.45 mm long. The female is 43-55 mm long by 0.67 mm wide with eggs of 60-67x25-35 µm. It has been reported in up to 18% of cattle in Alabama.

♦ *T. globulosa*, in cattle, sheep, goats, and many other ruminants in Europe, Asia, Africa, Australia and southern South America. The males are 40-70

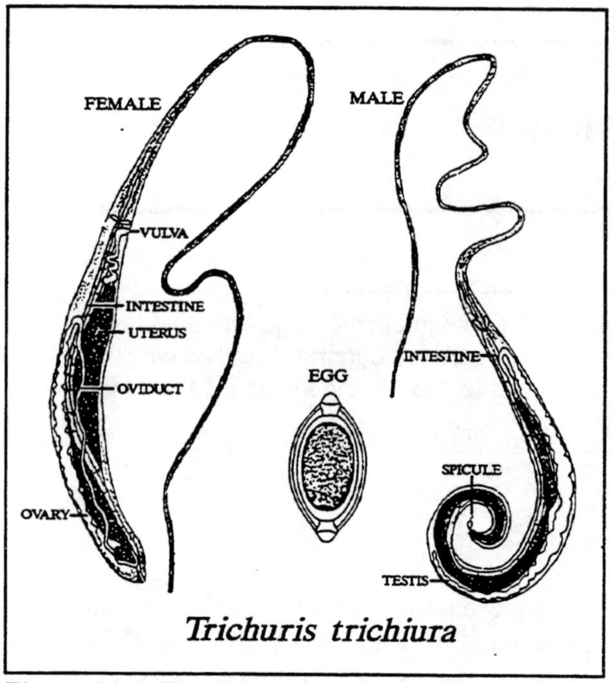


**Figure 22.2.** The whipworm of humans.

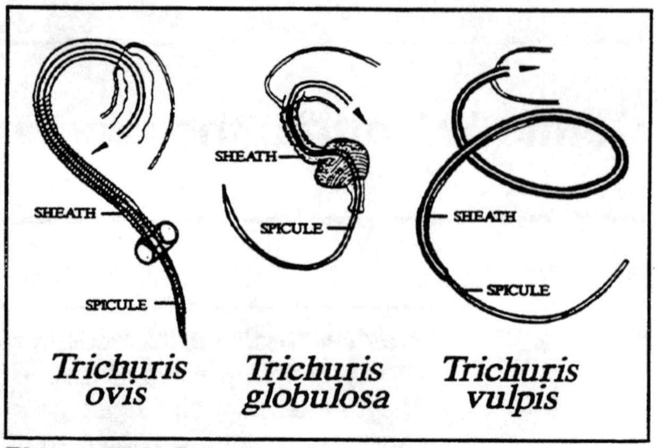


**Figure 22.3.** Spicules of some representative whipworms.

mm long by 0.71 mm wide with a pointed spicule 3.8-5.7 mm long. It can be distinguished from *T. ovis* because this latter has a small dilation at the very distal end of the sheath whereas the dilation in *T. globulosa* is larger and sub-terminal (Figure 22.3). The females are 42-60 mm long by 0.87 mm wide with eggs of 68-72x32-36 μm.

♦ *T. suis*, a cosmopolitan species of pigs that can also infect humans[1]. The males are 30-40 mm long with a spicule 2-2.35 mm long. The females are 30-50 mm long with eggs of 50-56x21-25 μm. It has been reported in up to 14% of pigs in Wisconsin.

♦ *T. vulpis*, a cosmopolitan species of canines that can also infect humans[2]. The males are 45-75 mm long with a spicule 7.6-11 mm long (Figure 22.3). The females are 45-75 mm long with eggs of 72-90x32-40 μm. It has been reported in about 40% of stray dogs in New Jersey and we see it in about 20% of fecal exams of dogs brought to the Ohio State University veterinary hospital.

♦ *T. campanula*, a parasite of the felines that occurs in the American continent. The males are 21.5 mm long by 0.33 mm wide with a spicule 1.2-1.5 mm long. The females are 17-31 mm long by 0.42 mm wide with eggs of 78-81x31-36 μm. It is uncommon in the U.S.A.

♦ *T. leporis* and *T. sylvilagi* of rabbits, hares, cottontails, and squirrels. The males are 19-21 mm long. The females are 17-21 mm long with eggs of 60-65x29 μm. The spicule is 2-2.3 mm long in *T. leporis* and 6-8 mm long in *T. sylvilagi*.

♦ *T. trichiura*, a cosmopolitan species of humans that also infects apes and monkeys. The males are 30-45 mm long with a spicule 2.5 mm long. The females are 35-50 mm long with eggs of 50-54x22-23 μm. This species is morphologically identical to *T. suis*. Its presence is spotty in the U.S.A. and reaches an average prevalence of about 2%. Its prevalence is much higher in many tropical and temperate countries.

## 3. Biology

The trichurids are oviparous worms. Each female lays about 2000-5000 eggs per day that leave the intestine with the stools of the host. These eggs contain a zygote that must mature in the external environment to a first stage larva which is the infective stage. For maturation, they need adequate temperature, humidity, shade, and oxygen. The eggs of *T. suis*, for example, develop the fist stage larva in 18 days at 37.5C (99F), in 54 days at 22C (71F), and in 210 days at 6-24C (21-75F). The eggs of *T. vulpis* develop in 12-15 days at 37C and in 35 days at 22C. Desiccation and direct sunlight will kill the eggs rapidly but in a humid and shady environment they can survive for up to 6 years.

When larvated eggs are ingested by an appropriate host, the L1s hatch in the small intestine, penetrate the intestinal wall where they remain for 3-10 days, and then they return to the lumen and move to the large intestine. The adults live in the cecum but they will invade the colon and even the rectum and final portions of the small intestine in massive infections. The adult worms thread their anterior end between the enterocytes and probably feed on tissue fluids, cells digested outside the worm's body, and small amounts of blood[3].

Eggs are first found in the stools of the host at about 3 months of the infection in ruminants, 41-45 days in pigs, 70-90 days in dogs, and 30-90 days in humans. The life span of the worms is 4-5 months in pigs, about 16 months in dogs, and up to 5 years in humans.

## 4. Medical importance

*Trichuris* infections are more prevalent in young hosts than in old ones. This is probably a manifestation of immunity since the risk of infection must be the same in young or old domestic animals. In most cases the infected host has few parasites that do not cause clinical manifestations. In heavy infections, trichuriasis causes **diarrhea** that may becomes watery, mucoid, and stained with blood. The animals fail to gain weight or **lose weight**, and may develop a hypochromic microcytic **anemia**.

The affected mucosa shows edema, hiperhemia, and frank inflammation, with the parasites hanging from their cephalic end. Microscopically, there are pyknotic nuclei, coagulation necrosis, and nodules containing pus or inflammatory cells around the parasites. The lymphatic tissue appears congestive and concentrations of lymphocytes are found even in areas without worms.

The physiopathology of trichuriasis is not clear since the parasite does not seem to cause direct damage to the intestinal cells and they absorb only 0.005 ml of blood per worm per day. The histopathology[4] suggests that an immune reaction to products of the parasite may be an important factor. The loss of weight, and possibly the anemia, may be a consequence of malabsorption due to the alteration of the intestinal mucosa.

The U.S. Department of Agriculture estimated in 1965 that pig trichuriasis caused an annual loss of about $ 700,000.

## 5. Diagnosis

The signs of trichuriasis are little characteristic so the clinical suspicion of the infection is based on the age of the animals and the prior knowledge of the presence of the infection in the area. Confirmation is obtained by the finding of the typical eggs of the parasite in coprologic exams. The presence of eggs in the feces tends to be cyclic so a single negative exam does not rule out the infection. Three exams every other day is recommended before declaring the animal free of infection. In heavy infections, the patient may suffer rectal prolapse with worms hanging from the mucosa of the everted rectum.

**Table 22.I. CHARACTERISTICS OF SOME COMMON TRICHURIDS**

| SPECIES | HOSTS | MALES | | FEMALES | |
|---|---|---|---|---|---|
| | | Size (mm) | Spicule (mm) | Size (mm) | Eggs (µm) |
| *T. ovis* | Ruminants | 50-80x0.5 | 4.8-6.9 (*) | 37-70x1 | 70-80x30-42 |
| *T. discolor* | Ruminants | 45-59x0.5 | 1.45 (*) | 43-55x0.7 | 60-67x25-35 |
| *T. globulosa* | Ruminants | 40-70x0.7 | 3.8-5.7(*) | 42-60x0.9 | 68-72x32-36 |
| *T. suis* | Pigs, occ. humans | 30-30 | 2.0-2.3 | 30-50 | 50-56x21-25 |
| *T. vulpis* | Canines, occ. humans | 45-75 | 7.6-11.0 | 45-75 | 72-90x32-40 |
| *T. campanula* | Felines | 21x0.3 | 1.2-1.5 | 17-31x0.4 | 78-81x31-36 |
| *T. leporis* | Lagomorphs | 19-21 | 2.0-2.3 | 17-21 | 60-65x29 |
| *T. sylvilagi* | Lagomorphs | 19-21 | 6.0-8.0 | 17-21 | 60-65x29 |
| *T. trichiura* | Humans, apes | 30-45 | 2.5 | 35-50 | 50-54x22-23 |

(*) see text.

**Summary:**

1. The trichurids are medium to large size nematodes of the large intestine of ruminants, pigs, domestic carnivores, lagomorphs, and primates.

2. Their anterior half is markedly more slender than their posterior half what have earned them the common name of whipworms.

3. The infection is acquired by ingestion of larvated eggs containing an infective L1.

4. They reach the adult stage without migrating outside the intestine.

5. When abundant, they may cause severe disease, particularly in young hosts.

## REFERENCES


1. Beer R.J.S. 1976. The relationship between *Trichuris trichura* (Linnaeus 1758) of man and *Trichuris suis* (Schrank 1788) of the pig. Res. Vet. Sc. 20:47.

2. Barriga O.O. 1982. Trichuriasis. In Steele J.H. (ed), *CRC Handbook Series in Zoonoses, Section C: Parasitic Zoonoses,* Vol II, CRC Press, Boca Raton, Florida, 339-345.

3. Lee T.D.G. and Wright K.A. 1975. The morphology of attachment and probably feeding site of the nematode *Trichuris muris* (Schrank, 1788) Hall, 1916. Can. J. Zool. 56:1889-1905.

4. Powers K.G., Todd A.C. and McNutt S.H. 1960. ??? Am. J. Vet. Res. 21:262-

# Chapter 23

# PHYLUM PLATYHELMINTHES: THE FLATWORMS

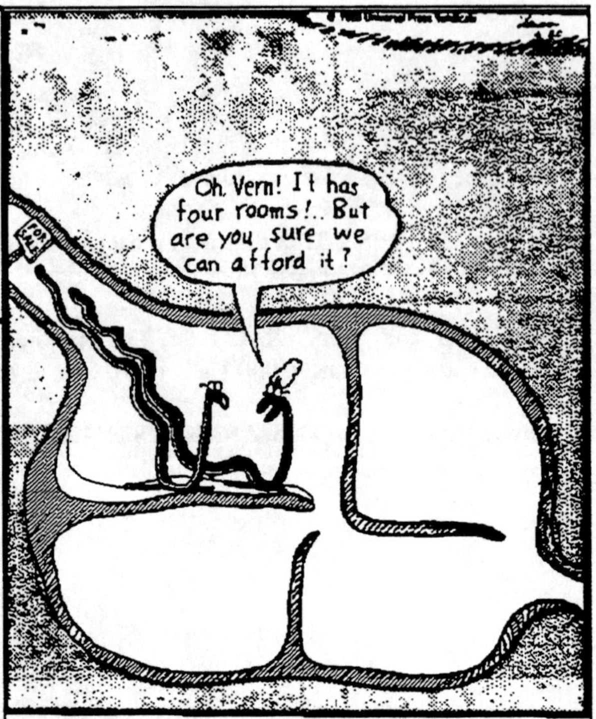
Oh, Vern! It has four rooms!.. But are you sure we can afford it?

Tapeworms in a cow's stomach

**Preview**. The platyhelminthes or flatworms are worms with a solid, commonly flattened body, and no anus. They contain two important parasitic groups, the Trematodes or flukes, and the Cestodes or tapeworms. These have complex life cycles that include definitive and intermediate hosts.

The **Platyhelminthes** (from Gr *platus*= flat, and *helmis*= parasitic worm) are worms with a solid body and without an anus. Different from the arthropods or nematodes, their body is filled with a connective tissue conventionally called **parenchyma**. The only cavities observed on a cross section of the body are the lumens of the hollow organs (digestive and genital tracts, mostly). In the species with a digestive apparatus, the gut is a blind tube with a mouth but without an anus.

They have soft, whitish or transparent bodies that are usually dorso-ventrally flattened which accounts for their common name, **flatworms**. They vary in size from almost microscopic to several meters in length. The respiratory and circulatory systems are absent, the digestive, excretory and nervous systems are simple, but the genital system is highly developed. With few exceptions, they are hermaphrodite. All parasitic species have complicated life cycles with definitive and intermediate hosts.

The platyhelminthes are divided into three classes: the **Turbellaria** (planarias and relatives) which are free-living, aquatic or semi-aquatic organisms; the **Trematodes** (flukes) which are all parasitic; and the **Cestodes** (tapeworms) which are all parasitic. Only the two last classes are of importance to veterinary medicine.

# THE CLASS TREMATODA OR FLUKES

**Preview.** The Trematodes or Flukes of domestic animals or humans are leaf- or pear-shaped parasites of the intestine, liver, lungs, or blood vessels. All have complicated life cycles involving one or two intermediate hosts, the first always being a snail. Many are little pathogenic in moderate infections but some may cause severe disease.

## 1. Morphology

The **Trematodes** (from Gr *trema*= perforation, and the suffix *ode*= like, referring to the suckers) of veterinary importance are organisms from a few millimeters to several centimeters long, some are thin and translucent whereas other are thick and fleshy. Most are leaf-shaped but a few are pear-shape. They do not posses pigments of their own but are often stained reddish, yellowish, or greenish by host's materials.

The general morphology of the digenetic trematodes is depicted in Figure 23.1. The most visible external feature is a couple of suckers, one surrounding the mouth at the anterior end (**oral sucker**), and the other somewhere on the ventral surface (**ventral sucker**). They act as attachment organs. The relative position and size of the suckers are useful criteria in the identification of some species. The body is filled with a loose connective tissue (**parenchyma**) that resembles an embryonary mesenchyma. Unstriated muscle fibers occur in longitudinal or circular bunches close to the body surface, dorso-ventrally in the body, or arranged around the suckers. This gives the flukes considerable mobility.

The body covering (**tegument**) is an anucleated cytoplasmic syncytium. This cytoplasm is connected with the cytoplasm of nucleated tegumental cells located among the parenchymal cells, just underneath the muscle layers. The syncytium contains mitochondria, ribosomes, endoplasmic reticulum, vacuoles, and, in some trematodes, rigid spines. The tegument is known to have functions in absorption, osmoregulation, excretion, and protection against host enzymes and immunity.

The **digestive system** consists of a mouth surrounded by the oral sucker, the esophagus, sometimes a pharynx, and two ceca. As a rule, the ceca are simple blind tubes but may be branched in some

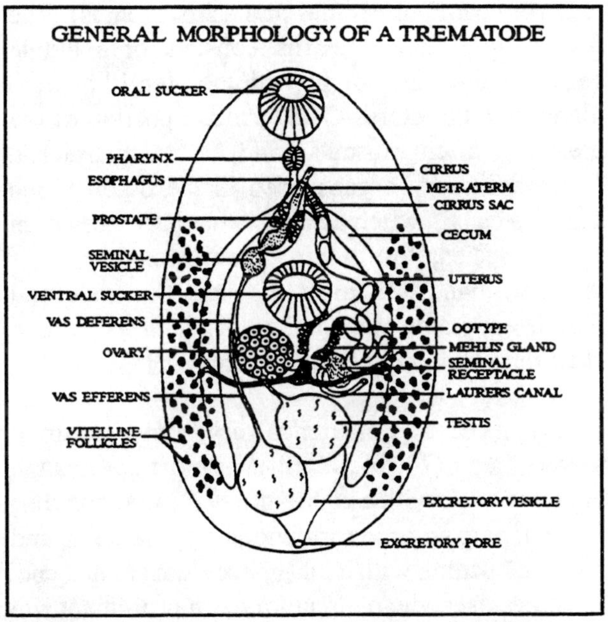


**Figure 23.1.** General morphology of a Digenea Trematode.

species (e.g., *Fasciola*). The ceca are involved with digestion, absorption, and secretion. Undigested food and secretions are regurgitated through the mouth.

The **excretory system** consists of two lateral convoluted tubes that usually open into an excretory gland at the posterior end of the fluke. The main tubes branch into secondary tubules than end in ciliated cells. Although the structure of the secretory system is important for the classification of some groups, it is difficult to observe.

The **nervous system** consists of a pair of ganglia located behind the oral sucker that originate three pairs of nerve trunks (dorsal, lateral, and ventral) that run forward, and three that run backward.

The trematodes do not have identifiable respiratory or circulatory systems.

With few exceptions (e.g., the schistosomes) the trematodes are hermaphrodite. The **male genital system** is composed of one to many testes (most commonly, two), vas deferens, a seminal vesicle, a prostate gland, a cirrus sac, and a cirrus or penis. The cirrus or its sac may be absent in some species (e.g., the paramphistomes and schistosomes). The **female genital apparatus** consists of a single ovary, oviduct, the ootype with the Mehlis' or shell gland, and the uterus. The terminal portion of the uterus is often muscular and called metraterm. Three accessory organs open in the oviduct: the Laurer's canal, which acts as a copulatory organ in some species, the seminal receptacle, and the vitelline glands. In most digenea, the male and female apparatus open to the outside in a common chamber called the genital atrium.

The **eggs** of the trematodes vary from very small to very large (20 to 200 μm). In most species the eggs are oval, with a rather thin wall that contains a developing embryo surrounded by yolk cells, and have an opening with a lid (**operculum**) at one end. In some cases, the operculum has a prominent rim (e.g., *Heterophyes, Opisthorchis, Paragonimus*). In other cases, the wall presents external processes (e.g., *Schistosoma*) (Figure 23.2).

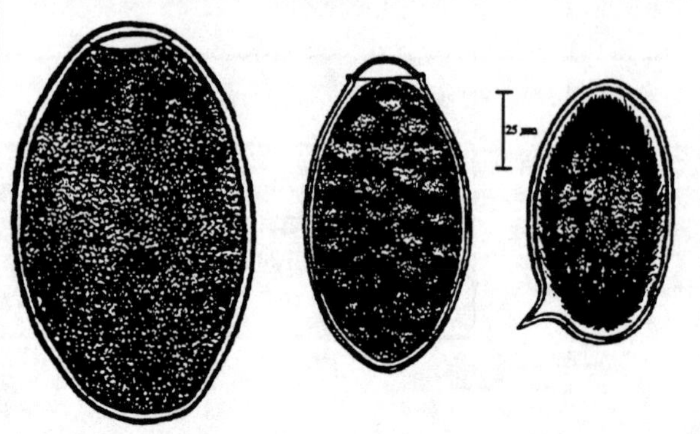


**Figure 23.2.** Morphology of some representative eggs of trematodes.

The shape of the testes or ovary ( round, oval, solid, branched, etc.), the relative position of the testes (side by side, tandem, or diagonal), the position of the ovary relative to the testes (anterior or posterior), and the distribution and location of the vitelline glands are important criteria for identification of some trematodes. The size, shape, color, and content of the eggs passed by the host often permit the identification of the infecting fluke in thefecal exam.

## 2. Identification and classification

The trematodes of the domestic animals or humans are identified by their flattened or pear-shape body, the presence of ventral suckers, and their solid body filled with a connective tissue. More than 8,000 species are known which are distributed into three orders: Monogenea, Aspidogastrea, and Digenea. The first two orders are parasites of cold-blooded vertebrates and will not be discussed here. The **Digenea** (from Gr *di*= two, and Lat *genesis*= generation, referring to the alternation of sexual and asexual generations in the definitive and intermediate hosts) include all the species parasitic in domestic animals or humans, as well as parasites of birds and fish.

There are close to 100 families of Digenea, and about 15 of them contain parasites that infect domestic birds or mammals. Accurate identification of trematode families is based on the observation of subtle characteristics of well prepared adult or pre-adult specimens which is definitively the province of the specialist, and of limited use to a practicing veterinarian. A description of the families of veterinary importance based on characters easy to observed by a non-specialist appears in Table 23-I.

In all host species, trematodes are particular abundant and varied in Asia where identification of species becomes difficult. They are less varied and, consequently, easier to identify in the rest of the world. The best conduct for a practicing veterinarian is to try to identify the trematodes found in his/her practice by the host, tissue location, and a few readily observed features of the parasite. With this purpose, we will arrange the common trematodes of veterinary importance by host and tissue location (intestine, liver, lungs, and blood vessels) rather than by systematic position. The summarized descriptions given below and in Table 23.II, and the accompanying figures may assist in the preliminary identification. In consulting the figures, important features to notice are the size and shape of the specimen, shape and location of the vitelline glands, testes, and ovary, and relative size and location of the suckers. Faced with an unfamiliar trematode, the practitioner should consult a specialist. Those who enjoy a challenge will find an account of many species of digenea of fish, birds, and mammals in Soulsby's book,[1] and comprehensive keys for the identification of the trematodes of North America north of Mexico in Schell's monograph.[2] Yamaguti's[3] book contains comprehensive keys to the genera of trematodes and lists of the species known until the early 1950s. Skrjabin[4] edited comprehensive keys to the digenetic trematodes of domestic animals and humans. Dawes wrote a classic monograph on trematodes[5] which unfortunately is dated by now.

### A. Common trematodes of ruminants

#### a. Digestive tube.

About 10 genera of trematodes, all belonging to the family Paramphistomatidae, occur in the rumen and reticulum of ruminants. Most are small (< 10 mm long), pear-shape, with the oral sucker at the thinner end and the ventral sucker at the thicker end, and with clear and large (> 100 um) eggs. The life cycle is like in *Fasciola* (see below). The most common genera of paramphistomes are *Paramphistomum* and *Cotylophoron* (Figure 23.3).

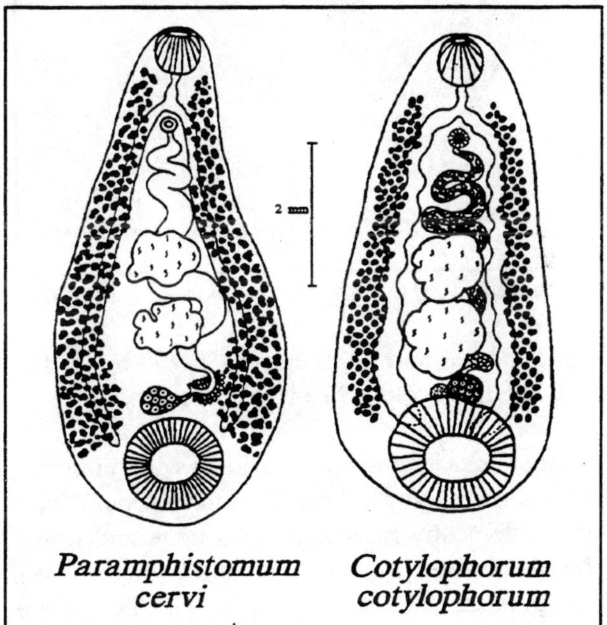


**Figure 23.3.** Two common intestinal flukes or ruminants.

#### b. Liver.

*Fasciola hepatica* is the most common liver fluke of ruminants (Figure 23.4). It occurs world wide. *F. hepatica* is medium sized (20-40 mm long by 10-15 mm wide at its widest), leaf-shape, greenish-brown, with a conic anterior end and lateral shoulders, and with branched ceca. The eggs are yellowish and large (130-150 by 65-90 um). It infects ruminants, pigs, equines, rabbits, humans, and many other mammals. Its life cycle is described under Biology.

*Fasciola gigantica* is more prevalent in tropical regions. It is similar to *F. hepatica* but longer (25-75 by 12 mm), with a smaller anterior cone and reduced shoulders, a longer esophagus and more

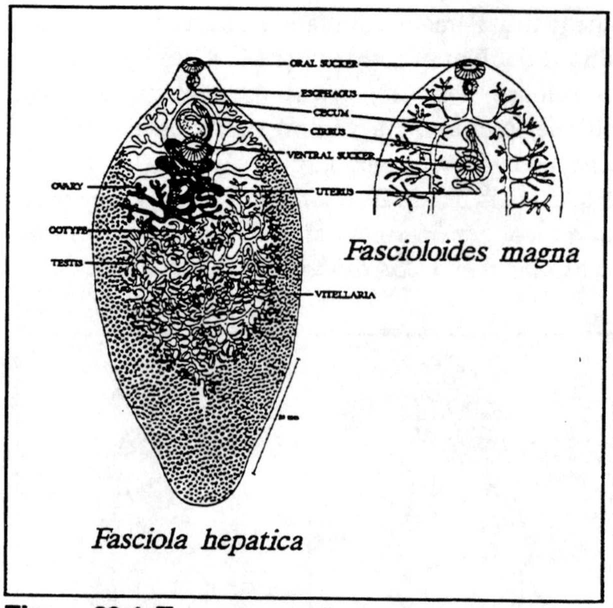


**Figure 23.4.** Two common liver flukes or ruminants.

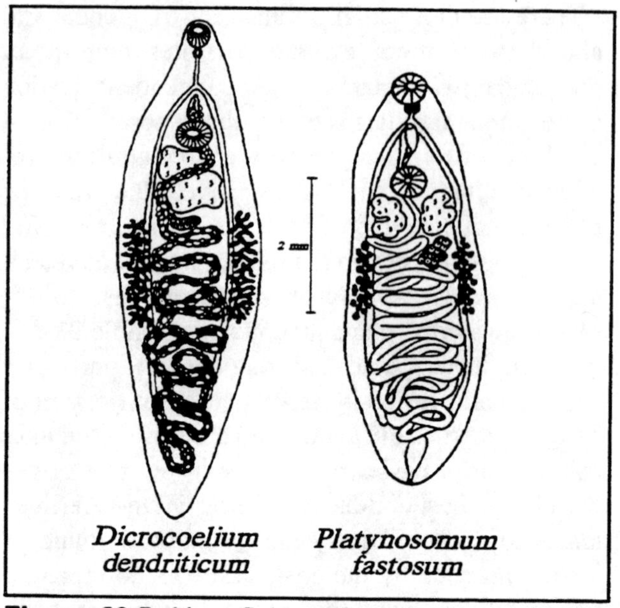


**Figure 23.5.** Liver flukes of ruminants and other hosts (*D. dendriticum*) and of carnivores (*P. fastosum*).

branched ceca, and larger eggs (155-200 by 90-105 um). The life cycle is like in *F. hepatica.*

*Fascioloides magna* is a parasite of wild ruminants that occurs in North America and Europe. It also infects domestic ruminants. It is large and fleshy (25-100 mm long, 11-26 wide, and 2-4 mm thick), oval, pinkish, and with large eggs . The life cycle is like in *F. hepatica* but it infects several genera of aquatic snails (*Lymnaea, Fossaria, Pseudosuccinea, Stagnicola*).

*Dicrocoelium dendriticum* is a widespread parasite of ruminants and, occasionally, pigs, dogs, rabbits, rodents, and man. It is small (< 10 mm long), lanceolate, with small, brown eggs (Figure 23.5). The miracidia develop inside the eggs until they are ingested by the first intermediate host, land snails of several genera (e.g., *Cionella, Zebrina*). The cercariae pass out in slime balls and are eaten by ants *Formica*. The ants with metacercariae in their hemocele are ingested by the definitive host while grazing.

**c. Lungs**

The only trematodes in the respiratory apparatus of ruminants are *Schistosoma nasalis* in the nasal veins of bovines, goat, and horses in India, and rarely *Paragonimus* sp. as an incidental parasite, and *F. hepatica* as an erratic parasite (see descriptions below).

**d. Blood**

*Schistosoma* spp. and *Ornithobilharzia* spp. are members of the family Schistosomatidae, the only trematodes of veterinary importance that have separated sexes. They are 5-25 mm long and live in the blood vessels of the host. The males are 1-2 mm wide, flattened, and with the lateral borders folded ventrally forming a groove to hold the female that is very thin and cylindrical (Figure 23.5). The eggs are 70-280 by 40-85 um, have no operculum, and frequently bear an apical spine. In *Schistosoma*, the males have 10 or fewer testes, and the females have the ovary in the anterior third of the body and a few eggs in the uterus. In *Ornithobilharzia*, the males have 30 or more testes, and the females have the ovary in the posterior half of the body and only one egg at a time in the uterus.

The miracidia infect different genera of aquatic snails, and the cercariae penetrates the skin of the definitive host without encysting previously. Several species of *Schistosoma* and *Ornithobilharzia* occur in ruminants in Africa and Asia.

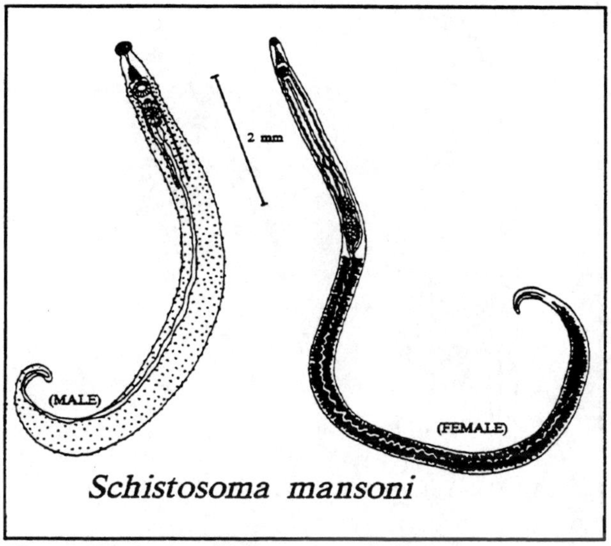


Figure 23.6. A schistosome of humans.

**B. Common trematodes of pigs**

**a. Digestive tube**

*Fasciolopsis buski* is a large and thick fluke of pigs and humans in the Far East. It is large (up to 75 by 20 mm), oval, and with unbranched ceca. The life cycle is like in *F. hepatica* but using *Segmentina* and *Hippeurus* snails.

**b. Liver**

Pigs are readily infected by *F. hepatica* or *D. dendriticum* (see above). *Clonorchis* (syn. *Opisthorchis*) *sinensis* is a small trematode of humans, pigs, and domestic carnivores in Asia. It is about 16 by 4 mm, elongated, translucent reddish, with small, yellowish brown eggs that have a distinct rim around the operculum . It uses several genera of aquatic snails as first intermediate host, and fish as second intermediate hosts.

**c. Lungs**

*Paragonimus* sp. affects pigs and other species. Because *Paragonimus* is of particular importance in domestic carnivores, it is described with the lung flukes of carnivores.

**d. Blood**

*Schistosoma incognitum* and *S. japonicum* occur in the mesenteric veins of pigs in Asia.

**C. Common trematodes of equines**

**a. Digestive tube**

The paramphistomes *Gastrodiscus* spp. and *Pseudodiscus* spp. occur in the colon of horses in Asia.

**b. Liver**

*Fasciola, Fascioloides* and *Dicrocoelium* (see above) can infect the liver of equines.

**c. Lungs**

*Schistosoma nasalis* (see above) is found in the nasal veins of horses in India.

**d. Blood**

*Schistosoma* spp. occur in the portal and mesenteric veins of equines in Africa and India, and in the nasal veins in India.

**D. Common trematodes of carnivores**

**a. Digestive tube**

*Alaria* spp. occur in the intestine of carnivores worldwide. They are small (< 10 mm long), with the anterior half of the body flat and wide, and the posterior half conical (Figure 23.7). The eggs are dark yellow and large (> 100 um). Mice, rats, snakes, and birds may act as paratenic hosts.

*Nanophyetus salmincola* is a very small, oval, whitish fluke of carnivores that occurs in the N.W. of the United States and the E. of Siberia (Figure 23.7). It is particularly important because it transmits the rickettsiae of Salmon poisoning and Elokomin fluke fever.

*Heterophyes heterophyes* is a very small (< 2 mm), pear-shaped trematode of the intestine of carnivores or humans in Asia, the Middle East, and adjacent countries of Europe. The eggs are small, light brown, thick shelled, and with a rim around the operculum.

*Cryptocotyle* spp. are tiny flukes (< 2 mm) of the intestine of aquatic birds and carnivores in North America, Europe, and Japan.

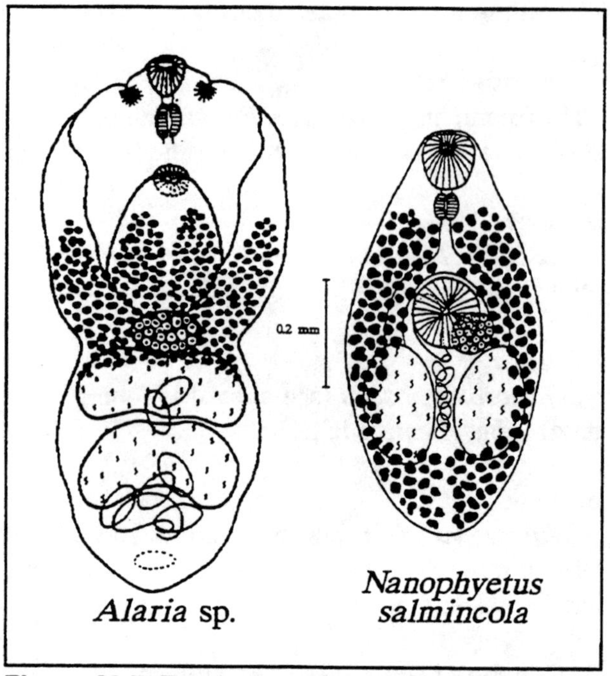


**Figure 23.7.** Two intestinal flukes of carnivores.

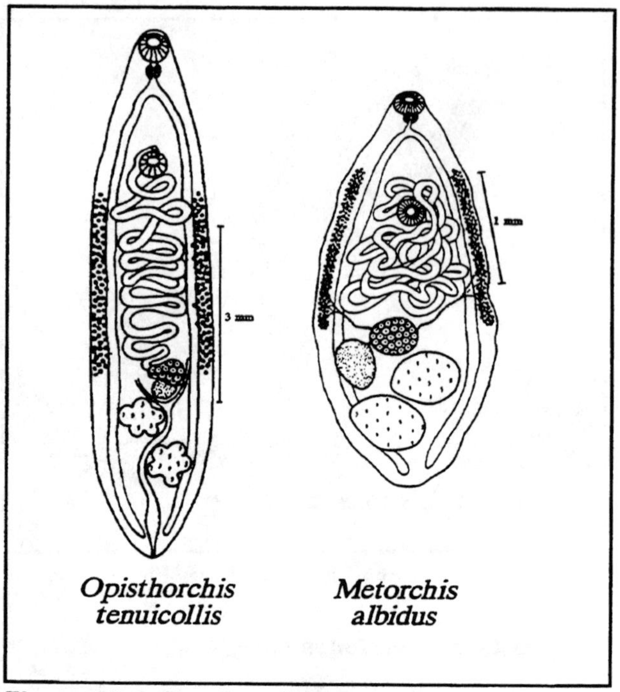


**Figure 23.8.** Two liver flukes of carnivores.

**b. Liver**

Several trematodes of the family Opisthorchiidae occur in the bile duct of carnivores. They are small (up to 12 by 2 mm), translucent reddish, lanceolate or oval, and with small, thick-walled, brown eggs which have a distinct rim around the operculum and are passed with a miracidium already formed. Species of *Opisthorchis* occur in Asia, Europe, and North America (Figure 23.8). The genera *Amphimerus, Metorchis,* and *Parametorchis* occur in North America.

*Platynosomum* (Figure 23.4) is common in Malaysia, Central and South America, the Caribbean, and Florida.

*Concinnum* is occasionally reported from the pancreatic and bile ducts of cats and wild carnivores in the United States.

**c. Lungs**

*Paragonimus* spp. are small (up to 16 by 8 mm), tick-bodied, reddish, oval flukes that live in pairs in the lungs of carnivores and other animals (including pigs and humans) in different parts of the world. Their eggs are rather large, yellowish brown, and with a rim around the operculum. *P. westermani* is the common species in Asia, and *P. kellicotti* occurs in North America (Figure 23.9). The life cycle involves aquatic snails (*Pomatiopsis* in the United States) and crabs or crayfish (the crayfish *Cambarus* in the United States).

**d. Blood**

*Schistosoma* spp. occur in the portal and mesenteric veins of dogs in Asia, and *Heterobilharzia* sp. in the mesenteric veins of wild and domestic carnivores in North America, along the coast of the Gulf of Mexico.

**E. Common trematodes of fowl**

**a. Digestive tube**

*Echinostoma* (Figure 23.10) and *Echinoparyphium* are cosmopolitan, narrow but fleshy flukes of the large or small intestine of chicken, ducks, and other birds. They are small (< 20 mm), with a collar of spines around the oral sucker.

*Notocotylus* are small flukes (< 5 mm) of the cecum and rectum of the fowl, duck, goose, and

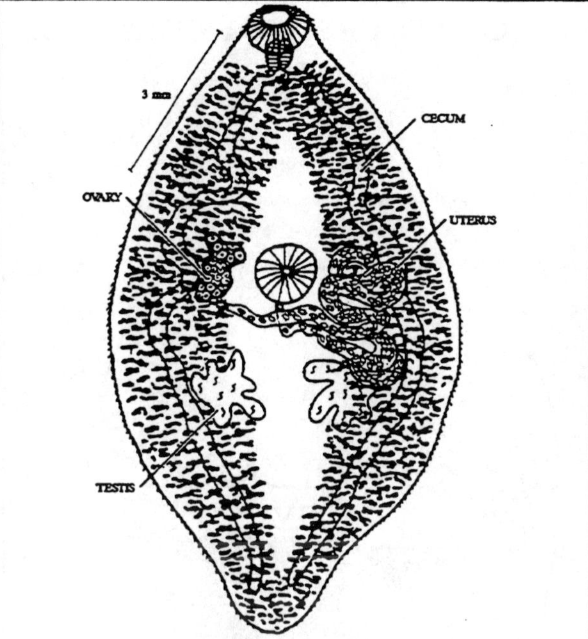


*Paragonimus kellicotti*

**Figure 23.9.** The American lung fluke of carnivores.

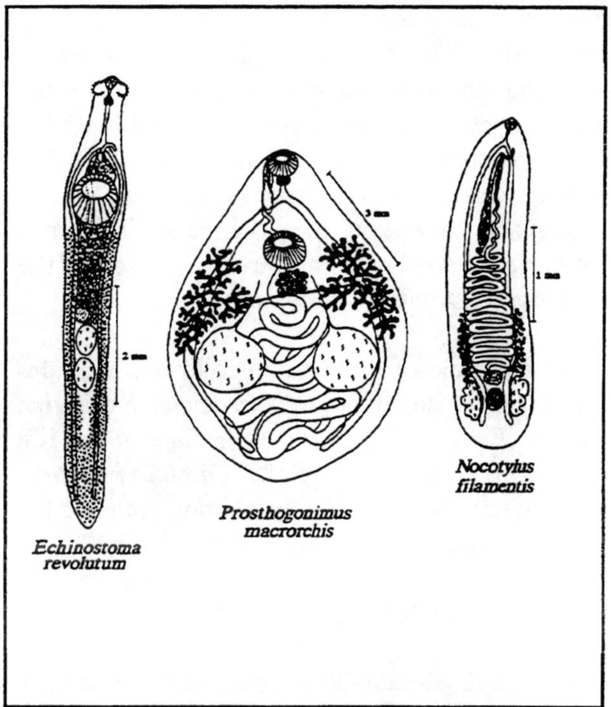


**Figure 23.10.** Some trematodes of fowl.

wild aquatic birds (Figure 23.10). They lack a ventral sucker and their small eggs (about 20 um long) are prolonged by a long filament at either pole.

*Prosthogonimus* spp. are parasites of the large intestine and urogenital system (see below).

**b. Urogenital ducts**

*Prosthogonimus* spp. are found in the bursa, oviduct and posterior intestine of the fowl, duck, and other birds. They are pear-shape, less than 10 mm long, and with small eggs (Figure 23.10).

**F. Common trematodes of humans**

**a. Digestive tube**

*Fasciolopsis buski* (see above) is a trematode primary of humans in the Far East.

A number of other flukes of domestic animals (*Opisthorchis, Echinostoma, Heterophyes,* etc) may also infect the intestine of humans.

**b. Liver**

Cases of infection with *Fasciola, Dicrocoelium,* and *Opisthorchis* are occasionally found in humans.

**c. Lungs**

*Paragonimus* sp. is encountered with some frequency in humans in the Far East, and rarely in other areas.

**d. Blood**

*Schistosoma japonicum* (in the Far East), *S. mansoni* (in Africa and tropical Latin America), and *S. haematobium* (in Africa and the Middle East) are primarily parasites of humans that can also infect other mammals.

**3. Biology**

Virtually all digenetic trematodes require a snail as a first intermediate host. This is so consistent that most authorities believe that the digenea were originally parasites of snails, and only later in evolution they invaded vertebrates.[6] In most species, the juvenile parasites that leave the snail encyst in a second intermediate host, often a fish. Some species encyst on aquatic plants (see table 23.II). The definitive host acquires the infection while feeding, and the fluke reaches adulthood in this host. As an exception, the juvenile schistosomes that leave the snail penetrate directly the skin of the definitive host without encysting.

The life cycle of the digenea follows a well defined pattern with only minor deviations in different species (Figure 23.11). We will discuss the life cycle of the common liver fluke, *Fasciola hepatica*, as a general model, and will mention some of the most common exceptions (see table 23.II).

### 3.1. Egg formation and maturation

The adult *F. hepatica* live in the bile ducts of their definitive host. The biflagellate sperms are deposited in the female genital apparatus through the cirrus which is inserted in the metraterm or Laurer's canal of the same or a different specimen. As the ova pass down the oviduct, they are fertilized by the sperms stored in the seminal receptacle, surrounded by vitelline cells contributed by the vitelline glands, and subjected to the secretion of the Mehlis' glands. This secretion lubricates the uterus for the passage of the eggs, forms a lipoprotein membrane (homologous with the vitelline membrane) around the vitelline cells, and stimulates sperm activity. The eggshell is formed by droplets of protein secretion from the vitellin cells that harden as the eggs pass down the uterus.

As compared to other parasites, trematodes lay comparatively few eggs: *Fasciola hepatica* produces 3000-3500 eggs per worm per day in cattle or sheep, *Opisthorchis viverrini* 900 in cats, and *Paragonimus kellicotti* 1000-2000 in cats. This is compensated, however, for the subsequent asexual multiplication in the first intermediate host.

The eggs of *F. hepatica* leave the host unembryonated and require humidity, oxygen, and

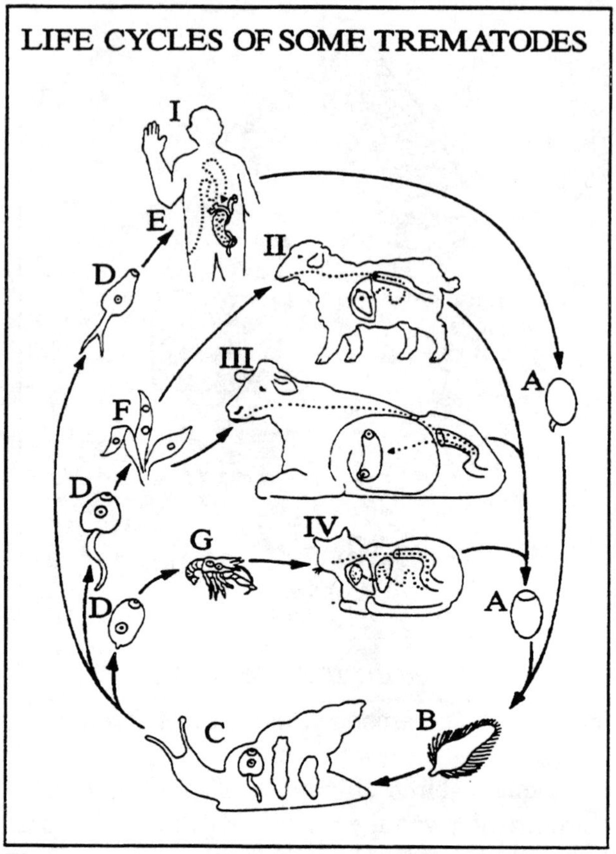


**Figure 23.11.** Life cycles of four representative trematodes. I; *Schistosoma*; II, *Fasciola*; III, *Paramphistomum*; IV, *Paragonimus*. A, egg; B, miracidium; C, stages in snail; D, cercaria, E, penetration in the host; F and G, metacercariae.

temperature to embryonate. They need to be immersed in water or in a water-saturate environment to develop but they will survive for a couple of months in feces with more than 60% water. Low oxygen tension does not kill the embryo but delays greatly the hatching of the eggs. Development occurs only between 10 and 30C (60 to 86F), hatching takes 2 or more months at 10C but only 8 days at 30C. Above 30C, development is inhibited. The eggs die in 24 days at 37C, and rapidly below the freezing point, particularly if they are embryonated. Under appropriate conditions, the ovum multiplies into a population of somatic cells and another of germ cells. The somatic cells form an oval embryo called **miracidium** (Figure 23.12) and the germ cells are preserved inside it. Hatching is stimulated by light which causes the miracidium to secrete substances that "unglue" the operculum, and push against it. Because the miracidium does not eat, it has only a few hours upon leaving the shell to swim around and find an appropriate snail before dying from exhaustion of its food reserves.

### 3.2. Development in the snail

A phase of asexual multiplication of pre-adult stages in a first intermediate host is very characteristic of the trematodes. This phenomenon is called **pedogenesis** (from Gr *paido*= child, juvenile, and Lat *genesis*= generation) and may compensate for the comparatively low fecundity of the adult flukes.

Location of the snail by the miracidium appears to occur by a combination of chemical attractants (in the snail mucus) and sheer luck. The miracidium contacts the snail by its apical papilla and penetrates it in about 30 minutes by a combination of mechanical boring and enzymatic dissolution of the snail tissues. Upon penetration, it loses its ciliated covering and becomes a sac-like organism with germ cells inside (**sporocyst**).

The sporocyst germ cells multiply into a population of somatic cells and new germ cells. The somatic cells originate 5 to 8 elongated embryos (**rediae**) that show parenchyma, muscles, an epithelium, a mouth, a simple intestine, nerve cells, an excretory system, a birth pore, and germ cells inside. When fully developed, the rediae escape from the sporocyst and invade the snail hepatopancreas. Depending on the number of infecting miracidia, the nutritional state of the snail, and the prevalent temperature, 30 to 350 rediae may occur inside a single snail.

The rediae germ cells, in turn, multiply to form a juvenile fluke with a tail (**cercaria**), and leave a remnant of germ cells that will form the genital apparatus of the adult fluke. The cercariae have the same organs as the adult fluke except a reproductive system. They also posses a number of cystogenous glands. From 10 to more than 2000 cercariae may be found in a single snail. Depending on the temperature, development of the cercariae may be completed in 3 to 7 weeks. Emergence of the cercariae appears to be caused by the physical activity of the snail which, in turn, is stimulated by fresh water, like that contributed by rains.

Multiplication of the flukes in the snail adds considerably to the biotic potential of the parasite. It has been calculated that a single miracidium of *F. hepatica* would generate about 320 cercariae, and experimental work has shown that each infected snail produces 418 cercariae as average. Depending on the number of parasites and the tissue damage produced during invasion, development, and emergence, the infected snail may die from the infection.

### 3.3. Encystment

The released cercariae swim around and, within 2 hours, attach to an aquatic plant by their ventral sucker, cast off their tails, and the cystogenous glands produce secretions that form a cyst shell around the cercaria. This encysted organism, about 0.2 mm in diameter, is called a **metacercaria**. They become infective for the definitive host in a couple of days. The survival of the metacercaria depends on the prevalent humidity and temperature. A relative humidity above 70% is necessary for prolonged survival. At 12-14C (53.6-57.2F), 100% of the metacercariae live for 6 months but only 5% for 10 months. Some may survive around the freezing point in winter, bu they die in hot, dry summers. They do not live more than 1 or 2 months in silage, and probably die promptly in dry hay. The longest survival reported in natural grasses is 9 to 11 months.

### 3.4. Development in the definitive host

When the metacercaria is ingested by an appropriate definitive host, the outer layers of the cyst are dissolved by the proteolytic enzymes of the host's digestive tract. The parasite, in turn, is activated by an adequate combination of temperature, low redox potential, $CO_2$, and bile to produce secretions that bore a hole in the inner layers. The exsheathed flukes eat their way through

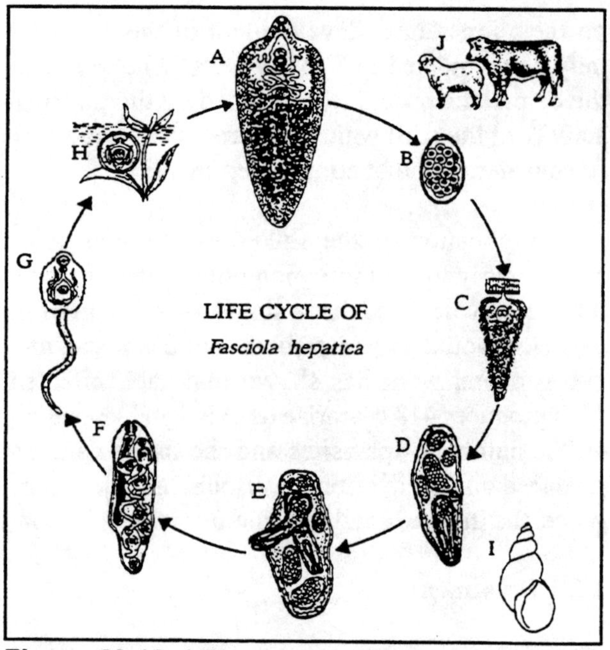


**Figure 23.12.** Life cycle of *Fasciola hepatica*. A, adult; B, egg; C, miracidium; D, sporocyst; E and F, first and second generation rediae; G, cercaria; H, metacercaria; I, *Lymnaea* snail (intermediate host); J, definitive hosts.

the intestinal wall and accumulate in the peritoneal cavity by the 3rd day. They seem to wander aimlessly around the abdominal cavity but many are seen eating their way into the liver parenchyma by the next day. At this time, the flukes are only 0.3 mm long. They keep tunneling into the organ and growing rapidly for 6 to 7 weeks, until they eventually penetrate the bile ducts. The flukes are 4 to 14 mm long and mature promptly at this time. The first eggs start appearing in the feces at 56 to 63 days of infection. The live span of adult trematodes in the definitive host is commonly counted in years. It is about 6 or more years for *F. hepatica* in sheep and may be longer for other trematodes in other hosts.

### 3.5. Variations in the life cycle

The life cycle of other species of trematodes may be somewhat different from that of *F. hepatica*. Some examples are listed in table 28.II. In some cases the eggs pass out already embryonated (e.g., *Dicrocoelium, Heterophyes, Opisthorchis, Platynosomum*), or may be eaten by the snail rather than invading it actively (e.g., *Cryptocotyle, Dicrocoelium, Methorchis, Notocotylus, Opisthorchis*). On occasions, the sporocyst forms a daughter or second generation sporocyst instead of rediae, or the rediae form a second generation of rediae. In most trematodes the cercariae encyst in a second intermediate host, either following ingestion by it, or after active penetration of its tissues. In the case of the schistosomes, the cercariae do not encyst but seek and penetrate the definitive host though the skin. Maturation of the cercariae to the infective stage can take from a few hours to a couple of weeks in different species.

There is little information on the development of the **intestinal trematodes** to the adult stage in the definitive host. In most cases, it appears that the metacercariae excyst in the intestine and the juveniles attach nearby and grow to adult in about a week. *Fasciolopsis* needs a longer time but it is not known to undergo migrations. In the cases studied, the young paramphistomes attach, sometimes very deeply, to the mucosa of the anterior part of the small intestine and remain there for 4 to 7 weeks. At this time, they initiate a migration to the rumen where they attach again and reach maturity at about 8 to 10 weeks of infection. *Alaria* is an exception to this pattern: the juveniles migrate through the peritoneal and pleural cavity, invade the lungs, reach the pharynx, and are swallowed to mature in the intestine. Transmammary (but not transplacental) transmission have been reported in *Alaria* infections of mice or cats.

Among the **liver trematodes**, many species reach the bile ducts through the common bile duct instead of the peritoneal cavity. *Fasciola* spp. and *Fascioloides*, however, wander through the peritoneal cavity and the liver parenchyma before reaching their adult location. The eggs leave with the bile and feces.

Among the **lung trematodes**, the only species important to veterinary medicine are *Paragonimus* spp (Figure 23.13). The juveniles excysted in the intestine penetrate the intestinal wall and wander in

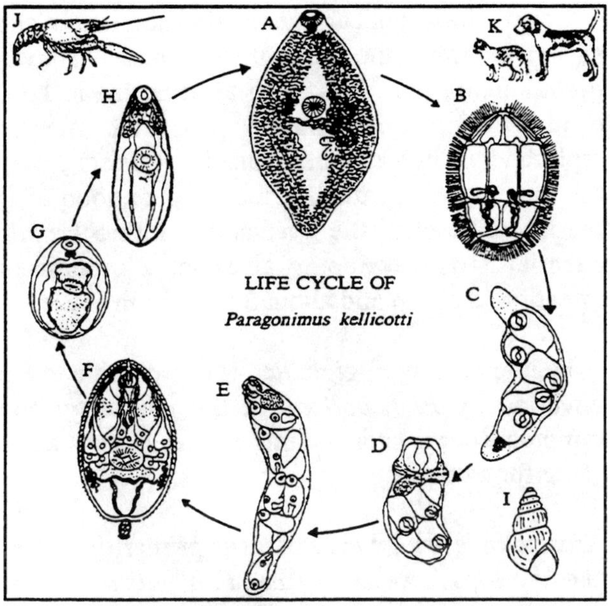


**Figure 23.13.** Life cycle of *Paragonimus kellicotti*. A, adult; B, miracidium; C, sporocyst; D and E, first and second generation rediae; F, cercaria; G, metacercaria; H, juvenile; I, *Pomatiopsis* snail (first intermediate host); J, *Cambarus* crayfish (second intermediate host); K, definitive hosts.

the peritoneal cavity for up to 2 weeks, then they go through the diaphragm and wander in the pleural cavity for a few days. Finally they enter the lung parenchyma and form a cyst near a bronchiole. Two worms are commonly found in each cyst. The eggs leave the lung by the bronchiole, are carried to the pharynx, swallowed, and pass out with the feces. Some eggs may remain in the lung or find their way to other organs.

The life cycle of all **blood trematodes** is supposed to be comparable to that of the schistosomes. The cercariae invade the skin of the definitive hosts, lose their tails, and are carried by the blood to the lungs. From there they are carried to the liver and are found in the portal vessels by the 8th day of infection. They form pairs in the portal vessels and move to their definitive location: the mesenteric veins in most species; vesical veins in *S. haematobium* of humans and *S. mattheei* of ruminants; and nasal veins in *S. nasale* of ruminants and equines. The eggs are deposited in the smallest veins close to the lumen of the respective organs. Many eggs work their way through the tissues to the lumen and then out but some remain in the tissues and form granulomas.

### 4. Medical importance

As a rule, trematodes are little pathogenic. Only in the case of intense infections they cause detectable symptoms in the host. Three major pathogenic mechanisms are claimed to explain the production of disease by trematodes: a) the movement of the worms in the host tissues and the suction of tissues into the suckers, both of which cause mechanical injury; b) the release of digestive enzymes outside the worm body which would cause inflammation and necrosis; and, c) the production of parasitic substances which are antigenic or toxic to the host. The last two mechanisms are largely speculative and have been verified only in a few cases.

The paramphistomes are an adequate example of **intestinal trematodes** which are alternatively pathogenic and apathogenic.[7] The preadult stages in the small intestine may cause severe disease whereas the adults in the rumen go generally unnoticed. Over 2,000 parasites in sheep and over 20,000 in cattle are necessary to produce fatal disease.

The activity of the juvenile paramphistomes in the intestinal mucosa causes superficial desquamation and necrosis, edema, hypertrophy of the mucosal glands, tracks of tissue destruction, congestion and hemorrhages around the parasites, and infiltration with mononuclear cells and a few eosinophils. The affected animals become progressively anorexic, the intestinal alterations interfere with the digestion and absorption, and the intestinal congestion and hemorrhages favor the loss of plasma proteins into the lumen which causes hypoproteinemia. As a result, the animals stop eating but drink water frequently, develop a fluid and fetid diarrhea that may contain blood and immature worms, lose condition and weight, and may develop a submandibular edema. The acute disease lasts about a week in small ruminants and 2 or 3 weeks in large ruminants. Mortality may be high (20 to 70%) and is attributed to starvation and pulmonary edema. Once the worms leave toward the rumen, reorganization of the submucosa and regeneration of the mucosa take place. Still, the survivors usually continue losing weight for a few weeks after recovery. For reasons unknown, clinical paramphistomiasis is rare in the United States.

The adult parasites are attached superficially to the epithelium and papillae of the rumen. Although the affected papillae appear anemic and atrophic, there are no signs of inflammation in the underlying tissues and the affected animals do no show symptoms of parasitism.

*Fascioliasis hepatica* is a common example of pathogenic **liver trematodes.**[8] In adult sheep, less than 100 flukes cause slight symptoms, about 200 to 700 cause chronic disease and deaths, about 700 to 1400 cause subacute disease and deaths, and larger numbers cause acute or peracute disease with many deaths. In cattle, about 600 flukes do not cause symptoms, about 1400 cause symptoms in 60% of the animals and an occasional death, and about 5000 cause lethal disease.

The penetration of the flukes through the intestinal wall and their migration in the peritoneal cavity does not result in symptoms, perhaps because the flukes are so small (< 300 μm) compared to the organs affected. Penetration in the liver, however, causes a traumatic hepatitis and points of hemorrhage that may be important in massive infections. The intrahepatic migration produces tortuous tracts that increase in size as the worms grow. Initially, the wall of the tracts show degenerate and necrotic hepatocytes and inflammatory cells, and the lumen is filled with fibrin, hepatocyte debris, blood, and inflammatory cells. Later in the infection, the tracts heal by fibrosis.

By the time that the flukes reach the bile ducts, extensive proliferation of the duct epithelium and fibrosis of the duct wall already started. The presence of the flukes in the ducts accelerates these changes and causes destruction and necrosis of the ductal wall with periductal inflammation that may extend to the surrounding parenchyma. Deposits of calcium in the hyperplastic ducts are characteristic of cattle fascioliasis.

Eosinophilia appears soon after infection and subsides after the migratory phase. Hyperglobulinemia (due mostly to an increase in IgG) occurs during the migratory phase but is soon replaced by a hypoalbuminemia that persists during the ductal phase. Jaundice may appear soon after the flukes reached the liver and a normochromic anemia starts developing at about 2 months of infection in sheep and about 3 months in cattle.

The infection by *F. gigantica* is comparable to the infection by *F. hepatica* but the pathology and symptoms occur later and this species is less pathogenic for cattle.

*Fascioloides magna* is a parasite primarily of deer that develops more slowly than *F. hepatica.* In deer, the flukes in the liver are enclosed in a thin fibrous cyst communicated with the bile ducts. In cattle, they are surrounded by a thick fibrous wall closed to the bile ducts that contains a black fluid. In sheep, the worms do not encysts and keep wandering in the liver causing extensive destruction.

*Dicrocoelium dendriticum* constitutes an example of the liver trematodes that reach the bile duct through the common duct. No traumatic hepatitis occurs in these cases but inflammation and fibrosis in the region of the portal triads is common and may extend to the liver parenchyma causing extensive cirrhosis. Although less severe than in fascioliasis *hepatica*, hyperplasia, fibrosis, and inflammation of the ducts occupied by the flukes may occur in intense infections.

The **lung trematodes**, *Paragonimus* spp., cause some traumatic injury and neutrophilic-eosinophilic inflammation during their migration to their final location, but without clinical expression. Once in the lungs, the flukes produce infarction and postinflamatory necrosis that cause the formation of a cavity in the organ. This cavity is soon walled by abundant connective tissue that forms a cysts around the parasites. Eggs are often found in the neighborhood of the flukes where they induce eosinophilic granulomatous reactions. Many pulmonary cases go clinically unnoticed but severe infections may result in chronic, intermittent cough with blood in the sputum, and, eventually, weakness and lethargy. *P. westermani* in humans (and presumably other species in other hosts) may migrate to the brain, and its eggs may spread by the circulation to other organs.[9,10]

The major pathogenic mechanism of the **blood trematodes** is the formation of chronic, granulomatous inflammations associated with the presence of eggs in the tissues. Infected animals develop multiple micro-abscesses at the location of the eggs. In severe intestinal infections, hemorrhagic enteritis, anemia, and emaciation are common. In severe nasal infections, purulent discharge, snoring, and dyspnea may occur. Animals with an acute enteric disease may die or develop a chronic disease. The nasal infection is usually chronic. Long standing infections cause the formation of abundant fibrous tissue. In humans, who have a longer life span than domestic animals, fibrosis of the liver is a major complication.

## REFERENCES


1. Soulsby, E.J.L. 1982. *Helminths, Arthropods and Protozoa of Domesticated Animals,* 7th ed.,Lea & Febiger, Philadelphia, 809 pp.

2. Schell, S.C. 1985. *Handbook of Trematodes of North America North of Mexico.* University Press of Idaho, Moscow, Idaho, 263 pp.

3. Yamaguti, S. 1958. *Systema Helminthum.* Vol I. *The Digenetic Trematodes of Vertebrates*, parts 1 and 2. Interscience Publishers, New York. 1554 pp.

4. Skrjabin, K.I. 1964. *Keys to the Trematodes of Animals and Man.* Translated from the Russian by H.P. Arai and R.W. Dooley. U. of Illinois Press, Urbana, Illinois, 351 pp.

5. Dawes, B. 1946. *The trematoda.* University Press, Cambridge, 644 pp.

6. Pearson, J.C. 1972. A phylogeny of life-cycles on the digenea. Adv. Parasit. 10:153-189.

7. Horak, I.G. 1971. Paramphistomiasis of domestic ruminants. Adv. Parasit. 9:33-72.

8. Sinclair, K.B. 1967. Pathogenesis of *Fasciola* and other liver flukes. Helm. Abstr. 36:115-134.

9. Yokogawa, M. 1965. *Paragonimus* and Paragonimiasis. Adv. Parasit. 3:99-158.

10. Yokogawa, M. 1969. *Paragonimus* and Paragonimiasis. Adv. Parasit. 7:375-387.

## TABLE 23.I. SOME FAMILIES AND GENERA OF TREMATODA OF VETERINARY IMPORTANCE

**1. Family Schistosomatidae**: small trematodes with separate sexes; males with a gynecophoric canal; non-operculated eggs, often with spine; parasites of the blood vessels of mammals or birds.
Genus *Schistosoma*: males with 10 or fewer testes; females with ovary in the anterior third of the body and a few eggs in the uterus,
Genus *Ornithobilharzia*: males with 30 or more testes; females with ovary in the posterior half of the body and only one egg at a time in the uterus.

**2. Family Notocotylidae**: small trematodes with tongue-like bodies and without a ventral sucker; testes parallel and ovary intertesticular, all at the posterior end of the body; eggs with long bipolar filaments, pass embryonated; parasites of the intestine.
Genus *Notocotylus*: 3 longitudinal rows of glands on ventral surface of body

**3. Family Paramphistomidae**: thick, pear-shaped trematodes with the ventral sucker at the posterior end; testes tandem or oblique; ovary posttesticular; non-spinous tegument; parasites of the intestine.
Genus *Cotylophoron*: with a muscular sucker enclosing the genital pore,
Genus *Paramphistomum*: no muscular sucker enclosing the genital pore.

**4. Family Diplostomidae**: anterior half of the body flat or spoon-shaped; posterior half cylindrical and containing the reproductive organs; parasites of the intestine.
Genus *Alaria*.

**5. Family Dicrocoelidae**: tongue-like, translucent trematodes; ventral sucker, testes and ovary in anterior half of the body; ovary posttesticular; eggs pass embryonated; parasites of the bile or pancreatic ducts,
Genus *Concinnum*: solid, parallel testes,
Genus *Platynosomum*: lobed, parallel testes,
Genus *Dicrocoelium*: slightly lobed, tandem testes.

**6. Family Heterophydae**: small but tick trematodes; spinous tegument; testes and ovary in posterior half of the body; ovary posttesticular; eggs pass embryonated; parasites of the intestine,
Genus *Apophallus*: solid, oblique testes; vitellaria in the posterior half of the body, long esophagus
Genus *Cryptocotyle*: lobed, oblique testes; vitellaria extending to anterior half of body,
Genus *Heterophyes*: solid, parallel testes; vitellaria in the posterior half of the body,

**7. Family Fasciolidae**: medium to large trematodes with flat, leaf-shape bodies; branched testes and ovary; ventral sucker in anterior fifth of the body; parasites of bile ducts or small intestine,
Genus *Fasciola*: medium size (15-30 mm) and thin; branched ceca; anterior end of the body ends in conical projection; suckers of comparable size; in bile ducts,
Genus *Fascioloides*: large size (> 30 mm) and thick; branched ceca; anterior end of the body rounded: in liver,
Genus *Fasciolopsis*: large (> 30 mm) and thick; non-branched ceca; ventral sucker much larger than oral sucker.

**TABLE 23.I. SOME FAMILIES AND GENERA OF TREMATODA OF VETERINARY IMPORTANCE**
(continuation)

**8. Family Opisthorchidae**: trematodes with flat, elongated, translucent bodies; testes and ovary in the posterior half of the body; ovary pretesticular; eggs pass embryonated; parasites of bile ducts or small intestine,
Genus *Clonorchis*: branched, tandem testes; vitellaria in middle third of the body,
Genus *Metorchis*: solid, oblique testes; vitellaria in the anterior half of the body,
Genus *Opisthorchis*: lobed, oblique testes; vitellaria in middle third of the body.

**9. Family Paragonimidae**: trematodes with oval, thick bodies; spinous tegument; lobed, parallel testes; lobed ovary on one side of the body; pretesticular uterus on the opposite side; abundant vitellaria all along the ceca; parasites of the lungs.
Genus *Paragonimus*.

**10. Family Nanophyetidae**: small (1 mm) but thick body; non-spinous tegument; vitellaria fill the sides and posterior part of the body; parasites of the small intestine.
Genus *Nanophyetus*.

**11. Family Prosthogonimidae**: small trematodes with spinous tegument; parallel testes in the middle of the body; lobed, pretesticular ovary; vitellaria in the anterior half of the body; eggs pass embryonated; parasites of the cloaca and oviduct of birds or the liver of mammals.
Genus *Prosthogonimus*.

**12. Family Opisthorchiidae**: small, oval or elongated trematodes with a translucent body; testes in the posterior part of the body; ovary pretesticular; vitellaria in a narrow band lateral to the ceca; small eggs with a rim around the operculum and an embryo when passed; parasites of the liver ducts.
Genus *Metorchis*: oval body; ovoid, oblique testes; vitellaria in anterior part of body,
Genus *Parametorchis*: oval body, lobed, oblique testes; vitellaria in anterior part of body,
Genus *Clonorchis*: body tapering anteriorly; branched, tandem testes; vitellaria in middle part of body,
Genus *Amphimerus*: very narrow tapering body; oval, tandem testes, vitellaria interrupted at the ovary,
Genus *Opisthorchis*: body evenly elongated; lobed, oblique testes; middle body, non-interrupted vitellaria.

**TABLE 23.II. CHARACTERISTICS OF SOME COMMON TREMATODES**

| GENERA | EGGS (µm)* | 1st INT. HOST | STAGES* | 2nd INT. HOST | IN THE DEFINITIVE HOST | | | PREPATENCY (days) |
|---|---|---|---|---|---|---|---|---|
| | | | | | MIGRATION | LOCATION | SIZE(mm) | |
| *Alaria* | 106-134x 64-99 | Aquatic snail *Helisoma* | Sp1-Sp2-Ce | tadpoles | peritoneal & thoracic cavity | small intestine | 3-6x 0.7-1.0 | 10 |
| *Apophalus* | 35-40x 19-24 | Aquatic snail *Flumenicola* | Sp-Re-Ce | Cyprinidae fish | none | small intestine | 0.5-1.0x 0.2-0.2 | 8 |
| Concinnum | 52-59x 33-38 | Land snail *Mesodon* | Sp1-Sp2-Ce | arthropod? | common bile duct? | pancreatic & bile ducts | 2.6-3.3x 1.1-1.4 | 50? |
| *Cryptocotyle* | 30-50x 16-25 | Marine snails | Sp-Re-Ce | marine fish | none | small intestine | 0.5-2.0x 0.2-0.9 | 10? |
| *Dicrocoelium* | 36-45x 22-30(E) | Land snail *Cionella*, etc | Sp1-Sp2-Ce | ants *Formica* | common bile duct | bile ducts | 6-10x 1.5-2.5 | 44-77 |
| *Echinostoma* | 90-125x 60-70 | Several aquatic snails | Sp-Re1-Re2-Ce | snails & frogs | none | small intestine | 5-20x 0.5-2.0 | 15-20 |
| Eurytrema | 50-60x 33-38 | Land snail *Bradibaena*, etc | Sp1-Sp2-Ce | orthoptera insects | pancreatic duct | pancreatic & bile ducts | 8-16x 5-8.5 | 80-100 |
| *Fasciola* | 130-200x 63-105 | Aquatic snail *Lymnaea* | Sp-Re-Ce | encysts on plants | peritoneal cavity | bile ducts | 15-75x 10-15 | 56-90 |
| *Fascioloides* | 110-170x 75-100 | Aquatic snail *Lymnaea*, etc | Sp-Re-Ce | encysts on plants | peritoneal cavity | bile ducts | 25-100x 10-30 | 210-225 |
| *Fasciolopsis* | 125-140x 70-90 | Aquatic snail *Segmentina*, etc | Sp-Re-Ce | encysts on plants | none | small intestine | 30-75x 8-20 | 30-90 |

(*) Ce = cercariae; E = eggs embryonated when passed; R = eggs with distinct rim around operculum; Re = rediae; Sp = sporocyst; numerals 1 and 2 indicate generations, e. g., Re1 = first generation of rediae, Re2 = second generation of rediae.

**TABLE 23.II. CHARACTERISTICS OF SOME COMMON TREMATODES (continuation)**

| GENERA | EGGS (µm)* | 1st INT. HOST | STAGES* | 2nd INT. HOST | IN THE DEFINITIVE HOST MIGRATION | LOCATION | SIZE(mm) | PREPATENCY (days) |
|---|---|---|---|---|---|---|---|---|
| *Heterophyes* | 26-30x 15-17(E,R) | Aquatic snail *Pironella*, etc | Sp-Re-Ce | several fish | none | small intestine | 1-2x 0.3-0.7 | 9 |
| *Metorchis* | 22-32x 11-18 | Aquatic snail *Amnicola* | Sp-Re-Ce | Cyprinidae fish | common bile buct | bile duct | 2.5-6.0x 1.0-1.5 | 28-35 |
| Nanophyetus | 64-97x 34-55 | Aquatic snail *Oxytrema*, etc | Re1-Re2-Ce | Salmonidae & other fish | none | small intestine | 0.1-2.5x 0.3-0.5 | 5-8 |
| *Notocotylus* | 20x12 | Aquatic snails *Stagnicola* | Sp-Re1-Re2-Ce | encysts on plants | none | cecum and rectum | 2-5x 0.6-1.5 | 22-70 |
| *Opisthorchis* | 26-35x 11-20(E,R) | Aquatic snail *Bithynia*, etc | Sp1-Sp2-Ce | Cyprinidae & other fish | common bile duct | bile & pancreatic duct, intestine | 6-8x 1-5 | 16-28 |
| *Paragonimus* | 75-120x 42-67(R) | Aquatic snail *Pomatiopsis*, etc | Sp-Re1-Re2-Ce | crayfish and crabs | peritoneal & thoracic cavity | lungs | 7.5-16x 4-8 | 56-150 |
| Paramphistomes | 114-176x 73-100 | Several aquatic snails | Sp-Re1-Re2-Ce | encysts on plants | small intestine | rumen | 8-13x 2-5 | 56-71 |
| *Platynosomum* | 34-50x 20-35(E) | Aquatic snail *Sublima* | Sp-Re-Ce | lizards | common bile duct | bile ducts | 4-8x 1.5-2.5 | 84 |
| *Prosthogonimus* | 22-32x 10-15 | Aquatic snails | Sp1-Sp2-Ce | nymphs of dragonflies | none | post. intestine, bursa, oviduct | 6-8x 1-5 | 7-20 |
| *Schistosoma* | variable | Several aquatic snails | Sp1-Sp2-Ce | none, cercarial penetration | skin, lungs, liver, veins | portal, mesenteric, nasal, or vesical veins | 5-22x 1-2 | 20-70 |

(*) Ce = cercariae; E = eggs embryonated when passed; R = eggs with distinct rim around operculum; Re = rediae; Sp = sporocyst; numerals 1 and 2 indicate generations, e. g., Re1 = first generation of rediae, Re2 = second generation of rediae.

# Chapter 24

# THE CLASS CESTODA OR TAPEWORMS

**Preview.** The Cestodes or Tapeworms of domestic animals or humans are narrow, flat, and commonly long parasites of the small intestine. All have complicated life cycles involving one, or sometimes two, intermediate hosts. The larval stages in mammals are usually vesicles of variable size located in diverse tissues. Although as a rule the adults in the intestine are little pathogenic, the larvae in the tissues may cause serious disease depending on their number or location.

## 1. Morphology

### 1.1. The adult parasite

The **Tapeworms** are elongated, narrow, and flat organisms, well deserving of their common name. The adult stages measure from a few milimeters to several meters in length and consist of three major parts: scolex, neck, and strobila (Figure 24.1).

The **scolex** is the anterior part of the worm that serves for adhesion to the host and locomotion (this latter, by offering an anchoring point toward which the entire worm can progress). To this purpose, it may bear **suckers** or **hooks**. In the species of veterinary importance, the suckers are four cup-like structures (**acetabula**) or a pair of elongated grooves (**bothria**). The hooks are disposed in one or more circles around an apical evaginable appendix called **rostellum**. The rostellum and hooks must not be very important to adhesion because they are missing in several quite successful species. The scolex is often called "head" but it lacks all the structures commonly associated with a head (mouth and organs of the senses). The name "holdfast" has been proposed but it is not common.

The **neck** is the portion between the scolex and the first segmentation of the strobila (see below). It may be from fairly long to almost indistinguishable short. It contains embryonary cells that constantly form new segments for the strobila.

The **strobila**, also called body or chain, is the rest of the tapeworm. It is formed by segments called **proglottides** (sing. **proglottis**) that are constantly being formed by the neck. They are pushed backwards and mature as new proglottides are produced. The newly formed proglottis (**inmature**) is barely more than a set of germinal cells enclosed in an envelop of somatic cells. As the proglottis tissues differentiate, these cells form the genital apparatuses and a few other organs, and the segment becomes a **mature** proglottis. After fertilization, virtually all the structures regress and the proglottis (now called **gravid**) becomes a sac full of eggs. By the time the eggs are formed, the gravid proglottides have moved to the posterior end of the tape

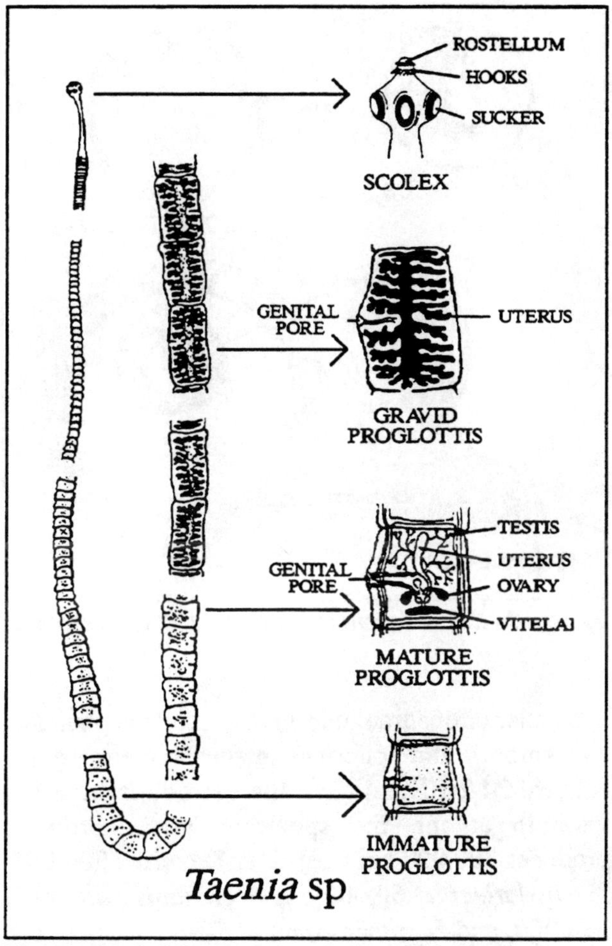


**Figure 24.1**. Morphology of a taenid cestode.

worm and are released from the strobila, or desintegrate. Most tapeworms have many proglottides. The smallest is *Echinococcus granulosus* with only 3, and the largest *Diphyllobothrium latum* with about 4,000.

The body covering of the cestodes is a **tegumentum** similar to that of the digeneic trematodes. Its surface coat is rich in carbohydrates and has a turnover rate of 6-8 hours. Because the cestodes do not posses distinct digestive, respiratory, or circulatory systems, all the corresponding functions are fulfilled by transport through the tegumentum. The bulk of the body is made of a mesenchymatic tissue (called **parenchyma**) in which bundles of longitudinal muscles, calcareous corpuscles (5-35 μm in diameter), and the organs are embedded.

The nervous system is formed by paired ganglia in the scolex, connected by trasversal comisures. These ganglia produce two longitudinal cords that run along the lateral borders of the stobila and are connected by comisures in each proglottis. The excretory system consists of a number of flame cells that take the excess fluid from the tissues and discharge it into a system of collecting vessels that run the length of the strobila.

All cestodes are hermaphrodites. The masculine organs mature and regress earlier than the femenine organs in a same progrotis. The **masculine genital apparatus** consists of one to many testes that discharge into a single vas deferens. At its distal end, the vas deferens often becomes muscular to form an evaginable copulatory organ, the cirrus. The cirrus is commonly enclosed in a sheath (cirrus pouch) and opens outside through a genital pore. During copulation, the cirrus introduces the sperm into the vagina of the same or a different proglottis, which also opens in the genital pore.

The activity center of the **feminine genital apparatus** is the ootype. It is a cavity surrounded by unicellular glands (Mehlis' gland) and connected by ducts to the ovary, vagina, vitelline glands, and uterus. Its function is to form the eggs. Each proglottis has a single ovary that may vary in size, shape, and location. The ovary produces the ova that are discharged into the ootype. The vagina is a duct that runs from the genital pore to the ootype. It carries the sperm and often has a seminal receptacle along its course. The vitelline glands are cells distributed in a single compact mass (vitellarium) or in scattered follicles. They contribute cells that provide the yolk and materials for the eggshell. The Mehlis' gland also supplies materials for the eggshell. Once formed, the eggs pass and accumulate inside the uterus.

In some groups, the uterus of the gravid proglottis becomes a sac filled with eggs (e.g., *Taenia* spp.); in others the uterus disappears and the eggs, single or in groups, are enclosed in hyaline egg capsules embedded in the parenchyma (e.g., *Dipylidium*); in still other groups the uterus develops a fibro-mus

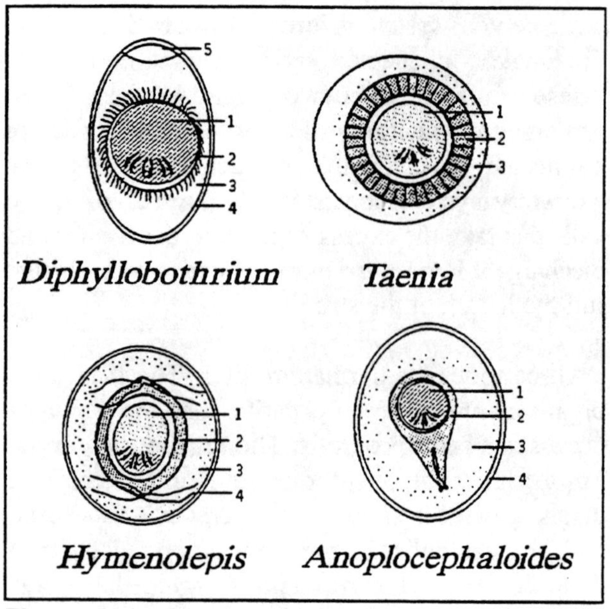


**Figure 24.2.** Common egg types in the cestodes.

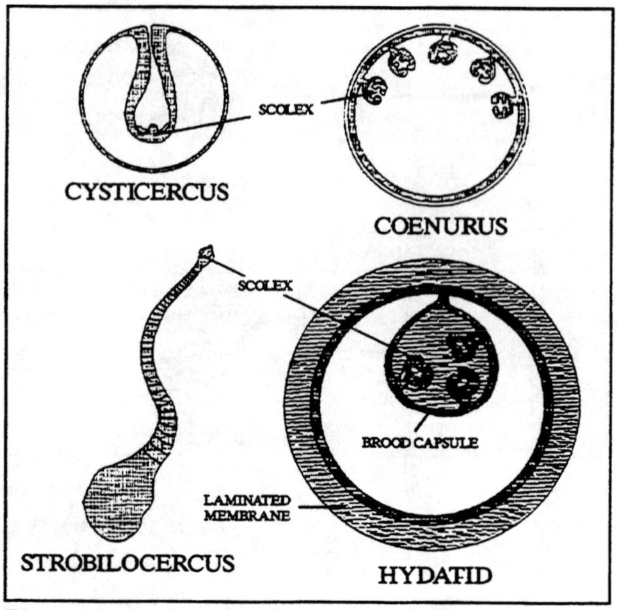


**Figure 24.3.** Common larva types in the cestodes.

cular hollow structure (the parauterine organ) that receives the eggs as the uterus degenerates (e.g., *Thysanosoma*). In some species, the eggs leave the proglottides through a preformed uterine pore (e.g., *Diphyllobothrium*). In others, the complete gravid proglottis explotes releasing the eggs into the intestine (e.g., *Hymenolepis*). In still others, the last proglottides detach from the strobila and pass out with the feces to desiccate and release the eggs in the external environment (e.g., *Taenia, Echinococcus*).

The mature cestode egg contains a multicellular embryo (**oncosphere** or hexacanth) that bears 6 hooks and is surrounded by 3 membranes. The hexacanth hooks are lost during infection and have no relationship with the rostellar hooks. The inermost membrane is called the embryophore. It is ciliated in the Pseudophyllidea, thick and made up of brick-like blocks in the Taenidae, pear-shaped in the Anoplocephalidae (where is called the "pyriform apparatus"), and smooth and spherical in the Hymenolepidae. The middle membrane is thick and semi-transparent. In the Taenidae, this layer is lost in the intestine. The outermost membrane is the capsule or shell. It is oval and operculate in the Pseudophyllidea, absent in the Taenidae, thick and triangular or quadrangular in the Anoplocephalidae, and smooth and spherical in the Hymenolepidae (Figure 24.2). Fertility in the cestode is high but variable among the species: *Taenia saginata* produces 700,000 eggs per day, *T. solium* 300,000, *T. hydatigena* 60,000, *Hymenolepis diminuta* 250,000, and *H. microstoma* 46,000.

### 1.2. The larval stages

The larval stage of the tapeworms is commonly called a **metacestode**. The scolex of the metacestode (which eventually will become the scolex of the adult tapeworm) is customarily called **protoscolex**. Four types of metacestodes are commonly found in mammals: cysticercus, strobilocercus, coenurus, and hydatid (Figure 24.3).

The **cysticercus** is a thin-walled vesicle filled with fluid that encloses a single invaginated scolex with its neck. It is commonly the size of a pea or smaller. The **strobilocercus** is similar to the cysticercus but bears an inmature strobila. The **coenurus** is a larger vesicle that contains several invaginated scoleces that arise individually from different points of its wall. It may grow up to the size of an apple. The **hydatid** is also a large vesicle that produces internal brood capsules which, in turn, originate internal, invaginated scoleces. Very characteristically, its wall has a laminated external layer. The hydatid grows slowly but it can reach the size of an apple or larger. A fifth type of metacestode that may require identification by a veterinarian is the **plerocercoide** of *Diphyllobotrium* spp. This is a white, 5-20 mm long larvae, with an pseudosegmented body, and a scolex similar to that on the adult (see Figure 24.13). It is found in the viscera or muscles of fish.

Other larval forms unlikely to be found by a practitioner are the cysticercoid, procercoid, and tetrathyridia. The **cysticercoid** consists of an almost solid vesicle with a solid tail, that contains an evaginated scolex. It occurs in invertebrates. The **procercoid** is a solid larvae with a spherical tail that bears the hooks of the oncosphere. It is the first larval stage of the Pseudophyllidae and is found in copepods. The **tetrathyridium** resembles an elongated plerocercoid but it bears an invaginated scolex with four acetabula. It is the second larval stage of *Mesocestoides* and is found in amphibia and reptiles, and occasionally in birds and mammals.

The life span of some representative cestodes is shown in Table 24.I..

## 2. Identification and classification

The adult cestodes of domestic animals or humans are easy to identify for their presence in the intestinal tract or associated ducts, their typical segmentation, and the presence of a scolex. In the large to medium-size species, the segmentation is well-evident to the naked eye. In the minute species (v.g., *Echinococcus granulosus, Hymenolepis nana, Davainea proglottina*), verification of the segmentation may required more careful examination but it is also unequivocal. The identification of genera and species will be discussed with the taxomony.

The larval cestodes of domestic animals or humans are also easy to identify because they constitute vesicles of variable sizes and typical morphology (see below). The cysticerci located in muscle or peritoneum may escape detection, however, when they are hidden among the tissue fat. Many larval cestodes were given independent scientific names before the relationship between the adult and the larva stages was known. Although we know better now, it is still common to use the old latin names for the larvae.

The classification of the cestodes is still object of controversy (for example, see Skrjabin et al.[1], Yamaguti[2], and Wardle et al.[3]). We will follow the ideas of Schmid[4] because they permit an easier identification of the worms, and this is the primary interest of the veterinary practitioner. The 4000 to 5000 cestodes currently described are distributed into 13 orders, but only the Cyclophyllidea and Pseudophyllidea contain species of veterinary importance. The **Cyclophyllidea** have 4 acetabula on the scolex, a compact vitellaria posterior to the ovary, no uterine pore, and produce non-operculated eggs. The **Pseudophyllidea** have 2 bothria on the scolex, scattered follicular vitellaria, a uterine pore, and produce operculated eggs.

**The order Cyclophyllidea** contains 13 families but only 6 contain parasites of veterinary importance:

### 2.1. Family Mesocestoididae

The only genus, *Mesocestoides*, contains many species of questionable validity. They are medium to large, narrow cestodes without rostellum or hooks but with well developed acetabula. The uterus is shaped as a sinous tube first but later develops a posterior parauterin organ. The genital pore open in the midventral line. This genus is easy to identify because it is the only of the common cestodes of veterinary importance that has acetabula *and* a ventral genital pore. They are parasites of predaceous birds or mammals.

♦ *M. corti* is found occasionally in domestic carnivores in North America and *M. lineatus* in Europe, Asia, and Africa. Either species has been reported from humans on a few occasions.

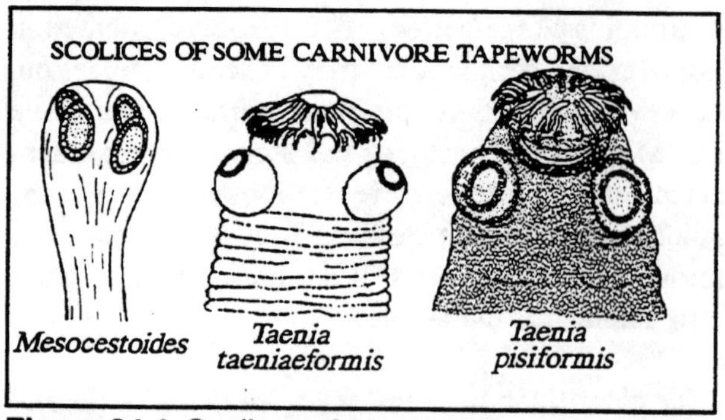


**Figure 24.4.** Scolices of some common cestodes of carnivores.

They may be up to 250 mm long by 0.3 cm wide. The eggs are 40-60x35-43 um, oval, with a pole thicker than the other, a thin middle membrane, and no outer membrane. This genus requires two intermediate hosts: the first is believed to be an oribatid mite or a beetle, the second is an amphibia, reptile, bird, or small mammal. The stage in the second intermediate host is a tetrathyridium which can multiply asexually (in the peritoneum, liver, or lungs) and produce massive infections. The final host is infected by ingestion of the intermediate host. Prepatency in dogs is at least 16 days.

### 2.2. Family Taenidae

The Taenidae is the largest and most important family of cestodes. It consists of large worms (except *Echinococcus* spp.) with a non-retractable rostellum bearing two rows of hooks (except *T. saginata*). They have a single set of genitalia with the genital pores on the border of the proglotis and alternating irregularly, numerous testes, and an ovary posterior. The inmature proglottides are wider than longer, the mature ones are roughly quadrangular, and the gravid progglotides are longer than wider. The gravid uterus is a tube along the center of the progglotis with lateral branches. The eggs are round or oval, about 30-40 um in diameter. The middle membrane is thick and radiated, and the outher membrane is often lost before observation. The larval stage is a cysticercus, strobilocercus, coenurus, or hydatid. The intermediate hosts of Taenidae are prey mammals whereas the definitive hosts are predaceous mammals.

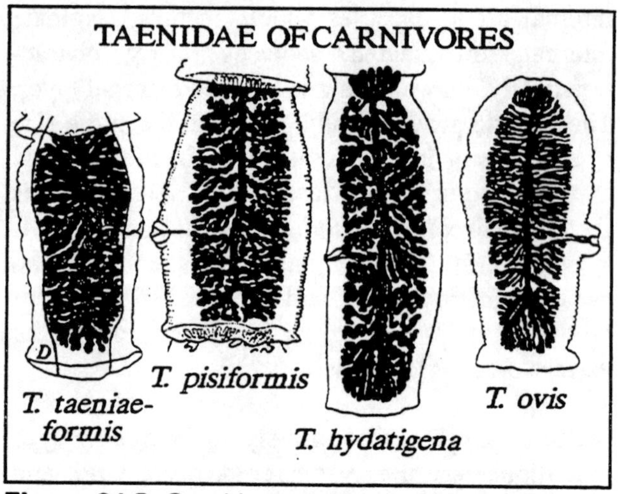


**Figure 24.5.** Gravid proglottides of some common cestodes of carnivores.

This family used to contain 5 genera of veterinary importance: *Taenia, Taeniarhynchus, Multiceps, Hydatigera,* and *Echinococcus*, but the first four are now assigned to the genus *Taenia*. Abuladze[5] lists 96 species and Schmidt[3] 108 species among these genera. The most common cosmopolitan, or nearly cosmopolitan, species of veterinary concern are the following:

♦ *Taenia pisiformis*. It is a large cestode of dogs and other canids, particularly coyotes. It is rarely found in cats (Figures 24.4 and 24.5). It most noticiable characteristic is the large size of the hooks of the first row on the rostellum . The proglottides are trapezoidal which gives the strobila a serrate appearance. The larvae is a cysticercus (*Cysticercus pisiformis*, from Lat *pissum*= pea, and *formis*= shape) about 6-13x4-6 mm found in the liver and peritoneal cavity of lagomorphs.

♦ *Taenia hydatigena*. It is possibly the largest cestode of dogs and other canids (Figure 24.5). The larva is a cysticercus (*C. tenuicollis*) from 0.5 to 5 cm in diameter, with a thin wall, and a protoscolex with a long neck. It is found in the liver or peritoneum of sheep, goat, and occasionally other ruminants or pig.

♦ *Taenia ovis*. It is a large cestode of dogs and other canids (Figure 24.5). The larva is a cysticercus (*C. ovis*) about 4-7x2-4 mm found in the muscles of sheep and goats.

♦ *Taenia* (syn. *Hydatigera*) *taeniaeformis*. It is a medium size (about 60 cm long) cestode of cats and other felids. Characteristically, it lacks a discernible neck (Figures 24.4 and 24.5). The larva is a strobilocercus (*Cysticercus fasciolaris*) found in the liver of rats or mice, occasionally in other small rodents, and rarely in lagomorphs. The presence of a strobilocercus used to define the genus *Hidatigera* in the past.

♦ *Taenia* (syn. *Multiceps*) *multiceps*. It is a large cestode of dogs and other canids. The mature progglottides are somewhat trapezoidal which gives the strobila a slightly serrate appearance. The larva is a coenurus (*Coenurus cerebralis*) that may reach 5 cm in diameter and contain 500-700 protoscolices forming clusters. It is found in the brain of sheep and goats, and rarely of other ungulates. The presence of a coenurus used to define the genus *Multiceps* in the past.

♦ *Taenia* (syn. *Multiceps*) *serialis*. It is a large cestode of dogs and other canids. The larvae is a coenurus (*C. serialis*) that may reach 4 cm in diameter and contain 400-500 protoscoleces distributed in radiating rows. It is found in the subcutaneous and intermuscular connective tissue of lagomorphs. Some authorities believe that all species in the old genus *Multiceps* should be assigned to a single species, and that the differences in the larvae of ungulates or lagomorphs are due to host influences.

♦ *Taenia solium*. It is a large cestode of humans (200-400 or more cm long) with the rostellum and the double row of hooks characteristic of the family (Figur24.6). The larvae is a cysticercus (*C. cellulosae*) of 6-8x4-6 mm found in the skeletal and cardiac muscles (but also brain and other organs) of pigs and, occasionally, dogs and humans.

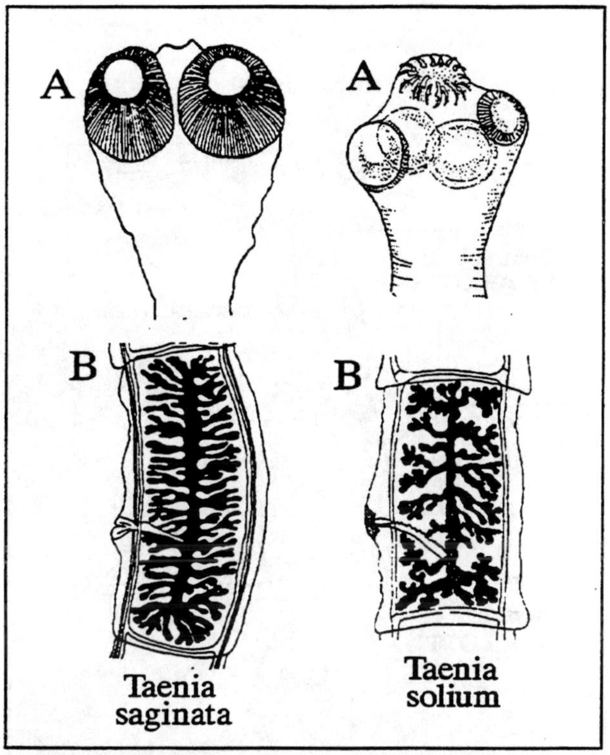


**Figure 24.6.** The common taenids of humans.

♦ *Taenia* (syn. *Taeniarhynchus*) *saginata*. It is a large (400-1000 cm long), unarmed (= without hooks) cestode of humans (Figure 24.6). The larvae is an unarmed cysticercus (*C. bovis*) about 7-10x4-6 mm found in the muscles of cattle and, occasionally, other bovids. *T. saginata* can be differentiate from *T. solium* because the former lacks rostellum and hooks on the scolex, has a muscular sphyncter in the vagina, a bilobed ovary in the mature proglottides, and 15 or more primary branches on each side of the uterus in the gravid proglottides (versus no sphincter, a trilobed ovary, and 12 or fewer branches in *T. solium*).

♦ *Echinocuccus granulosus*. It is a tiny cestode of dogs and other canids. It commonly measures 3-7 mm and bears only 3-5 proglottides (Figure 24.7). The gravid uterus develops lateral pouches but not real branches. The larva is an hydatid that may reach 10 or more cm and is found in the liver, lungs, or rarely other organs of sheep, goats, other ungulates, and occasionally humans. Although the hydatid may develop internal daughter cysts, exter-

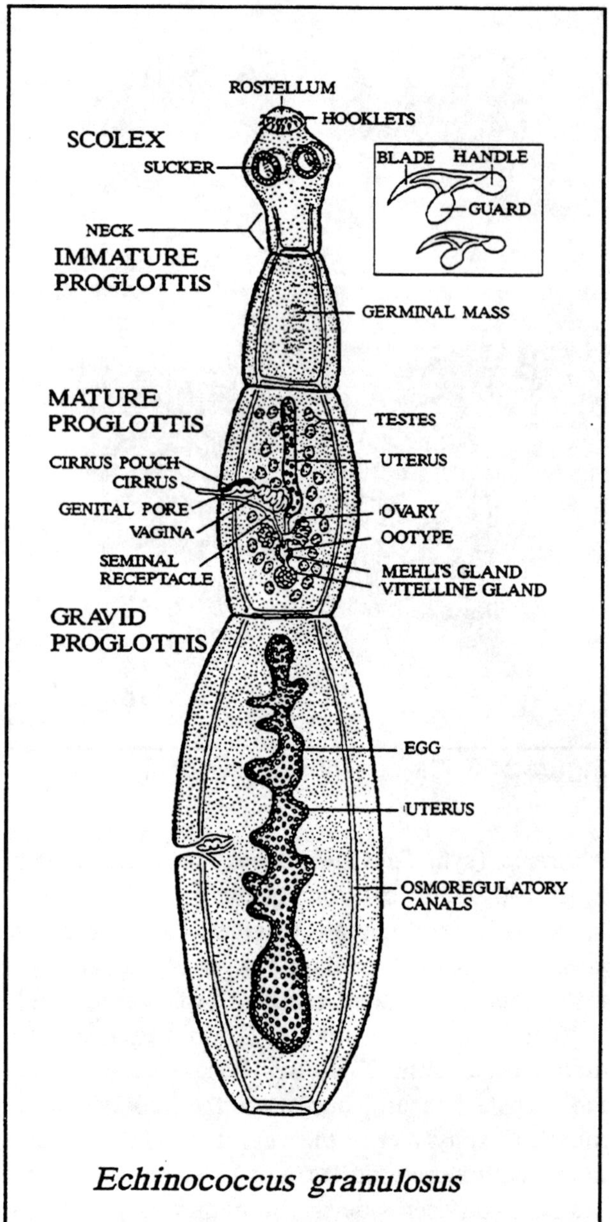


**Figure 24.7.** The worm that causes hydatidosis.

nally it is well contained by a dense layer of connective tissue formed by the host.

♦ *Echinococcus multilocularis*. It is also a tiny cestode of canids. The primary host is the fox but, different from *E. granulosus*, it may also infect cats. The gravid uterus is compact and does not develop lateral pouches. The larvae is called a multilocular or alveolar hydatid. Different from *E. granulosus*, the larvae of *E. multilocularis* is made up of small vesicles formed by external budding. This larva is poorly delimited by a loose connective tissue that does not restrict its infiltration into the surrounding tissues.

♦ Other less common Taenidae are *Taenia crassiceps* of wild and domestic canids and rodents in Europe and North America. *E. vogeli* of wild canids and rodents in northern South America, and *E. oligarthus* of wild felids and rodents in Central and South America. Abuladze[4] describes other species of restricted distribution that infect wild carnivores.

### 2.3. Family Davaineidae

These are small to medium size cestodes with a retractable, armed rostellum, and often armed acetabula. They can have a single or double set of genitalia per proglottis. The uterus is sacciforme in some species, develops a parauterin organ in others, or is replaced by egg capsules in still others. Only two of about two dozen genera are of veterinary importance: *Davainea* and *Raillietina*. In both there is a single set of genitalia per mature proglottis, the gravid proglottides are longer than wide, and the eggs develop in egg capsules.

♦ *Davainea proglottina* is a tiny tapeworm (0.5-3 mm long by 0.2-0.6 mm wide) with only 4-9 proglotides (Figure 24.8). The rostellum has 60-95 hooks. The acetabula are also armed with hooks. The eggs (28-40 μm in diameter) lie singly in eggs capsules. The adult worms infect the duodenum of gallinaceous birds. The cysticercoid infects several species of slugs.

♦ *Raillietina cesticillus* is the commonest tapeworm of chickens. It measures 4-10 cm long and 1.5-3 mm wide. It has a large scolex with a wide, prominent rostellum that bears 400-500 hooks (Figure 24.8). The acetabula are small and unarmed. The eggs (75-88 μm) lie singly in egg capsules. The adults are found in the anterior small intestine of chickens and other galinaceous birds. The cysticercoid infects several species of beetles.

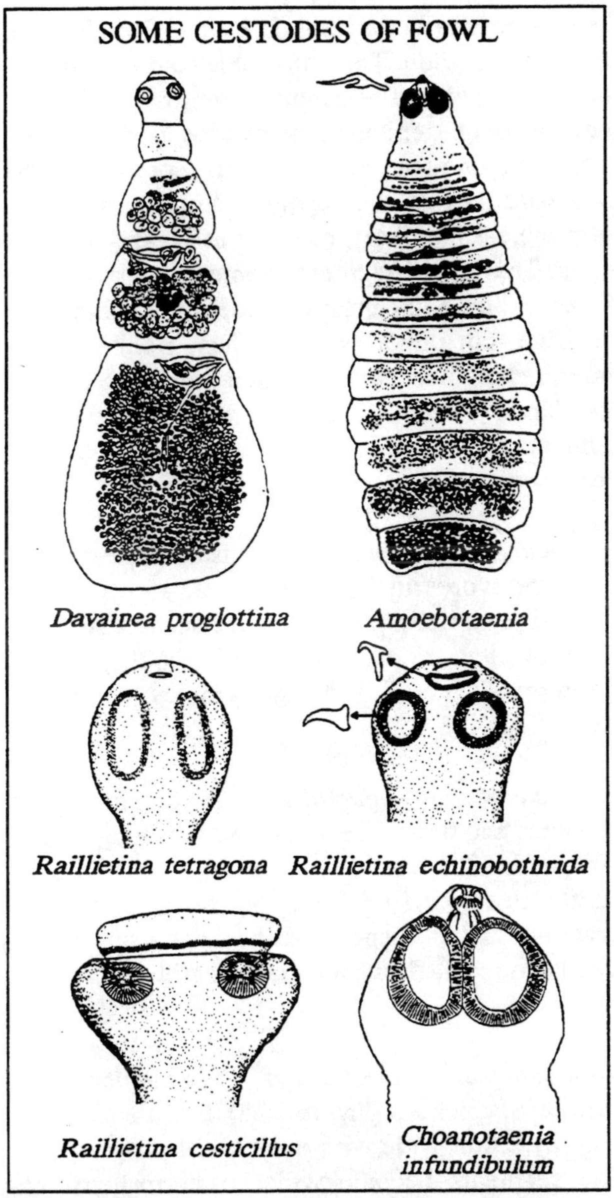


**Figure 24.8.** Some common cestodes of fowl.

♦ *Raillietina tetragona* measures up to 25 cm long and up to 4 mm wide. It has a narrow, inconspicuous rostellum that bears about 100 hooks 6-8 µm long, arranged in a single row (Figure 24.8). The acetabula are large, oval, and armed. The eggs develop in groups of 8-12 per egg capsule. The adults worms are found in the posterior small intestine of chicken and other gallinaceous birds. The cysticercoid infects ants.

♦ *Raillietina echinobothrida* resembles R. *tetragona*. It also measures up to 25 cm long by 4 mm wide but the rostellum is wider and bears about 200 hooks 10-13 µm long arranged in two rows. The acetabula are smaller, round, and armed. The eggs develop 6-12 per egg capsule. The cysticercoid develops in ants.

There are almost 300 other species of Raillietina, most of them in wild birds.

### 2.4. Family Hymenolepididae

This is a large family with many genera and hundreds of species. The only genus of some veterinary importance is *Hymenolepis*. *Hymenolepis* are small to medium size tapeworms with a narrow and translucent strobila. The acetabula are round and unarmed. The mature proglottides have 3 testes and a single ovary. The gravid proglottides are wider than long and develop a saccular uterus. Some authors have separated the many species of *Hymenolepis* into new genera,[3] but this redistribution is of no particular benefit to the veterinary practitioner.

♦ *Hymenolepis diminuta* is 100-600 mm long and 3-4 mm wide. The scolex is unarmed. The eggs are 60-80 µm in diameter with a thick internal membrane. The adults live in the small intestine of rats, other small rodents, and, occasionally, humans. The cysticercoids develop in fleas, flour beetles, and other insects.

♦ *Hymenolepis nana* is 5-40 mm long and 0.4-0.8 mm wide. The scolex bears 20-30 hooks 14-20 um long. The eggs are 44-62x30-55 µm, with a thick internal membrane, and 4-8 filaments growing from either pole of the oncosphere. The adults live in the small intestine of mice, other small rodents, and humans. The cysticercoids develop in fleas or flour beetles, but also in the intestinal villi of the definitive host. This last cycle appears to be the common one in humans. Epidemiological evidence suggests that the murine or human parasites are less infective

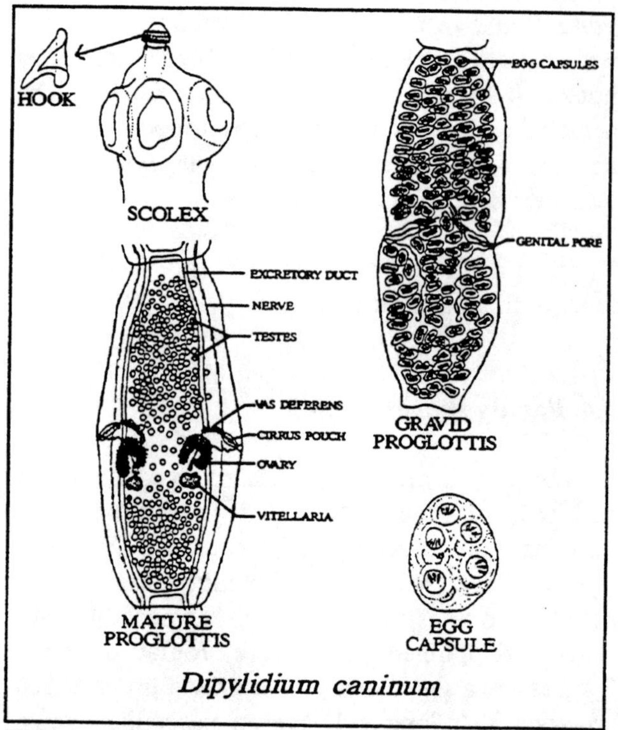


**Figure 24.9.** The most common cestode of dogs and cats.

for the heterologous host than for the homologous host.

♦ Many species of *Hymenolepis* can infect the small intestine of domestic birds. Most are less than 80 mm long, less than 1 mm wide, and translucent. With the exception of *H. carioca* which is unarmed, most have 8-35 rostellar hooks. The intermediate hosts are arthropods.

**2.5. Family Dilepididae**

This is also a large family with many genera and species. Only 5 genera are of veterinary concern. The diagnosis of the family has so many exceptions that it is more practical to study the species of veterinary importance individually.

♦ *Dipylidium caninum* is the most common tapeworm of dogs (Figure 24.9). It also infects cats and, occasionally, humans. It is up to 200-700 mm long by 2-3 wide. The retractable scolex bears 4-7 rows of hooks. The mature progrottides have a double set of genitalia side by side, with a genital pore opening on either lateral border, in the posteriar half of the segment. When gravid, the uterus breaks into eggs capsules each carrying 3-30 eggs. The gravid segments commonly pass in the feces and look like grains of rice when contracted, or like cucumber seeds when relaxed. The intermediate hosts are fleas that ingest the eggs at the larval stage. Some authors believe that the common tapeworm in cats is a different species, *D. sexcoronatum*.

♦ *Joyeuxiella* spp. are tapeworms of domestic and wild carnivores in Europe, Africa, and the Near East. The are similar to *Dipylidium* but smaller, with 14 or more rows of rostellar hooks, genital pores pre-equatorial, and eggs capsules with single eggs.

♦ *Choanotaenia infundibulum* is a parasite of chickens and turkeys. It is 50-230 mm long by 1-3 mm wide. The rostellum has 16-20 hooks in a single row. There is one set of genitalia per proglottis and each egg capsule carries a single egg. The intermediate hosts are the housefly and several beetles.

♦ *Amoebotaenia cuneata* (syn. *A. sphenoides*) is a parasite of chickens (Figure 24.8). It is about 4 mm long by 2 mm wide with only 12-24 proglottides. The segments become wider posteriorly which gives the worm a roughly triangular shape. The scolex has 12-14 rostellar hooks in a single row, and four prominents acetabula. There is a single set of genitalia per proglottis and the uterus is sacciform. The intermediate hosts are earthworms.

♦ *Metroliasthes lucida* is the common tapeworm of turkeys. It may be up to 20 mm long by 2 mm wide and rather fleshy. It lacks rostellum and hooks. The gravid proglottides exhibit a posterior uterus with two lobes side by side, and a medial parauterine organ anterior to the uterus. The gravid proglottides

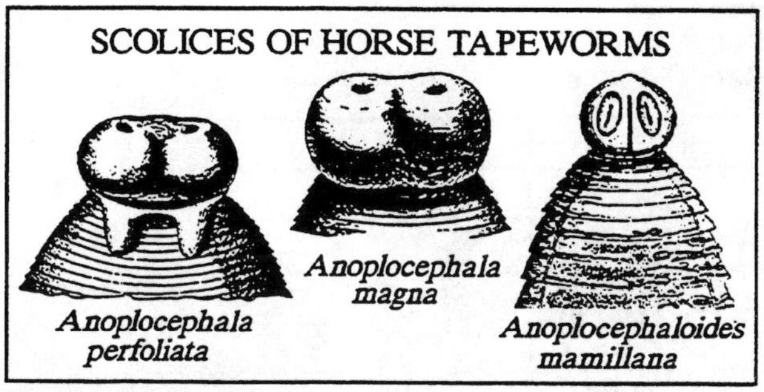

**Figure 24.10**. Common cestodes of horses.

are longer than wide. The intermediate hosts are grasshoppers.

### 2.6. Family Anoplocephalidae

Anoplocephalidae is also a large family of tapeworms that infect almost exclusively mammals. The scolex lacks rostellum and hooks. The proglottides are much wider than long, and carry a single or double set of genitalia according to the species. In most species, the embryos are enclosed in a pear-shape membrane with two crossed projections at the thinner pole (pyriform apparatus).

♦ *Anoplocephala perfoliata* is a fleshy cestode of up to 70 mm long by 12 mm wide. The scolex is small (2-3 mm wide) but wider than the first segments, with four projections into the strobila (lappets), and four cup-like acetabula directed forward (Figure 24.10). The neck is very short. The segments have a single set of genitalia. The adults are found in the large and small intestine of equines. The cysticercoids are found in oribatid mites.

♦ *Anoplocephala magna* has a fleshy body that may reach up to 800 mm long by 25 mm wide. The scolex is large (3-6 mm wide), wider than the first segments, without lappets, and with 4 cup-like acetabula directed forward (Figure 24.10). The neck is very short. The segments carry a single set of genitalia. The adults are found in the small intestine and, occasionally, stomach of equines. The cysticercoids are found in oribatid mites.

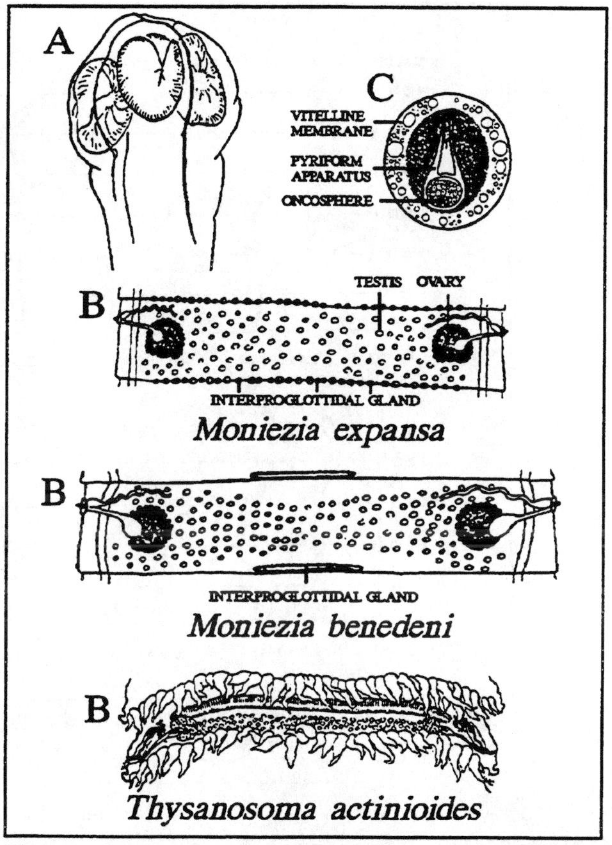

**Figure 24.11.** Some common cestodes of ruminants. A, scolex; B, mature proglottides; C, egg.

♦ *Anoplocephaloides* (syn. *Paranoplocephala*) *mamillana* has a fleshy body of up to 40 mm long by 6 mm wide. The scolex is very small (0.7 mm wide), narrower than the first segments, and with 4 acetabula directed laterally that have slit-like opennings (Figure 24.10). The segments carry a single set of genitalia. Like in *Anoplocephala* spp., the genital pores are unilateral, rarely alternating. The adults live in the small intestine and, occasionally, the stomach of horses. The cysticercoids develop in oribatid mites.

♦ *Moniezia expansa* is a fleshy worm of up to 1000-2000 mm long by up to 16 mm wide. The scolex is small ((0.4-0.7 mm) but has 4 prominent acetabula. The proglottides bear a double set of genitalia with the genital pores oppening at either lateral border. At the posterior border of each segment there is a transverse row of 12-30 interproglottidal glands that

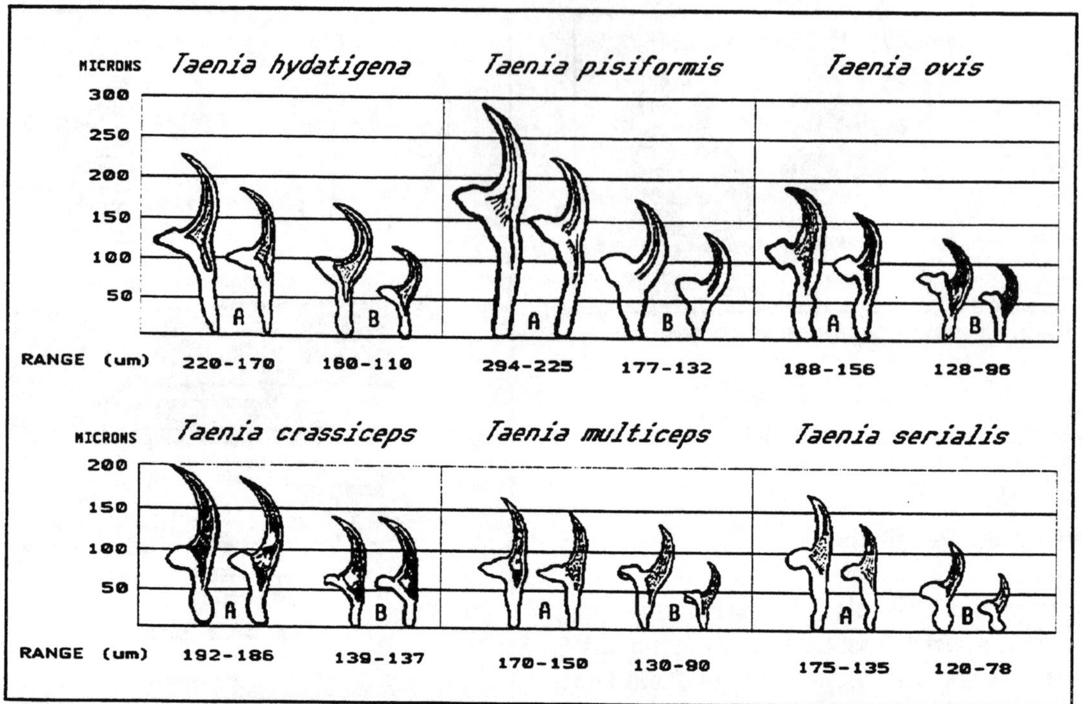


**Figure 24.12.** Sizes and shapes of the large (A) and small (B) rostellar hooks of some common cestodes of domestic carnivores.

occupies almost the complete width of the segment (Figure 24.11). The eggs have a pyriform apparatus.. The adults live in the small intestine of sheep and goats, but also infect cattle. The cysticercoids develop in oribatid mites.

♦ *Moniezia benedeni* is similar to *M. expansa* but it is more common in cattle than in small ruminants. It is somewhat broader (up to 26 mm wide), and the interprogglotidal glands are assembled in a continuous row that ocupies only the central third of the width of the segment (Figure 24.11).

♦ *Thysanosoma actinioides* is a delicate worm of up to 350 mm long by 8 mm wide. It has a double set of genitalia per proglottis. The posterior border of each segment has a conspicuous fringe of papillae (Figure 24.11) which has earned the common name of "fringed tapeworm" for this worm. The uterus develop several parauterine organs that enclosed several eggs devoid of a pyriform apparatus. The adults live in the small intestine, bile ducts, and pancreatic ducts of ruminants. The cysticercoids develop in insects of the order Psocoptera.

A common problem in veterinary medicine is the identification of the Taenid cestodes of dogs. Some species can be recognized by a few easily observable characteristics. For example, the small size of *Echinococcus*, the serrated strobila of *T. pisiformis*, the combination of bothria and a uterus in rosette in *Diphyllobothrium* or bothria and a uterus in spiral in *Spirometra*, the combination of acetabula and a ventral genital pore in *Mesocestoides*, etc. In other cases, however, accurate identification demands careful preparation and observation of mature proglottides which is beyond the usual needs and skills of a veterinary practitioner. Although not completely reliable, mesurements of the hooks is a simple and convenient first approach. Figure 24.12 may help with a preliminary identification.

**The order Pseudophyllidea** contains only two genera of veterinary importance.

◆ *Diphyllobothrium latum* is a very large cestode of the intestine of humans, domestic carnivores, bears, and other fish-eating mammals. It is from 2 to 10 or more meter long , 2 cm wide at the widest, and rather fleshy. The scolex is small (2-3 mm long and 1 mm wide), unarmed, looks like a spatula, and have a ventral and a dorsal suctorial grooves (bothria) (see Figure 24.14). The uterus is dark and coiled in a rossette in the middle of the mature proglottides which are wider than long, and square at the vey end. The uterus discharges the eggs through a uterine pore that is located in the mid-ventral line of the proglottid, a little behind the genital pore. The eggs are 67-71 x 40-51 µm, yellow-brown, operculated, and bear a little knob at the pole opposed to the operculum.

It requires two intermediate hosts: a freshwater copepod for the procercoids, and a fresh-water fish (pike, salmon, trout, etc) for the plerocercoid.

◆ *Spirometra* spp. are parasites of domestic and wild carnivores very similar to *Diphyllobothrium* but considerably smaller (< 1 m), with a tiny scolex (0.2-0.5 mm in diameter), and a uterus coiled in spiral. The eggs are 35-37 x 60-65, operculated, and pointed at both ends. The first intermediate hosts are copepods and the second are frogs and water snakes. A large number of amphibia, reptiles, birds, and even mammals (including humans) may also serve as second intermediate hosts.

## 3. Biology

### a. The Cyclophyllidea

The basic biology of the **Cyclophyllidea** cestodes follows a simple pattern: an (often prey) animal carrying the larval stage of the cestode in its systemic tissues is ingested by an (often predator) animal that will develop the adult stage in its small intestine (Figure 24.13). Every medically important cestode is transmitted by some variation of this pattern. The pattern is best explained by using a taenid cestode (e.g., *Taenia pisiformis*) as an example.

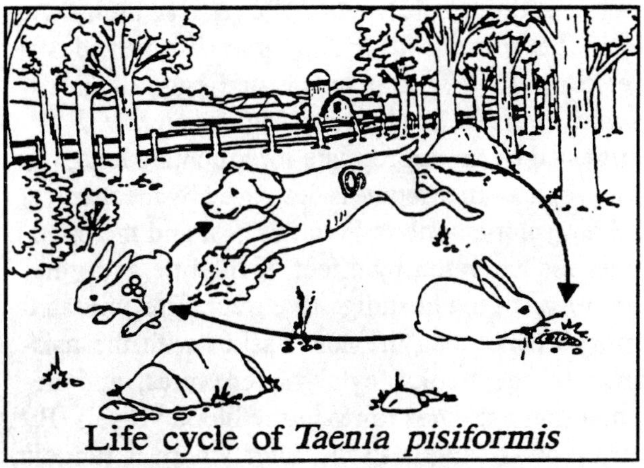


**Figure 24.13.** The life cycle of *T. pisiformis* in its ecological environment.

The larval stage (cysticercus) is found in the liverand peritoneal cavity of lagomorphs. When these cistycerci are eaten by a dog, the host tissues are digested and the metacestode is activated by the bile and enzymes in the digestive tract of the definitive host. As a result of this activation, the larva frees itself from its surrounding membranes, evaginates the proscolex, and attaches to the intestinal mucosa. The bile composition of the definitive host seems to determine whether this host is appropriate for further development or not. The parasite then starts to grow rapidly and forms the strobila. The young parasites are about 1-2 cm long by the end of the second week and attain maturity (eggs production) by the beginning of the third month of infection. The eggs leave the hosts inside the gravid proglottides. Free eggs in the feces are found only infrequently.

The eggs of the Cyclophyllidea are already infective when void and do not require a maturation period outside. This poses a particular problem of possible infection for a veterinarian examining animals that bear zoonotic cestodes (e. g., *Echinococcus*). The proglottides commonly desiccate and desintegrate in the external environment and release the eggss which are spread by rains and winds. The eggs appear to be quite resistant to changes of temperature but little resistant to changes of humidity. Eggs of *E. granulosus*, for example, survived -26C (-32F) for 54 days and 51C (124F) for 24 hours but died rapidly at < 25% relative humidity. Eggs of *E. granulosus* or *T. pisiformis* survived two weeks in 40% formaldehyde and eggs of *T. saginata* survived 22 (but not 70) days on hay.

Ingested by an appropriate intermediate host, the embryophore membrane is destroyed by mechanical and enzymatic actions from the host and the oncosphere is activated by effect of the bile and other conditions of the host digestive tract. The activated embryo penetrates the host tissues with the asistance of the hooks, cytolytic enzymes, and decementing enzymes to reach the blood vessels. By the blood it travels to the liver where it tunnels some more, chooses a place, its cells dedifferentiate, and then they differentiate again into a cysticercus.

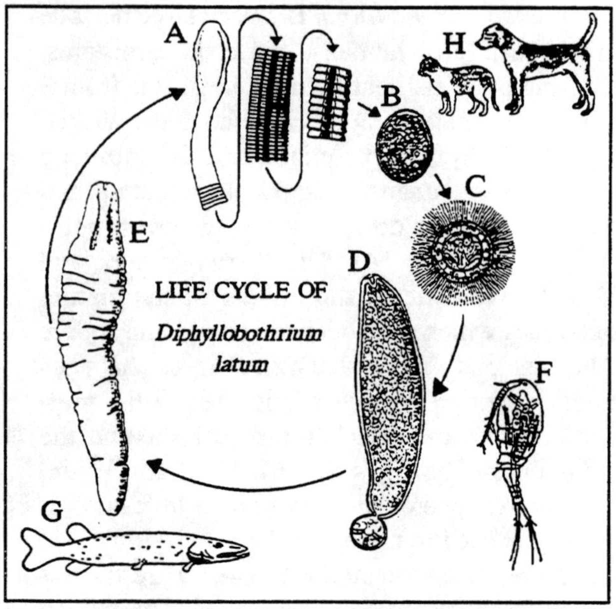


**Figure 24.14**. Life cycle of *D. latum*. Adult worm (A), egg (B), coracidium (C), procercoid (D), plerocercoid (E), first (F) and second (G) intermediate hosts, and definitive hosts (H).

### b. The Pseudophyllidea

The basic biology of a **Pseudophyllidea** is somewhat different from the Cyclophyllidea and in the early stages resembles that of the Trematoda (Figure 24.14).The Pseudophyllidea lay eggs that require an aquatic environment to develop a free swiming oncosphere surrounded by a ciliated embryophore (**coracidium**). The eggs die below -5C (23F) or above 30-35C (86-95F) but will keep for several weeks or months at 2-4C (36-39F). The coracidium of *D. latum* develops in 8-9 days at 18-20C (64-68F) but the variation among species is marked. Once formed, the coracidium responds to strong light producing a decementing enzyme that opens the operculum. The released coracidium swims around randomly until it is eaten by a copepod. High infectivity for the copepod lasts for only 36-48 hours at 18-20C. The infectivity appears to correlate with the energy reserves of the coracidium: it lasts longer at lower temperatures and shorter at higher temperatures.

Once ingested, the coracidium ciliated covering is destroyed by the copepod digestive enzymes and the free oncosphere penetrates the intestinal wall toward the hemocele. There the oncosphere (about 55 μm in diameter) develops into a **procercoid** in 2-3 weeks. The mature procercoid is a solid body about 0.5 mm long with the hooks of the oncosphere located at a caudal appendage (cercomere)

When the copepod is eaten by a fish, the procercoid penetrates the stomach wall into the peritoneal cavity and invades the muscles and connective tissue to mature into a **plerocercoid** in 7-30 days. The plerocercoid is a white, spindle-shaped organism, 5-20 mm long by 2-3 mm wide. It has a scolex with two bothria and a pseudosegmented body. If the second intermediate host is eaten by a larger fish, the plerocercoid passes unchanged to the the new host that acts as a transport host. The plerocercoid of *D. latum* survives 0C (32F) for 20 days and -5C (23F) for 3 days which permits its distribution wih the infected fish to almost any geographic area.

If an infected fish is eaten by an appropriate definitive host, the plerocercoid is released, attaches its scolex to the intestinal mucosa of the new host, and grows up to 30 proglittides per day to become an egg-bearing organism in 3-5 weeks.

#### 4. Medical importance

##### a. The adult parasite

As a rule, the infection by adult cestodes is essentially non-pathogenic. The study of large numbers of cases of *Taenia* infection in humans (which are more capable to communicate their disconfort than lower animals) has shown that fewer than a third of the patients present any sign attributable to the presence of the cestode. The objective symptoms recorded more often were nausea, abdominal discomfort, weakness, and anal pruritus. Changes of appetite or weight, constipation or diarrhea, or alterations of the hemogram (except in *Diphyllobothrium* infections, see below) were even less common. The major complaint was the revulsion of the patients who knew that they were carrying a large worm, and the untimely passage of proglottides that interfered with social activities. Despite this, vague digestive disturbances of domestic animals are often blamed on infections by adult cestodes.

**In ruminants**, *Moniezia* spp. are found in large numbers only in young ruminants. Massive infections are believed to cause diarrhea and poor condition. Intestinal obstruction has been recorded occasionally. Russian authors attribute considerable pathogenicity to these worms but this has not been substantiated in the USA. *T. actinioides* does not seem to cause overt disease normally although occasionally may cause obstruction of the bile flow. Condemnation of infected livers is a source of losses.

**In horses**, massive infections with *A. magna* can cause catarrhal or hemorrhagic enteritis in horses and *A.. perfoliata* can rarely provoke obstruction of the ileocecal valve. Both species have been blamed for intestinal perforations.

**In dogs and cats**, tapeworms do not seem to cause disease. I have collected 1.1 kg (2.4 lb) of *D. caninum* from a 13 kg (29 lb) dog and 5,500 specimens of *E. granulosus* from a 18 kg (40 lb) dog and both animals looked in perfect health. Dog infected with *D. caninum* often drag their anus over the floor what is interpreted as a sign of anal pruritus and is often attributed to the cestode infection.

**In chickens**, tapeworms are common in animals raised in free flocks but uncommon in confined birds. Only *C. infundibulatum* and *R. cistillus* have a chance to proliferate among confined fowl because they are transmitted by flies and beetles that breed in the litter. Neither is particularly pathogenic. *D. proglottina* is the most pathogenic: it penetrates deeply in the mucosa and may cause chonic infections with loss of condition or acute infections with hemorhagic or necrotic enteritis. *R. echinobothridia* is also pathogenic: it may provoke inflammatory nodules at the site of attachment. The other species may cause loss of condition only when the infections are massive.

**In humans**, the large tapeworms (*T. saginata, T. solium,* and *D. latum*) cause digestive disturbances in less than a third of the patients (see above). *D. latum* may trigger a pernicious-type anemia (see below) in predisposed people. Large numbers of *H. nana* in children may cause anorexia, epigastric pain with ot without diarrhea, and nausea or vomiting

The pathophysiology of the objective symptoms is obscure.[6] The strobila simply lies on the intestinal mucosa without awakening any discernible reaction from the host tissues. Although a large cestode can grow 5-20 cm per day, it is unlikely that the drain of nutrients becomes significant to a well-fed host. On the other hand, the large body of the worm may occlude mechanically vast portions of mucosa and interfere with its functions. The scolex can attach from very superficially (e.g., *D. latum*) to very deeply (e.g., *E. granulosus*) into the intestinal mucosa. In the last case, the hooks are embedded into the tissues and portions of mucosa are drawn into the suckers. Again, in most instances the tissue reaction to these insults is negligible. Only in the cases of *A. perfoliata* of horses and *R. echinobothridia* of chickens the scoleces may cause an intense inflammation with occasional hemorrhage, necrosis, and production of granulation tissue or fibrosis. Even then, hosts carrying numerous cestodes may not exhibit clinical manifestations.

Because the injection of cestode extracts may cause symptoms similar to the injection of histamine, it was speculated in the past that these parasites might produce toxins, or that their excretions or secretions might have a toxic effect on the host. The recent reports that cestode extracts may trigger complement activity by activation of the alternative pathway, and that infected hosts produce skin-sensitizing antibodies early in the infection[7] offer an alternative explanation for these findings.

Occlusion of the intestine in massive infections, or of the common bile duct or pancreatic duct by migratory tapeworms, is known to occur but only rarely.

Work with *Hymenolepis diminuta* have shown that the parasitism affects a number of biochemical parameters of the small intestine (reduction of bacterial content, lowering of the pH, increase of oxygen tension, changes in the gradient of carbohydrates and amino acids, modification of the oxidation-reduction potential). Similar changes have not been reported from humans or domestic animals. however.

*Diphyllobothrium latum* poses a special problem. This worm uses more vitamin B12 than other cestodes, and inhibits the binding of the host's intrinsic factor to the vitamin B12 (which is necessary for its absoption). In predisposed people, diphyllobothriasis may cause a pernicious-type anemia (macrocytic, megaloblastic) with low platelet and white cell counts, increased hemolysis, and reduced levels of plasma B12.

**b. The larval stages**

The larval stages of the tapeworms produce different pathologies during their diverse phases of development. During the invasion period, they cause tracks of necrosis of the involved tissues surrounded by a muff of inflammation. The lesion eventually heals by connective tissue. Unless massive or at a sensitive location (brain, eye), these lesions rarely have a clinical expression. Massive infection of sheep with eggs of *T. hydatigena* may cause a disease that resembles acute fascioliasis *hepatica*.

Once the larva has established, it grows quietly in its tissue of election causing only a slight peripheral inflammation. In most cases, pathology at this stage occurs only when the larvae grows enough to compress neighboring organs or obstruct conducts. The presence or severity of the disease in these cases depend largely on the location of the parasite. The hydatid of *E. granulosus*, for example, causes compression atrophy of the liver or lung tissues and may erode vessels causing small hemorrhages. This provokes clinical manifestations in humans but rarely in domestic animals. The coenurus of *T. cerebralis* causes pressure atrophy of the brain or spinal cord, and even erosion of the bones. Depending on the location, the affected animal may show nervous or motor signs. The location of the cysticercus of *T. solium* in the brain or eye may also cause signs correlated to its location.

Products of the hydatid of *E. granulosus* (and possibly other larvae) trigger IgE responses from the host who develops the subsequent allergy. This condition is of minor clinical importance normally but the accidental rupture of the larva, with a large and sudden discharge of allergens, may produce an anaphylactic shock. Furthermore, the metascolices that fall on a serosal surface (peritoneum, pleura) may originate new hydatids with production of a massive secondary hydatidosis.

The multilocular hydatid of *E. multilocularis* produces external buds that invade the surrounding tissues and, occasionally, may cause mestastases to other tissues. For all practical considerations, this larva behaves as an invasive tumor.

Observations with the cysticercus of *T. solium* and the coenurus of *T. cerebralis* have demonstrated that cestode larvae cause an important peripheral inflammation when they die (resulting from old age, treatment, or the host immune response). Apparently the increased discharge of antigenic substances from the degenerating parasite triggers severe tissue reactions in the host . This may result in clinical manifestations that were not evident during the life of the parasite. Eventually, the remains of the larva may calcify.

Occasionally, abnormal hosts ingest procercoids of *Spirometra* spp. with water containing infected copepods, or plerocercoids (sparganum) with the uncooked flesh of second intermediate hosts. The procercoid may develop into a sparganum, but the sparganus does not develop any further, in these hosts. The sparganum may, however, constitutes small nodules, sometimes around the eyes or migrating, in the subcutaneous tissue. The parasite in the nodules causes a severe eosinophilic inflammation and may become abscessed and surrounded by a fibrous capsule.

There are only two common clinical syndromes by tapeworm larvae in humans (hydatidosis and cysticercosis) and one in sheep (cenurosis). Other larvae are of rare occurrence or mostly non-pathogenic in their respective hosts or location.

**Hydatidosis** is the presence of hydatid larvae (of *E. granulosus*) in humans or domestic animals. Domestic animals apparently withstand the parasitism very well because sheep with about 50% of their livers replaced with parasite larvae do not show clinical manifestations. The livers must be condemned at the slaughterhouse, however, which constitutes a loss for the farmer.

The hydatid in humans occurs mostly in the liver (60-70%). less often in the lungs (20-30%), and rarely in other organs. In the liver, it causes vague pains and digestive disturbances, and sometimes jaudice. In the lung, it causes vague pains, frequent cough, and hemoptisis. Prompt surgical removal of the larva is indicated to prevent a possible rupture which may provoke an anaphylactic shock or the seeding of innumerable new larvae in the peritoneal or pleural serosas (secondary hydatidosis).

**Cysticercosis** is the presence of cysticerci in humans or domestic animals. Animals rarely show any symptom of cysticercosis but the presence of *C. cellulosae* (larva of *T. solium*) in the human brain or eye causes serious disease. Unless the larvae are numerous or located in particularly sensitive areas of the brain, symptoms occur only upon death of the cysticerci. The inflammation provoked by the death of the larvae causes motor (often convulsions), sensory, or mental disturbances, depending on the location of the parasite. A single parasite located in the aqueduct of Sylvius may cause hydrocephalus. In the eye, the cysticercus interferes with the vision when alive, and often triggers an iridocyclitis when it dies.

**Coenurosis** is the presence of coenurus larvae (of *T. serialis* or *T. multiceps*) in domestic animals. *C. serialis* does not cause overt disease although it may produce gross deformation of the body of rabbits when it grows under the skin. Massive infections with *C. cerebralis* may cause a meningoencephalitis in small ruminants during the invasive period. More often, there are no clinical manifestations until the larvae grows enough to compress the surrounding tissues. The signs depend on the location of the coenurus. In the parietal location, the affected animal often turns in circles toward the same side and losses the vision on the opposite side. In the frontal lobe, the animal holds its head low and steps high. In the spinal cord, the patient may develop a progressive paralysis of the hind limbs.

## TABLE 24.I. LONGEVITY OF SOME REPRESENTATIVE CESTODES

### A. CYCLOPHYLLIDEA

| Species | Egg | Larva | Adult Prepatency | Adult Patency |
|---|---|---|---|---|
| *Hymenolepis diminuta* | 11-60 days | as host | 17 days | as host |
| *H. nana* | 25 days | as host | 11-16 days | 12-24 days |
| *Moniezia expansa* | ? | 2-5 months | 30-50 days | 3 months |
| *Raillietina cesticillus* | ? | as host | 12 days | 70 days |
| *Echinocuccus granulosus* | up to 1 year | 10-12 years | 35 days | as host? |
| *Taenia saginata* | several months | several years | 40-60 days | up to 10 years |
| *T. crassiceps* | up to 200 days | 8 years | 35-42 days | at least 9 months |

### B. PSEUDOPHYLLIDEA

| Species | Egg | Coracidium | Procercoid | Plerocercoid | Adult Prepatency | Adult Patency |
|---|---|---|---|---|---|---|
| *Diphyllobothrium latum* | 8 months | 24-48 hours | 1-2 months | years | 15-18 days | 20 years |
| *Spirometra mansonoides* | up to 4 years | 24 hours | 1 month | as host | 11-20 days | 2 years |

## REFERENCES

1. Skrjabin, K.I. et al. (eds.). 1951-1985. *Osnovy Tsestodology (Essentials of Cestodology).* 11 volumes. Akademiya Nauk SSSR. Many volumes translated into English by the Israel Program of Scientific Translations and published by the US Department of Agriculture and the US National Science Foundation, Washington, D.C.

2. Yamaguti, S. 1959. *Systema Helminthum. The Cestodes of Vertebrates*, vol. 2. Interscience, New York, 860 pp.

3. Wardle, R.A., McLeod, J.A, and Radinovsky, S. 1974.*Advances in the Zoology of Tapeworms*, 1950-1970. University of Minnesota Press, Minneapolis, 274 pp.

4. Schmidt, G.D. 1986. *Handbook of Tapeworms Identification.* CRC Press, Boca Raton, Florida, 675 pp.

5. Abuladse, K.I. 1970. *Taeniata of Animals and Man and Diseases Caused by Them.* Volume IV of *Essentials of Cestodology* by K.I. Skrjabin (ed). Translated into English by the Israel Program of Scientific Translations. US Department of Agriculture and US National Science Foundation, Washington, D.C., 549 pp.

6. Rees G. 1967. Pathogenesis of adult cestodes. Helminth. Abstr. 36:1-23.

7. Barriga O.O. and Al-Khalidi NW. 1986. Humoral immunity in the prepatent primary infection of *Echinococcus granulosus.* Vet. Immunol. Immunopath. 11:375-389.

## Chapter 25

# THE PHYLUM PROTOZOA

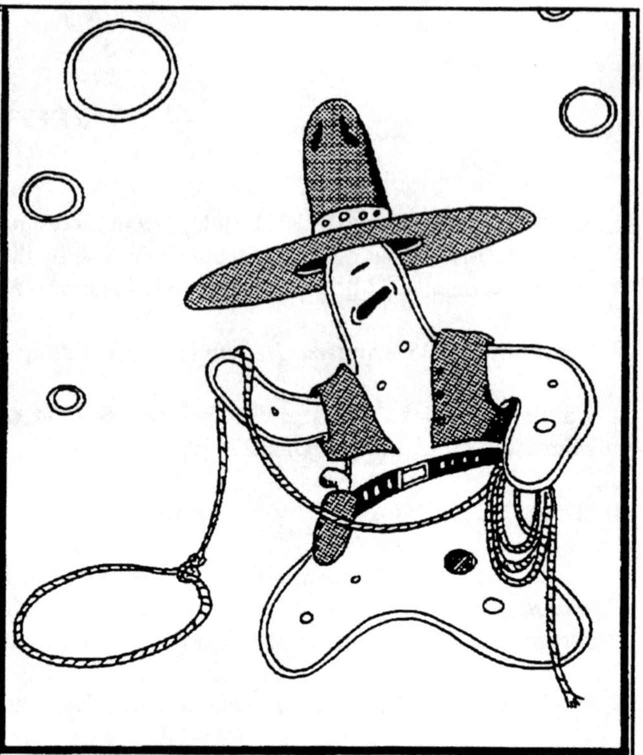

"Well?... Where are those macrophages?"

### 1. Structure

The protozoa are eukaryotic organisms that concentrate all the functions necessary for independent life into a single cell. Their body varies in size from about 4 to about 100 or more µm and is contained by the typical three-layered cellular membrane characteristic of most cells. The external surface of the cellular membrane is covered by the carbohydrate portion of the glycoproteins and glycolipids of the cell membrane. This layer of oligosaccharides has been called **surface coat** and has important functions in the recognition of the host by the parasite, and the defense of the parasite from host's immunity. The stages of the protozoa that must spend time in a dry external environment often deposit a wall underneath the cell membrane that protects them from desiccation. These protected stages are commonly called **cysts** or **oocysts.**

The cytoplasm commonly presents a thin peripheral portion **(ectoplasm)** that is more dense and gives the cell some rigidity, and a more massive central portion **(endoplasm)** that is more fluid. Like in the typical eukaryotic cells, the nucleus is contained by a double membrane that bears pores. In most protozoa, it is vesicular and contains one or more nucleoli.

Internally, the parasitic protozoa may exhibit the same organelles that are characteristic of all animal cells (Figure 25.1). For example, they may have a digestive vacuole that degrades particulate materials which may enter the cell, storage vacuoles that store crystalloid proteins, lipids, or carbohydrates (glycogen or amynopeptine), a contractile vacuole that expels indigestible remnants and regulates the water balance, mitochondria to produce energy, free

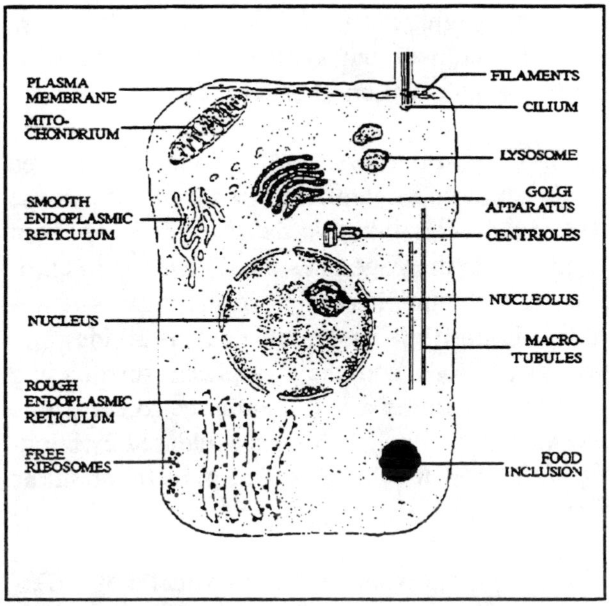


**Figure 25.1.** Morphology of a typical animal cell.

or endoplasmic ribosomes to synthesize proteins, smooth and rough endoplasmic reticulum, a Golgi apparatus, lysosomes, organelles for locomotion (cilia or flagella), a cytoskeleton of microtubules and microfilaments, etc. Because the parasitic protozoa may be highly adapted to their host envi ronment, some species lack some of these organelles, or may show special organelles. For example, the cytoskeleton of the Apicomplexa forms an apical complex characteristic of this group. We will discussed the specialized organelles in the corresponding places.

## 2. Identification and classification

The generic identification of the protozoa is based on the fact that they are single-cell organisms. Veterinarians often need to identify the transmission stages (cysts or oocysts) in the feces (e.g., intestinal coccidia, *Giardia).* Less often, they may need to recognize vegetative, mobile stages (trophozoites) in their natural habitat (e.g. *Giardia* in intestinal content, trypanosomes in blood, or *Tritrichomonas* in genital secretions). In these cases, the task consists of distinguishing the protozoa from other single-cell structures that may be present in the sample. Because of the wide variety in morphology among the protozoa and the contaminants, we will discuss the identification of specific protozoa with each group. In a few cases, the accurate identification of the parasite or the disease may require histopathologic or serologic techniques (e.g., toxoplasmosis, chronic babesiosis) that require sending samples to specialized laboratories.

As a group, the only feature common to all protozoa is their single-cell nature which is an inconsequential biological characteristic. Many protozoa are only remotely related so to make a rational classification of the group is difficult. The current classification was arranged by a committee of expert protozoologists,[1] and expanded in a recent comprehensive textbook.[2] Although it is solidly based on the latest scientific information, it is fairly complex and not particularly useful to the veterinary practitioner. We will use here a simplified version that retains the nomenclature that is familiar to veterinarians and physicians. The protozoa parasitic in higher mammals can be separated into four classes: Mastigophora, Sarcodina, Ciliophora, and Apicomplexa.

The **Mastigophora** (from Gr *mastix* = whip, and *phoros*= bearing, referring to the flagellum) are protozoa with one to many flagella (see respective section). They are also called **Flagellata** or **flagellates.** Most species of veterinary importance are extracellular parasites. *Trypanosoma cruzi* and *Leishmania* spp. constitute notable exceptions to this rule. The Mastigophora reproduce asexually by longitudinal binary fission.

The **Sarcodina** (from Gr *sarx*= flesh, and *odes* = like, because they look like a blob of protoplasm) are protozoa that produce pseudopods (see respective section). They are also called **Rhizopoda** (from Gr *rhiza* = root, and *podium* = foot, referring to the pseudopods) or **amoebae** (from Gr *amoibe*= change, referring to their changing shape). All species in domestic animals are extracellular parasites. They reproduce asexually by binary fission.

The **Ciliophora** (from Lat *cilium* = eyelash, and Gr *phoros*= bearing) are covered by cilia (see respective section) but their identifying characteristic is the presence of one or more large nuclei **(macronuclei)** and a small nucleus (**micronucleus**). The former regulates the metabolism of the cell and the latter is in charge of reproduction. The ciliophora are also called **Ciliata** or **ciliates** and are customarily defined as protozoa with **cilia.** Since the difference between cilia and flagella is only a matter of number and size, however, this is not an exclusive characteristic of the group. All parasitic species are extracellular. They reproduce asexually by transverse binary fission, o by a primitive form of sexual reproduction (conjugation).

The **Apicomplexa** are parasitic protozoa that bear an **apical complex** (see respective section) at its anterior end, and are devoid of flagella, cilia, or pseudopods. In the past they were called Sporozoa because the sporocysts involved in the transmission of some coccidia (see respective section) were considered homologous to the spores of fungi. However, sporocysts are neither homologous to the fungal spores nor present in all Apicomplexa. The Apicomplexa are intracellular parasites at least at some stage of their lives. They reproduce by alternation of asexual fission or budding, and sexual syngamy.

### 3. Reproduction

Most parasitic protozoa reproduce by fission, some by budding, a few by syngamy, and even fewer by conjugation. Fission and budding are asexual processes but syngamy and conjugation imply the intervention of sexes.

**Fission** is just the division of the nucleus followed by division of the cytoplasm. In **simple fission** the protozoa divides into two daughter cells of about equal size: in the flagellates the division is longitudinal to their major axis but in the ciliates is traversal. In **multiple fission** the nucleus divides into several portions and the cytoplasm surrounding each portion forms a cell membrane to constitute several daughter cells which are released by bursting of the mother cell. This strategy is found in the coccidia.

**Budding** is the production of two nuclei of different size followed by the division of the cytoplasm to form two cells also of different size. The smaller cell is called a bud. This occurs in *Babesia*, for example.

**Syngamy** (from Gr *sun* = together, and *gamos* = union, marriage) is the formation of gametes that later fuse to form a zygote. Commonly, the masculine gamete is smaller and called **microgamete** whereas the feminine gamete is larger and called **macrogamete**. Syngamy is characteristics of the Apicomplexa.

**Conjugation** is the interchange of micronuclear material by two different organisms. It occurs in the ciliates.

# THE CILIOPHORA OR CILIATES AND THE SARCODINA OR AMOEBAE

These two groups of protozoa are not related but since they are of limited veterinary importance, we will discussed then together in a single chapter.

## THE CILIOPHORA

The **Ciliophora** (from Lat *cilium*= eyelash, and Gr *phoros*= bearing) are recognized by the presence of one or more large nuclei (**macronuclei**) that regulates the metabolism of the cell, and a small nucleus (**micronucleus**) in charge of reproduction. They are also called **Ciliata** or **ciliates**. The Ciliophora are customarily defined as protozoa with cilia (singular, cilium) but since the only difference between cilia and flagella is that the former are shorter and more numerous, this is not an exclusive characteristic of the group. All parasitic species are extracellular. They reproduce asexually by transverse binary fission, or by a primitive form of sexual reproduction (conjugation) in which two individuals exchange micronuclear material instead of forming and fusing gametes.

The **cilia** are distributed in longitudinal or diagonal rows along the body of the parasite. The lines formed by the ciliary basal granules (called ciliary rows or kineties) can be observed by phase contrast or stained with silver and constitute a major criterion for classification.

Most ciliates are free-living organisms. Only three groups are of some veterinary importance: *Balantidium coli*, the ciliates of the ruminants, and the ciliates of the equines.

♦ *Balantidium coli* is a very common parasite of the large intestine of pigs that rarely infects humans and other primates, and has been occasionally reported in rats and dogs.[3]

The trophozoites are oval to pear-shaped, 30-150 by 25-120 µm, with a funnel-shaped mouth (cytostome) at one end and a small triangular anus (cytopyge) at the other end (Figure 25.2). Two contractile vacuoles (to expel excess water) and numerous food vacuoles are often observed in its interior. The macronucleus is large and kidney-shaped, the micronucleus is small and commonly hidden in the concavity of the macronucleus. Occasionally the micronucleus may be absent. The body is covered by numerous cilia of similar length. The trophozoites can survive outside the host for up to 5 days at room temperature.

The cysts are spherical to ovoid, 40 to 60 um in diameter (Figure 25.2). They have a double membrane containing a motile parasite covered by cilia. The cysts may survive for 2 or more weeks outside the host.

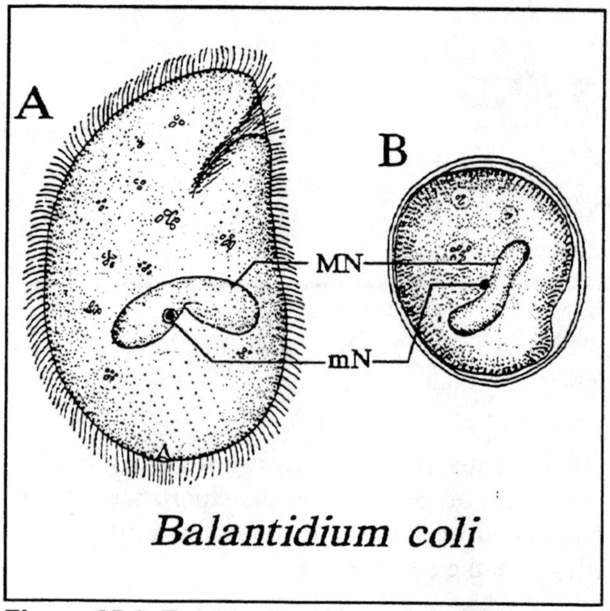


**Figure 25.2.** Trophozoite (A) and cyst (B) of *Balantidium coli.* MN, macronucleus; mN, micronucleus.

Infection occurs by ingestion of cysts or trophozoites. The parasite is non-pathogenic in pigs although it may invade the mucosa damaged by other pathogens. It is pathogenic but uncommon in humans and other primates. In these, it may cause deep and extensive ulcers that result in a mucous diarrhea stained with blood similar to that caused by amebiasis.[4] The trophozoite can be demonstrated by direct smears of diarrheic feces, and the cysts by conventional flotation of formed feces. The pig infection does not need treatment. The human infection responds well to tetracyclines (50 mg/kg/day for 5 days).

♦ **The ciliates of the ruminants**. The rumen and reticulum of the ruminants contain a large and enormously varied population of ciliates. It may reach to a million individuals per ml, and include perhaps 100 species. Most belong to the order Entodiniomorphida. Although they are true parasites because they depend on their host for survival, they do not cause harm. On the contrary, they may provide up to 20% of the protein and 20% of the volatile fatty acids available to their host. Furthermore, some species degrade cellulose and other carbohydrates for which the host lacks enzymes.

Ruminants are born without ciliates and acquire the infection with the forage contaminated with the saliva of older animals when they start eating solid food. The ruminant ciliates are not passed in the feces because they do not form resistant cysts and the trophozoites are killed by the acidity of the stomach. Although the association ruminant-ciliates is often presented as an example of mutualism, it is not so because the host survives quite well without the parasites.[5,6]

♦ **The ciliates of the equines**. Similarly to the ruminants, the equines posses a large and varied population of ciliates in their cecum and colon. Occasionally, some appear during fecal exams in horses and the practitioner wonders about its significance. The equine ciliates are not pathogenic but little else is known about their importance for the host.

## THE SARCODINA

The **Sarcodina** (from Gr *sarx*= flesh, and *odes*= like, because they look like a blob of protoplasm) lack flagella and cilia but produce temporary projections of the cytoplasm called **pseudopods.** The protozoan fixes the distal end of the pseudopod to a substrate and then retrieves it into the body pulling the entire cell forward. The pseudopods are also used for phagocytosis so these organisms often show foreign materials in cytoplasmic vacuoles. The sarcodina are also called **Rhizopoda** (from Gr *rhiza*= root, and *podium*= foot) referring to the characteristic pseudopods, or **amoebae** (from Gr *amoibe*= change) referring to their changing shape. All species of veterinary interest are extracellular parasites. They reproduce asexually by binary fission.

Although amoebae are common in the digestive tract of mammals, they are rarely pathogenic for domestic animals and only one species is common and consistently pathogenic for humans.

♦ *Entamoeba histolytica* is a 12-30 µm amoeba of the large intestine of humans and other primates. It

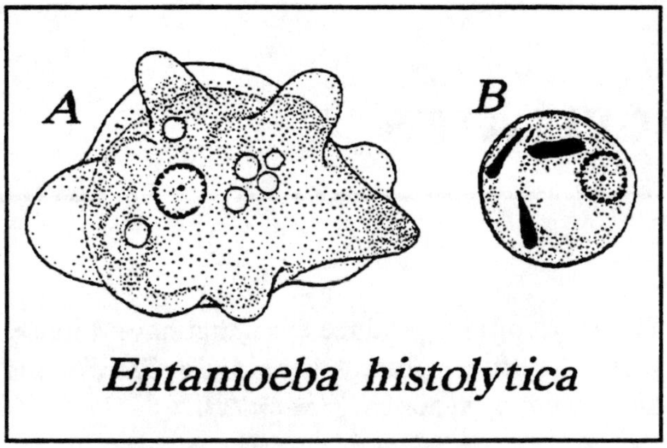


**Figure 25.3.** Trophozoite (A) and cyst (B) of *Entamoeba histolytica.*

may cause from diarrhea to intestinal ulcerations with dysentery. The parasites that reach the liver by the circulation may cause necrosis of the organ. In human medicine, *E. histolytica* must be distinguished from the apathogenic *E. coli.* The former has a central nucleolus whereas the latter has the nucleolus off center.

Both species have been reported infrequently from domestic carnivores, pigs, and rats in which they do not appear to cause natural disease. There is no evidence that amebiasis *histolytica* is a zoonotic infection. Most human cases can be traced to contamination by other humans.

♦ *Naegleria* and *Acanthamoeba* are free-living amoebae that rarely invade mammalian tissues.[8] They have been found in cases of human meningoencephalitis, and in lungs, liver , and pancreas of immunoincompetent humans, dogs, and cattle.

## REFERENCES

1. Levine, N.D. (chairman) et al. 1980. A newly revised classification ofthe Protozoa. J. Protozool. 27:37-59.

2. Lee, J.J., Hutner, S.H. and Bovee, E.C. 1985. *An Illustrated Guide to the Protozoa*. Soc. Protozool., Lawrence, Kansas, 629 pp.

3. Zaman, V. 1978. *Balantidium coli*. In Kreier J.P. and Baker J.R. (eds), *Parasitic Protozoa*, 2nd ed., vol. 3, Academic Press, New York, 43-63.

4. Walzer, P.D., Judson, F.N., Murphy, K.B. et al. 1972. Balantidiasis outbreak in Truk. Am. J. Trop. Med. Hyg. 22:33-41.

5. Dehority, B.A. 1993. The rumen protozoa. In Kreier J.P. and Baker J.R. (eds), *Parasitic Protozoa*, 2nd ed., vol. 3, Academic Press, New York, 1-42.

6. Dehority, B.A. 1993. *Laboratory manual for classification and morphology of rumen ciliate protozoa*. CRC Press, BocaRton, Florida, 120 pp.

7. Martinez-Palomo, A. 1993. Parasitic amebas of the intestinal tract. In Kreier J.P. and Baker J.R. (eds), *Parasitic Protozoa*, 2nd ed., vol. 3, Academic Press, New York, 65-141.

8. John, D.T. 1993. Opportunistically pathogenic free-living amebae. In Kreier J.P. and Baker J.R. (eds), *Parasitic Protozoa*, 2nd ed., vol. 3, Academic Press, New York, 143-246.

# Chapter 26

# THE MASTIGOPHORA OR FLAGELLATES

The **Mastigophora** (from Gr *mastix*= whip, and *phoros*= bearing, referring to the flagellum), **Flagellata**, or **flagellates**, are protozoa with one to many flagella and with one or more identical nuclei. This last characteristic distinguish them from the Ciliophora which possess a macronucleus and a micronucleus. A flagellum is a hair-like organelle formed by a central core (axoneme) enclosed in an outer sheath. The axoneme is composed of nine peripheral and two central fibrils that arise from a basal granule (**blepharoplast**) located in the cytoplasm. In some species, the microtubules form one or more longitudinal rods called **axostyles** that act as a central skeleton to permit movement. In many flagellates, the Golgi apparatus (**parabasal body**) or bundles of microtubules (**medial bodies**) that stain intensely with hematoxylin accumulate in discrete areas of the cytoplasm. A few species have a cellular mouth or cytostome. Most flagellates of veterinary importance are extracellular parasites. *Trypanosoma cruzi* and *Leishmania* spp. constitute notable exceptions. The Mastigophora reproduce asexually by longitudinal binary fission.

Numerous flagellates may inhabit the digestive tract of domestic animals. Only three families, however, contain members pathogenic for the species of veterinary importance: Hexamitidae, Trypanosomatidae, and Trichomonadidae.

## FAMILY HEXAMITIDAE

The **Hexamitidae** are piriform, bilaterally symmetrical flagellates of the digestive tract. They have eight flagella and two nuclei, and may have adhesive disks, medial bodies, axostyles, or cytostomes. The nuclei are vesicular and located side by side. The Hexamitidae produce cysts that have 4 nuclei when mature. Important genera are *Giardia* and *Spironucleus* (synonym *Hexamita*).

### ♦ *Giardia*

**a. Morphology and identification**

*Giardia* are flagellates of the anterior portion of the small intestine of vertebrates.[1] They are pear-shape, bilaterally symmetrical organisms, with the dorsal aspect convex and the anterior part of the ventral aspect concave forming an adhesive disk. They differ from *Spironucleus* in that *Giardia* is larger, has smaller nucleoli, and possesses medial bodies and an adhesive disk.

In the past, many species of *Giardia* were described and named according to their host (e.g., *G. canis, G. bovis, G. caviae*, etc.). Only three morphological types are accepted nowadays: *G. intestinalis* (syn. *G. lamblia*) of humans, domestic animals, and others mammals; *G. muris* of rodents, birds, and reptiles; and, *G. agilis* of frog tadpoles. *G. intestinalis* is almost twice longer than wide (about 10-19 µm long x 5-12 µm wide x 2-4 µm thick), with fang-shaped transverse medial bodies, and the adhesive disk occupying less than half the body length (Figure 26.1). *G. muris* is more circular (about 7-13x5-10 µm), with small round medial bodies, and the adhesive disk occupying more than half the body length.[2]

**b. Medical importance**

The taxonomy and host specificity of *Giardia* are still far from resolved. Some cross infections, isoenzymes studies, and antigenic comparisons suggest that the same species infects humans, carnivores, ruminants, equines, pigs, beavers, muskrats, and other laboratory animals but dissenting reports exist.[3] The most common mecha-

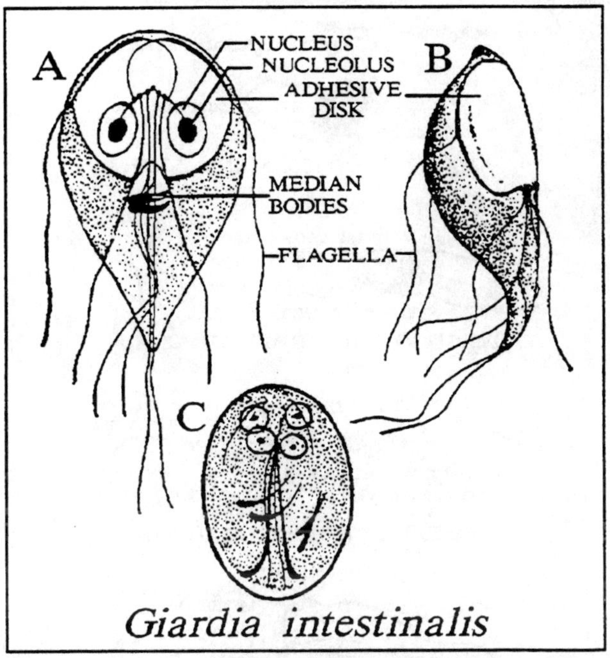


**Figure 26.1.** Ventral (A) and lateral (B) view of the trophozoite and mature cyst (C) of *Giardia intestinalis*.

nism of infection in humans is direct or waterborne transmission of cysts from another human. Waterborne transmission from animal sources, however, has been suspected in several cases. The zoonotic nature of human giardiasis has not been resolved yet.

*Giardia* is found in about 4% of the humans stools presented for fecal exam in the United States. In surveys throughout the world, it has been found in 20-35% of dogs, 10-15% of cats, 5-90% of calves, 6-80% of lambs, 17-32% of foals, and 7-44% of piglets.[4] In all cases, the infection rate is considerably higher in young individuals.

Giardiasis is frequently asymptomatic but it may cause disease in humans, domestic carnivores, and, possibly, farm animals. The symptoms in humans are from intermittent soft feces to continuous or chronic diarrhea, sometimes with mucus or high fat content (steatorrhea), and weight loss. The parasite attaches to the mucosal cells but rarely causes discernible lesions beyond some villus atrophy. The symptoms are probably caused by biochemical alterations of the cells or their environment. The symptoms in infected domestic carnivores are similar to those in humans. Experimental infection in calves produced slight diarrhea but successful treatment of diarrhea in farm animals with anti-*Giardia* drugs has been taken as demonstration of the *Giardia* etiology of the diarrhea.

**c. Diagnosis and treatment**

The infection is diagnosed by the demonstration of trophozoites in soft or diarrheic feces, or bi- or tetranucleated cysts (7-10x8-13 µm, Figure 26.1) in formed feces. The parasites pass intermittently in the feces so three exams every other day are necessary before declaring a patient free of giardiasis.

Metronidazole (25 mg/kg twice a day for 5-7 days for dogs; 10-25 mg/kg twice a day for 5 days for cats; 5 mg/kg three times a day for 10 days for horses), quinacrine (1 mg/kg twice a day for 5 days for calves), dimetridazole (50 mg/kg daily for 5 days for calves), or furazolidone (4 mg/kg, twice a day for 5 days for dogs or cats) are effective.

### ♦ *Spironucleus*

*Spironucleus* and *Hexamita* are parasites of the small intestine of primates, rodents, birds, and cold-blooded vertebrates. Their taxonomy is still confusing. The species pathogenic for laboratory rodents, turkeys, and pigeons, commonly called *Hexamita*, belong to the genus *Spironucleus*. They differ from *Giardia* in that they are smaller (usually <11x5 µm for *Spironucleus* versus >11x5 µm for *Giardia*) and do not have adhesive disks or medial bodies.

*S. muris* (trophozoite of 2-3x7-9 µm, cysts of 3-4x6-7 µm) lives in the small intestine and cecum of rats, mice, golden hamster, and wild rodents. It may cause diarrhea (Figure 26.2).

*S. meleagridis* (trophozoite of 2-5x6-12 µm) lives in the small intestine of turkey poults and in the cecum of older turkeys. It also infects other birds. In birds younger than 10 weeks, it may cause a catarrhal enteritis with foamy, watery diarrhea that may kill 7-80% of the birds within 1-2 weeks of the first deaths. The birds that recover remain stunted and often carriers of the infection..

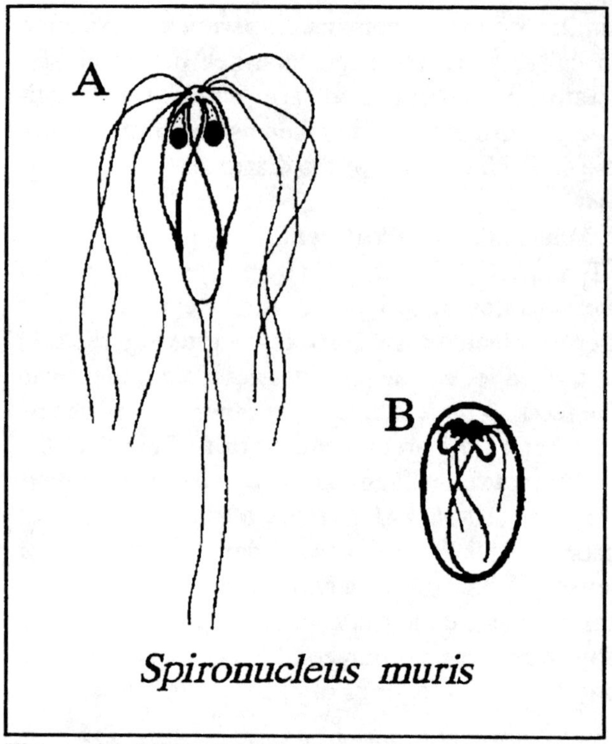


**Figure 26.2.** Trophozoite (A) and inmature cyst (B) of *Spironucleus muris.*

*S. columbae* (trophozoite of 3-7x5-9 μm) occurs in the small and large intestine of pigeons. I may cause catarrhal enteritis.

## FAMILY TRYPANOSOMATIDAE

The **Trypanosomatidae** are flagellates with a single flagellum and a single nucleus. They are mostly parasites of the blood or tissue fluids. A few species have intracellular stages. Four forms may occur during their development: **trypomastigote** (formerly trypanosome), with a flagellum that arises from the posterior end and is attached to the body by an undulating membrane; **epimastigote** (formerly crithidial), with the flagellum arising near the nucleus and a diminutive undulating membrane; **promastigote** (formerly leptomonad), with the flagellum arising from the anterior end and no undulating membrane; and micromastigote or **amastigote** (formerly leishmania), with a short intracellular flagellum, or without a flagellum (Figure

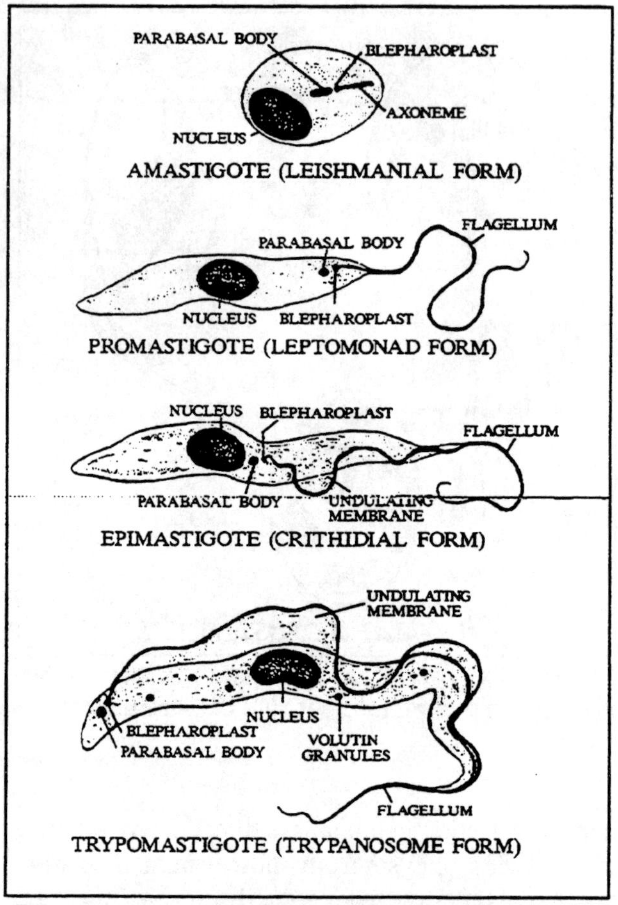


**Figure 26.3**. Forms of the trypanosomes.

26.3). The most important genera are *Trypanosoma* and *Leishmania.*

### ◆ *Trypanosoma*

The trypanosomas are parasites of particular relevance to Africa and Latin America. Some species are transmitted by the bite of the vectors (group Salivaria) and others by contamination of the host's skin or mucosas with the vector feces (group Stercoraria).In the vertebrate host, trypomastigotes and occasionally epimastigotes occur in the blood or body tissues, and amastigotes inside the cells in those species that invade host cells (*Trypanosoma cruzi*). The four forms may occur in the invertebrate host (vector) or in culture, .

◆ *T. gambiense* and T. *rhodesiense* are the agents of the **sleeping sickness** of humans in Africa. They are transmitted biologically by the bites of *Glossina* flies (tsetses). Wild ruminants and carnivores are reservoirs of the parasites. The human infection has diminished tremendously in the last decades but still there are about 10,000 cases per year..

◆ *T. congolense* and *T. brucei* infect ruminants, equines, pigs, and domestic carnivores, and *T. vivax* ruminants and equines, in Africa causing a progressive and often fatal disease (**nagana**). They are transmitted biologically by the bites of tsetses. These and other trypanosomas negate the full use for livestock of the area of distribution of the flies (about latitude 15°N to 15°S in Africa). This area comprises about 7 million square km (4.5 square miles) of excellent land that could support 150 million heads of high quality cattle per year.

◆ *T. evansi* infects ruminants, equines, pigs, and domestic carnivores in Africa (north of the area of tsetses), Asia, and Central and northern South America and *T. viennei* infects cattle and horses in Central America and northern South America. They produce a progressive disease (**surra**, morriña, derrenguera). They are transmitted mechanically by horseflies, and in the case of *T. evansi*, also by vampire bats.

◆ *T. equiperdum* infects equines in parts of Africa, of Asia and in Mexico, Central America and northern South America. causing a venereal disease called **dourine**. It is transmitted by coitus.

◆ *T. cruzi* exists in the Americas where it causes **Chagas' disease** in 18 million people. Chagas' disease has an acute phase of little clinical transcendence. With time, however, cross reactivity of the parasite antigens with host's muscle and nervous tissue causes damage of hollow viscera (heart, esophagus, colon) which eventually leads to death. Cases have been reported in domestic carnivores . A number of wild mammals are reservoirs of the infection. The disease is transmitted biologically by the feces of infected kissing bugs.

Other trypanosomas infect humans (*T. rangeli*) in Latin America, or cattle (*T. theileri*) or sheep (*T. melanophagium*) throughout the world, but are not pathogenic.

### ◆ *Leishmania*

The *Leishmania* are trypanosomatidae that exist in the form of amastigotes of 2-5x1-3 μm in the mammalian host, and as promastigotes in the vector or in cultures.. They are transmitted biologically with the bite of sand flies (*Phlebotomus* in the Old World and *Lutzomyia* in the Americas). All *Leishmania* live in the macrophages and monocytes of the mammalian host. They cause large accumulation of mononuclear cells, multiply in them, and destroy them together with the surrounding tissues. The released parasite invade new cells to repeat the cycle of multiplication and release.

The taxonomy of *Leishmania* is complicated. Several species that cause similar diseases have been gathered in complexes.

◆ *Leishmania tropica* complex. It includes the species *L. tropica* and *L. major* in the Middle East, southwest Asia, north Africa, and south Sahara , and *L. aethiopica* in Ethiopia and Kenya. They cause chronic cutaneous ulcers that heal to retracting fibrous tissue in 2-10 months (**Old World cutaneous leishmaniasis**). *L. major* and *L. aethiopica* are zoonotic infections with local rodents acting as reservoirs. *L. tropica* is commonly transmitted from person to person but dogs may act as reservoirs.

◆ *Leishmania mexicana* complex and *L. braziliensis* complex. There are at least 5 species in the *L. mexicana* complex and 3 in the *L. braziliensis* complex. Both complexes are distributed unevenly from southern Texas to northern Argentina. Rodents and marsupials (sloth), and occasionally dogs, are reservoirs of the infection.

Most species of the *L. mexicana* complex cause a cutaneous ulcer similar to that of the Old World cutaneous leishmaniasis (**American cutaneous leishmaniasis**). In a small proportion of patients, the cutaneous lesions are very chronic and, with time, may invade the mucous membranes. The species of the *L. braziliensis* complex have a much greater tendency to produce invasion of the mucosas with destruction of the nasal septum, palate, or pharynx which results in considerable mutilation (**mucocutaneous leishmaniasis** or spundia).

◆ *Leishmania donovani* complex. It includes the species *L. donovani* in southern Asia, *L. infantum* in southern Europe, middle Asia, and north Africa, and *L. chagasi* from Mexico to northern Argentina but particularly in northeastern Brazil. Domestic and wild canids are the main reservoirs of *L. infantum* and *L. chagasi* but the classic *L. donovani* from India has no known animal reservoir.

The species of the *L. donovani* complex infect the systemic reticuloendothelial tissues of humans, particularly of the spleen, lymph nodes, liver, and bone marrow, causing a consumptive disease (**visceral leishmaniasis** or kala-azar) Without treatment, the patient dies within a year. Infected dogs may develop the visceral disease but most often they show only cutaneous lesions.

## FAMILY TRICHOMONADIDAE

The **Trichomonadidae** are pear-shaped, bilaterally asymmetrical flagellates of the digestive or genital tracts. They have one to six flagella, one directed posteriorly and attached to the cytoplasm by an undulating membrane, a single nucleus at the anterior end, and a single, thick axostyle. A rod with transverse striations (**costa**) runs along the union of the undulating membrane with the body. The costa is characteristic of this family. A **parabasal body** is located close to the blepharoplast. Some genera have a **pelta**, a crescent-shaped bundle of microtubules that crown the axostyle. They do not produce cysts. The members of this family swim in a typical spiraling manner. Important genera are *Tritrichomonas, Trichomonas,* and *Histomonas*.

### ◆ *Tritrichomonas*

Members of the genus *Tritrichomonas* have three anterior flagella, a posterior flagellum that trails behind the body, and no pelta. There are a number of *Tritrichomonas* in the large intestine of many mammals and birds but none is pathogenic. Only *T. foetus* is of veterinary importance.

◆ *T. foetus* (10-25x3-15 μm, Figure 26.4) is a venereal parasite of cattle. It is transmitted by coitus or by artificial insemination.

In the cow, the parasites multiply in the vagina for the first two weeks and then invade the uterus, sometimes disappearing form the vagina. They cause the corresponding **vaginitis** and **endometritis** that are not very apparent. The endometritis commonly causes early **abortion** (1-16 weeks) which is often overlooked by the owner and taken as failure to conceive. The parasites clear spontaneously within 20 weeks of a primary infection or within 10 weeks of a secondary infection. When the fetal membranes are retained, an overt catarrhal or **purulent endometritis** may develop. The entire fetus may be retained and macerated causing a **pyometra**. In the bull, the parasite invades the glans and prepuce producing a low grade inflammation of little clinical expression. The parasites remain in the bull for all its useful life.

Diagnosis is done by observation of the parasites in washings of bull smegma, mucus of the anterior part of the vagina, or aborted materials. Culture of these fluids for 4-7 days makes the diagnosis more efficient. The parasites are recognized by their size, shape, and jerky motion. Giemsa or Wright stain facilitates observation of their morphology. The trichomonas may be difficult to find, however, and since the infection of a bull may spread the infection to many cows, many experts require six negative exams and two mounts of virgin heifers that remain negative for three exams before declaring a bull negative.

Since the females eliminate the infection spontaneously, commonly by the third estrus, and develop considerable resistance to the reinfection, they are rarely treated. Treatment of the male is not recommended. Valuable bulls may be left to mount only resistant cows. Metronidazole is effective but it requires local (rubbing the glans and prepuce for 15-20 minutes) and systemic treatments.

## ◆ *Trichomonas*

Members of the genus *Trichomonas* have a medium size pelta, four anterior flagella, and a posterior flagellum that does not trails behind the body. There are a number of *Trichomonas* in the mouth of several animals but they are not pathogenic. The only pathogenic species are *T. vaginalis* that infects the vagina of women and the urethra of men, and *T. gallinae* (Figure 26.4) that causes an inflammation of the mouth and sinuses of young pigeons with production of abundant caseous exudate.

## ◆ *Histomonas*

There is a single species, *H. meleagridis*. *H. meleagridis* is an atypical trichomonad. It infects the cecum and liver of chickens, turkeys, and other gallinaceous birds. In the cecal lumen and in cultures, it is ameboid, 5-30 µm in diameter, with ecto- and endoplasms, numerous food inclusions, and a single short flagellum (Figure 26.4). A parabasal body, a pelta, and an axostyle have been demonstrated by electron microscopy. In the tissues (cecal wall or liver), there are three forms, all devoid of flagellum: a large (8-17 µm in diameter), ameboid parasite, with a basophilic cytoplasm and many food inclusions; a large (12-21 µm), ameboid parasite with a basophilic cytoplasm without inclusions, and: a small (4-11 µm), ameboid parasite with a acidophilic cytoplasm that contains small granules. This pleomorphism makes it difficult to identify in fixed tissue sections. Its round shape, size, and pseudopod formation facilitates identification in fresh samples.

Although very common in chickens, *H. meleagridis* is rarely pathogenic for this species. It causes severe disease (**black-head**) in turkeys, however, particularly in birds 3 to 14 week old. The infection is acquired by ingesting fresh trophozoites with the

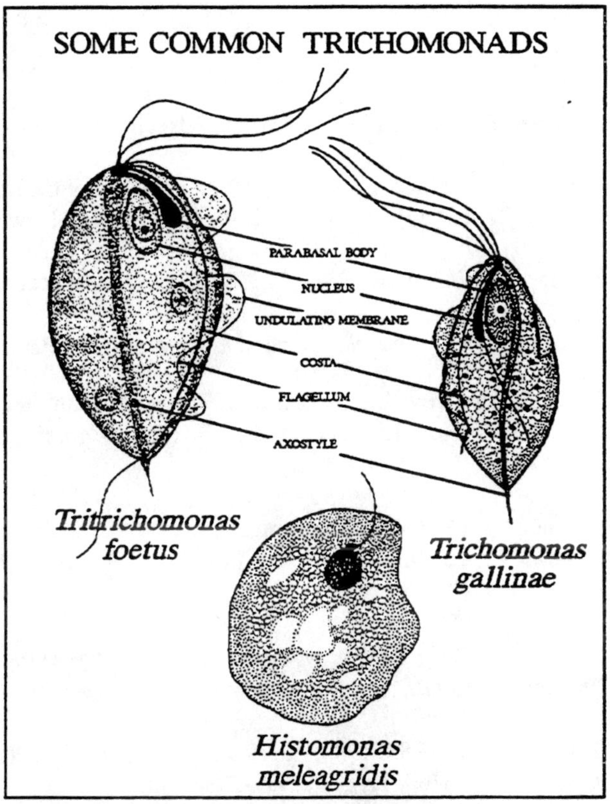


Figure 26.4. Some common trichomonads of domestic animals.

food or water, trophozoites inside the eggs of the nematode, *Heterakis gallinarum*, or the protozoa or the infected nematode eggs in earthworms. The parasite produces inflammation and ulcers in the ceca, and very characteristics circular, yellow-green areas of necrosis, about 1 cm in diameter, in the liver. The incubation period is 15-21 days and death may occur within 1-2 weeks.

Proper turkey management (separation from chickens, separation of poults from adults, prompt removal of the droppings) has reduced considerably the importance of this disease in the last decades. Furazolidone and dimetridazole and other drugs can be used in the feed as curative or preventive.

## REFERENCES

1. Meyer, E.A.(ed.). 1990. Giardiasis. Elsevier, Amsterdam, 368 pp.

2. Kulda, J. and Nohynkova, E. 1978. Flagellates of the human intestine and of intestine of other species. In Kreier JP (ed), *Parasitic Protozoa*, vol 2, Academic Press, New York, 1-138.

3. Kasprzak W & Pawlowski A. 1989. Zoonotic aspects of Giardiasis: a review. Vet. Parasit. 32:101-108.

4. Xiao, L. 1994. *Giardia* infection in farm animals. Parasitol. Today 10:436-438.

5. Logan-Henfrey, L.L., Gardiner, P.R. and Mahmoud, M.M. 1992. Animal trypanosomiasis in sub-Saharan Africa. In Kreier, J.P. and Baker, J.R. (eds), *Parasitic Protozoa*, 2nd ed., vol. 2, Academic Press, New York, 157-276.

6. Gardiner, P.R. and Mahmoud, M.M. 1992. Salivarian trypanosomes causing disease in livestock outside sub-Saharan Africa. In Kreier, J.P. and Baker, J.R. (eds), *Parasitic Protozoa*, 2nd ed., vol. 2, Academic Press, New York, 277-314.

7. Dusanic, D.G. 1991. *Trypanosoma (Schizotrypanum) cruzi*. In Kreier, J.P. and Baker, J.R. (eds), *Parasitic Protozoa*, 2nd ed., vol. 1, Academic Press, New York, 137-194.

8. Lainson, R. 1983. The American leishmaniases: some observations on their ecology and epidemiology. Trans. R Soc. Trop. Med. Hyg. 77:569-596..

# Chapter 27

# THE APICOMPLEXA OR SPOROZOA

The **Apicomplexa** are all parasitic protozoa characterized by the lack of locomotor organelles (flagella, cilia, or pseudopods) and by the presence of an apical complex at the anterior end.

The **apical complex** can be seen only with the electron microscope. It is composed of one or more polar rings, a conoid, subpellicular tubules, rhoptries, and micronemes (Figure 27.1).

The **polar ring** is a circular arrangement of microtubules at the anterior end of the parasite. The **conoid** is a hollow cone of spirally arranged microtubules that can protrude through the polar ring. The **subpellicular microtubules** are longitudinal arrangements of microtubules that originate from the polar ring and run backward under the cellular membrane. The **rhoptries** are club-like structures that reach inside the conoid. The **micronemes** are small rod-like structures in the anterior part of the parasite, around the rhoptries. Some Apicomplexa have one or more **micropores** which are invaginations of the outer cellular membrane through an opening of the inner membrane.

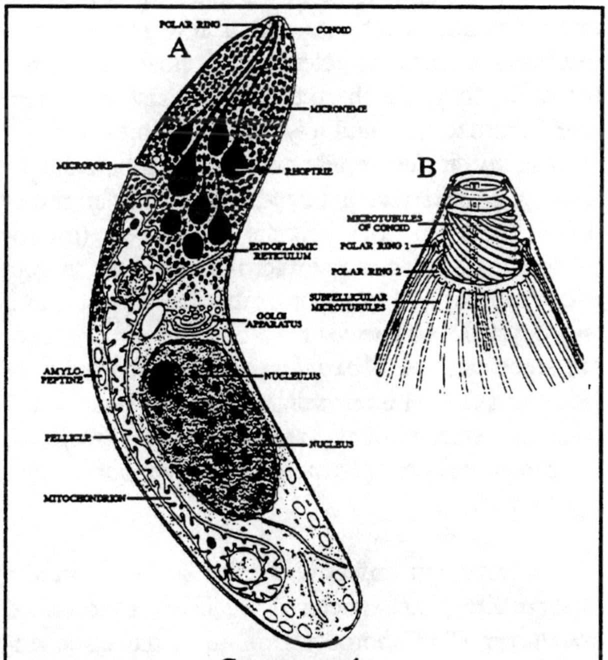


*Sarcocystis* sp.

**Figure 27.1**. Morphology of the trophozoite of an Apicomplexa (A) and details of the apical complex (B)

The functions of the apical complex are not completely understood yet. The conoid is believed to be related to penetration of host cells. The rhoptries are thought to produce enzymes to assist penetration. The subpellicular microtubules probably cause flexing of the parasite or ripples of its membrane for locomotion. The micropores appear to be feeding organelles. The apical complex is particularly well developed in the motile stages of the Apicomplexa. Not all its elements are present in all species (see below).

There are about 4500 Apicomplexa species, all parasitic, distributed into more than 60 families.[1] Only three orders are of veterinary importance, however: the Coccidia proper or Eucoccidiida, the Piroplasmida, and the Haemosporida. Their characteristics will be discussed with the corresponding group. Another group, the Gregarines, may become significant in the future. These are parasites of invertebrates and may turn to be important for the biological control of mosquitoes and other vectors.

# THE ORDER EUCOCCIDIIDA OR COCCIDIA PROPER

The **Coccidia** are parasites of the intestine of humans and many domestic animals.[2,3] A few live in extraintestinal locations, and a few infect extra-intestinal tissues of intermediate hosts. Morphologically, they are characterized because the infective sporozoites multiply by multiple division (merogony) in the vertebrate host, the motile stages have a conoid and a three-layered cellular membrane (pellicle), the original male cell (microgamont) produces many microgametes; the zygote is not motile; and the sporozoites are enclosed in a sporocyst. Most species have only a definitive host but some can use (*Toxoplasma*), and others require (*Sarcocystis*), an intermediate host. The genera that concern veterinarians are *Eimeria, Isospora, Cryptosporidium, Toxoplasma, Neospora,* and *Sarcocystis*.

The common infective forms of the coccidia (**sporozoites**) are enclosed inside a cyst called **sporocyst**. The sporocysts, in turn, are often enclosed in a larger cyst called **oocyst**. The general structure of an *Eimeria* oocyst appears in Figure 27.2. Because of the importance of the oocysts for the diagnosis of coccidial infections, it is convenient to review here the morphological differentiation of the oocysts of the genera of veterinary importance.

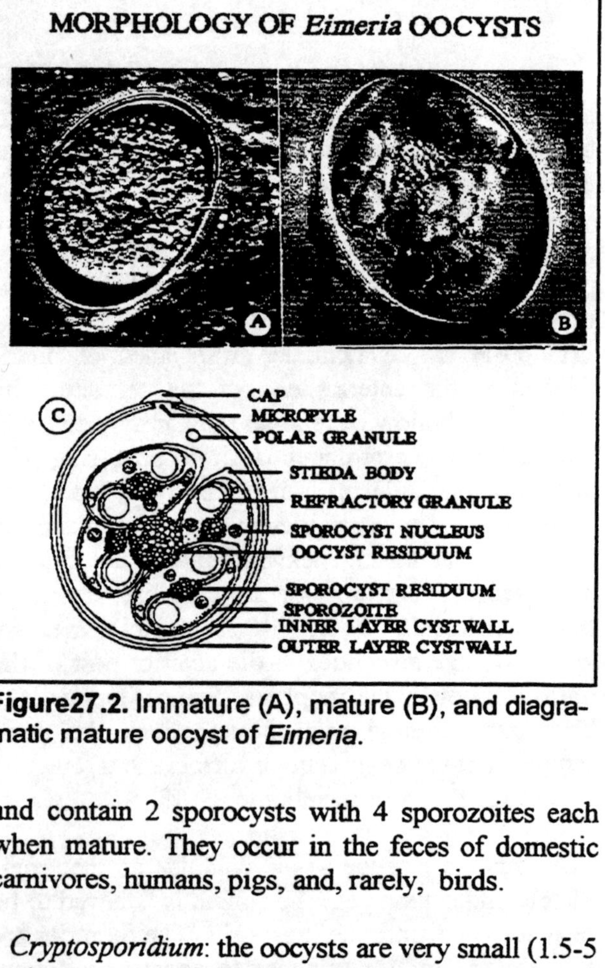


**Figure27.2.** Immature (A), mature (B), and diagramatic mature oocyst of *Eimeria*.

*Eimeria*: the oocysts are generally of medium or large size (>12 µm), pass in the feces unsporulated, and contain 4 sporocysts with 2 sporozoites each when mature. They occurs primarily in the feces of birds, ruminants, pigs, and rarely, other species.

*Isospora*: the oocysts are generally of medium or large size (>12 µm), pass in the feces unsporulated, and contain 2 sporocysts with 4 sporozoites each when mature. They occur in the feces of domestic carnivores, humans, pigs, and, rarely, birds.

*Cryptosporidium*: the oocysts are very small (1.5-5 µm), pass in the feces already sporulated, and contain 4 sporozoites that lack a sporocyst. In the feces of many mammals and birds.

*Toxoplasma*: the oocysts are small (10-12 µm), pass in the feces unsporulated, and contain 2 sporocysts with 4 sporozoites each when mature. In the feces of cats.

*Neospora*: The life cycle of *Neospora caninum* is not known entirely yet and oocysts have not been found so far.

*Sarcocystis*: the oocysts are medium size (12-21 µm) but they often break in the intestine so the individual sporocysts (10-20 µm) are found in the feces; they are passed sporulated and each sporocyst (2 per oocyst) contains 4 sporozoites. In the feces of carnivores or humans.

## THE GENUS *Eimeria*

*Eimeria* are parasites primarily of birds, rodents, lagomorphs, ruminants, pig, and, occasionally, equines. They infect mostly intestinal cells. Their exact location in the intestine varies depending on the species.

### a. Identification and classification

In veterinary medicine, the coccidia are usually identified by observation of the morphology of the oocysts passed by the infected host. *Eimeria* is characterized by the presence of four sporocysts in the oocyst, each containing two sporozoites.

With the **immature oocysts**, important criteria are the host, the size and shape of the oocyst, the thickness of the wall, and the presence or not of a micropyle. Study of mature oocysts provides more morphological information (see Figure 27.2) so it is often preferred. The elements commonly observed in a **mature oocyst** are the shape (ovoid, ellipsoidal, rounded, etc.), size, thickness and structure of the wall (one or two layers), presence of a polar granule, a micropyle (with or without a cap), and a oocyst residuum (left over material). The structures to observe in the **mature sporocysts** are the shape, size, presence of a knob at one end (Stieda body), and a sporocyst residuum. In the **sporozoites** one can observe their shape, size, and the presence of a refractory globule at one end.

To obtain sporulated oocysts, samples of feces are mixed with 3-5 volumes of 2.5% potassium bichromate and incubated at room temperature for 2-14 days (depending on the species) in a Petri dish, in layers of a few millimeters. The potassium bichromate prevents the growth of other micro-organisms and the thin layer permits the oxygenation of the oocysts.

The information in Figures 27.3 to 27.6 and in Tables 27.I to 27.IV. may permit the identification of the oocysts of some important *Eimeria* of domestic animals. The manual by Sloss et al.[4] is highly recommended for this purpose.

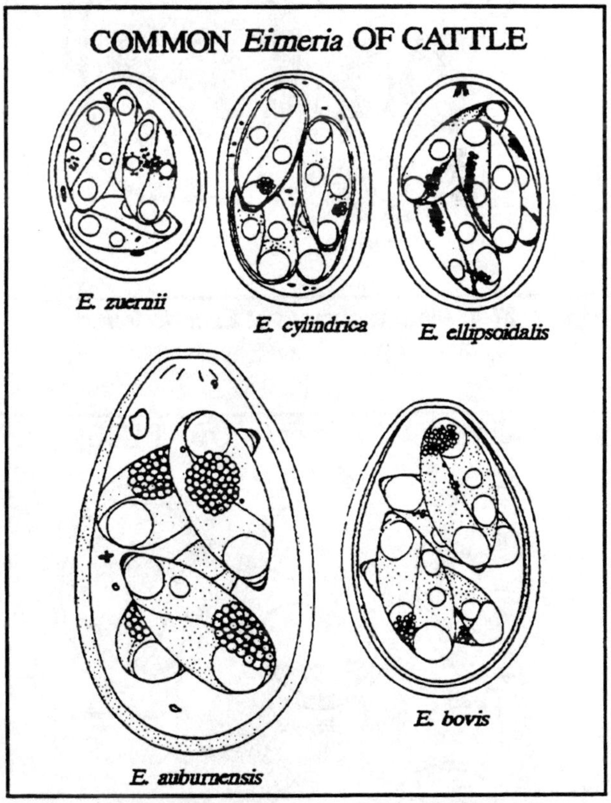


**Figure 27.3.** Mature oocysts of *Eimeria* found commonly in cattle.

Besides the species listed in the Tables, goats are infected with several *Eimeria* species. The most pathogenic are *E. christenseni*, *E. arloingi*, and *E. alijevi* of the small intestine. *E. leuckarti* is occasionally found in the small intestine of horses but its pathogenicity is questionable. Several *Eimeria* infect rabbits, *E. flavescens*, *E. irresidua*, and *E. magna* of the small intestine, and *E. stiedai* of the

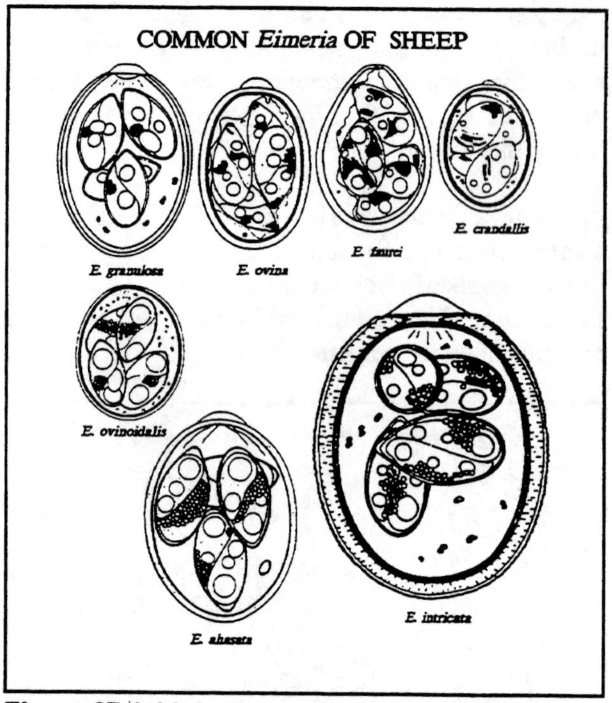


**Figure 27.4.** Mature oocysts of *Eimeria* found commonly in sheep.

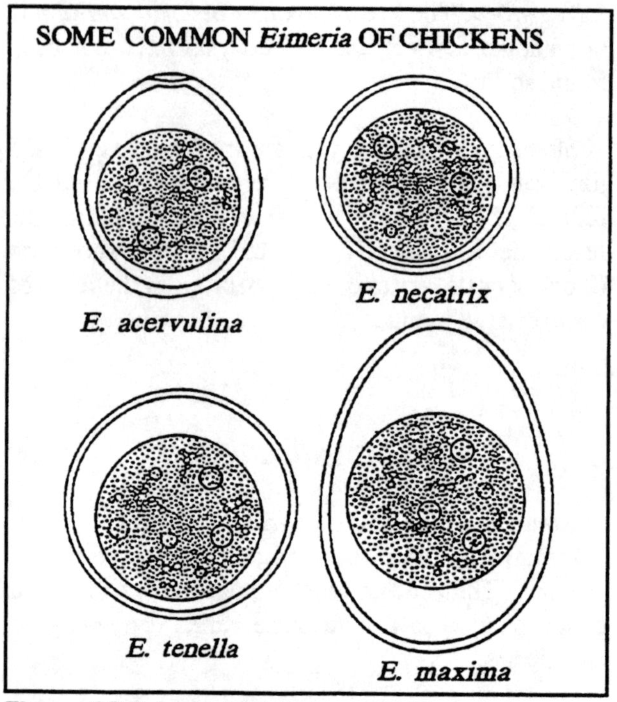


**Figure 27.6.** Immature oocysts of *Eimeria* found commonly in chickens.

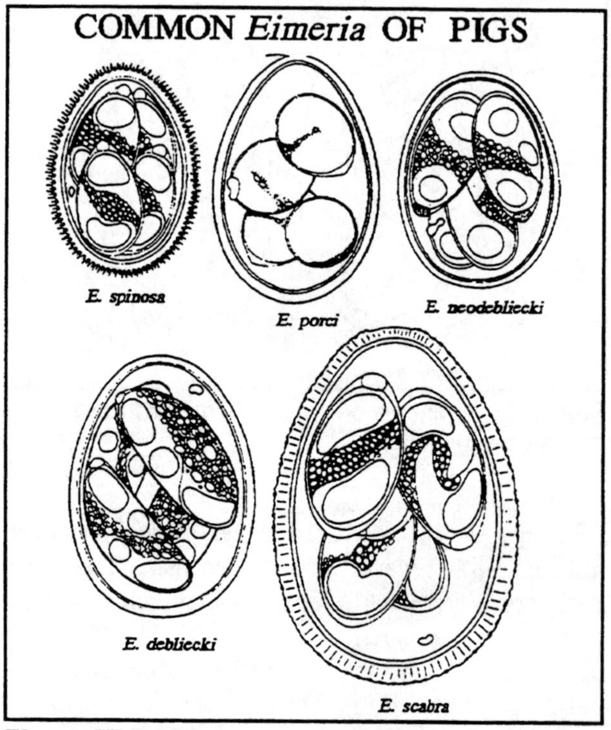


**Figure 27.5.** Mature oocysts of *Eimeria* found commonly in pigs.

bile ducts are the most pathogenic. Turkeys are also affected by several *Eimeria* but *E. adenoides* of the small intestine and ceca is the most pathogenic.

Some coccidial species simply cannot be differentiated by oocyst morphology alone. In these cases, additional criteria for the identification of species are the location of the lesions in the organ (e.g., ileum, ceca, Figure 27.7), the location of the parasites in the tissues (epithelium, lamina propria), even the location of the parasite inside the host cell (above or below the nucleus), and details of the biology of the parasite.

**b. Biology**

Infection occurs by ingestion of mature ( sporulated) oocysts. The biochemical conditions of the host's digestive tract activate the sporozoites that leave the sporocyst and invade host cells. In the cell, the sporozoites reproduce by multiple fission forming a rosette of tiny parasites called **schizont**

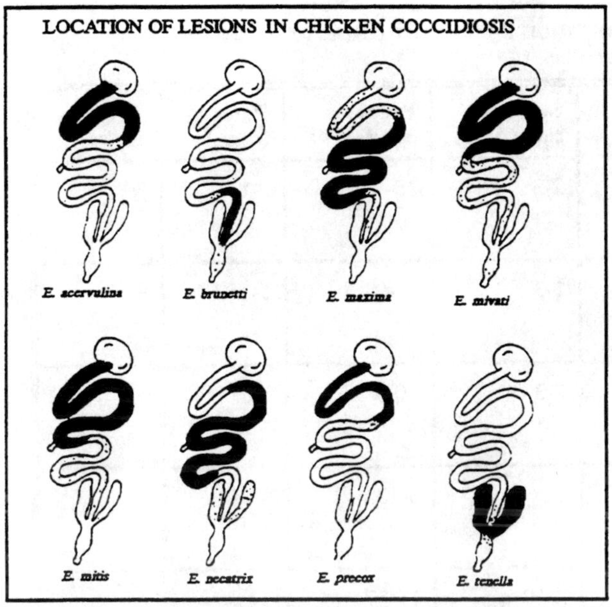


**Figure 27.7**. Typical location of the lesions of common *Eimeria* of chickens.

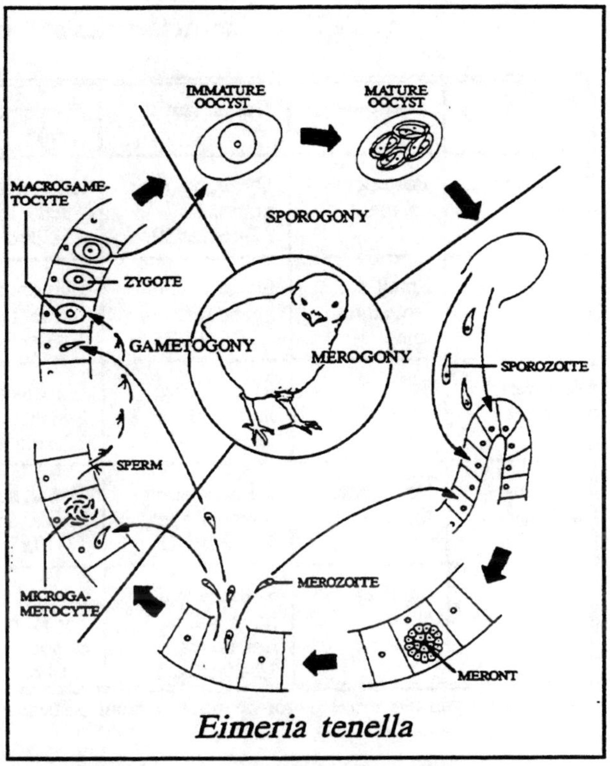


**Figure 27.8**. Life cycle of a typical *Eimeria*.

or **meront** (from Gr *skhizo*= split, or *meros*= part). Each individual parasite is called a **merozoite**. A meront can have several hundreds or a few thousands of them. The growing meront bursts the host cells after 2-3 days and each merozoite invades a new host cell to form a second generation meront. This new meront has a few hundreds merozoites that also burst the host cell after 2-3 days. This process of asexual reproduction is called **schizogony** or **merogony** (from Lat *gonia*= generation).

The merozoites of the second generation invade new host cells but, whereas some will form a third generation meront, most become sexual cells. The majority will turn into female cells (**macrogametes**) but a few will turn into male cells (**microgamonts**). The male cells mature and divide to form many biflagellate **microgametes**. The microgametes break out of the host cells, search for the macrogametes, and fertilize them. Each resulting zygote lays down a resistant wall around itself to become an oocyst, breaks out of the host cell, and passes out in the feces starting about a week after infection. This process of sexual reproduction is called **gametogony**.

Inside the oocyst, the zygote, which is non-infective, divides into four cells. Each cell will form a **sporocyst** (from Gr *sporos*= seed), and each sporocyst will develop two sporozoites inside. The oocyst containing four sporocysts which, in turn, contain two sporozoites is commonly called ***Eimeria*-type.** The sporozoites are the infective elements for the new hosts. This process of sporozoite formation is called **sporogony** and usually takes about 2 days at room temperature.

Figure 27.8 shows the life cycle of a chicken coccidia.

Because the life cycle of the coccidia ends in the formation of oocysts (which implies the departure of the parasites), the infection is self-limiting and normally resolves spontaneously after a few days or weeks. Some animals, however, may remain passing some oocysts for a longer time and are the responsible for the persistent contamination of the pastures or premises.

## Table 27.1. Characteristics of some common species of *Eimeria* of cattle

| Species | Location | Oocyst (µm)* | Sporocyst (µm)* | Sporulation (days) | Prepatency (days) | Patency (days) | Pathogenicity |
|---|---|---|---|---|---|---|---|
| *E. auburnensis* | Posterior small int. | Ovoid, pg, mp, no res, 32-46x19-30 | Ellipsoidal, Stieda, res, 15-23x6-11 | 2-3 | 16-24 | 2-8 | ++ |
| *E. bovis* | Small & large intestine | Ovoid, mp, no pg, no res, 23-24x17-23 | Ellipsoidal, Stieda, res, 13-18x5-8 | 2-3 | 16-21 | 5-15 | +++ |
| *E. cylindrica* | ? | Ellipsoid, pg, no mp, no res, 16-34x12-19 | Ellipsoidal, no Stieda, res, 12-16x4-6 | 2-3 | 10 | 10 | + |
| *E. ellipsoidalis* | Small intestine | Ellipsoidal, pg, no mp, no res, 12-32x10-29 | Ovoid, small Stieda, no res, 11-17x5-7 | 3 | 8-13 | ? | ++ |
| *E. zuernii* | Small & large intestine | Subspherical, pg or not, no mp, no res, 12-29x10-21 | Ovoid, small Stieda, res or not, 7-14x4-8 | 2-10 | 15-17 | 11 | +++ |

(*) pg = polar granule, mp = micropyle, res = residuum, Stieda = Stieda body

## Table 27.II. Characteristics of some common species of *Eimeria* of sheep

| Species | Location | Oocyst (µm)* | Sporocyst (µm)* | Sporulation (days) | Prepatency (days) | Patency (days) | Pathogenicity |
|---|---|---|---|---|---|---|---|
| *E. ahsata* | Small intestine | Ellipsoid, pg, mp, no res, 23-48x17-30 | Ellipsoid, no Stieda, res 12-22x6-10 | 1.5-3 | 18-21 | 10-12 | +++ |
| *E. crandallis* | Small intestine | Subspherical, pg, mp, no res, 18-28x15-20 | Ovoid, no Stieda, res or not, 8-13x6-9 | 1-3 | 13-20 | ? | + |
| *E. faurie* | Small intestine | Ovoid, pg, mp, no res, 25-37x18-28 | Ovoid, no Stieda, res, 11-17x7-9 | 1-4 | ? | ? | + |
| *E. granulosa* | ? | Piriform, pg or not, mp, no res, 22-37x17-26 | Ovoid, no Stieda, res, 17-22x9-14 | 3-4 | ? | ? | ? |
| *E. intricata* | Sm.& lg. intestine | Ellipsoid, pg, mp, no res, 39-59x27-47 | Ovoid, no Stieda, res. | 3-12 | 20-27 | 5-11 | + |
| *E. ovina* | Small intestine | Ellipsoid, pg, mp, no res, 23-36x15-24 | Ovoid, Stieda or not, res, 11-17x6-9 | 2-4 | 19-29 | 10 | ++ |
| *E. ovinoidalis* | Sm. & lg. intestine | Subspherical, 2 pg, mp, no res, 16-30x13-22 | Ellipsoid, Stieda, res, 10-14x4-8 | 1-4 | 9-15 | 7-28 | +++ |

(*) pg = polar granule, mp = micropyle, res = residuum, Stieda = Stieda body

**Table 27.III. Characteristics of some common species of *Eimeria* of pigs**

| Species | Location | Oocyst (µm)* | Sporocyst (µm)* | Sporulation (days) | Prepatency (days) | Patency (days) | Pathogenicity |
|---|---|---|---|---|---|---|---|
| *E. debliecki* | Small intestine | Ovoid, pg, no mp, no res, 20-30x14-19 | Ovoid, Stieda, res 13-20x5-7 | 10 | 6.5 | 4.5 | + |
| *E. neodebliecki* | ? | Ellipsoid, pg, no mp, no res, 17-26x13-20 | Ovoid, Stieda, res, 9-14x5-8 | 13 | 10 | 6 | ? |
| *E. porci* | ? | Ovoid, pg, mp, no res, 18-27x13-18 | Spherical, Stieda, res, 8-12x6-8 | 9 | 5-7 | 6 | ? |
| *E. scabra* | Posterior sm. int. | Ellipsoidal, pg, mp, no res, 25-45x18-28 | Ovoid, Stieda, res, 14-18x7-9 | 9-12 | 7-11 | 4-8 | + |
| *E. spinosa* | Posterior sm. int. | Ovoid, pg, no mp, no res, 14-26x12-21 | Ovoid, Stieda, res 10-14x5-7 | 9-22 | 7 | ? | + |

(*) pg = polar granule, mp = micropyle, res = residuum, Stieda = Stieda body

**Table 27.IV. Characteristics of some common species of *Eimeria* of the chicken**

| Specie | Location | Oocyst (µm)* | Sporocyst (µm)* | Sporulation (days) | Prepatency (days) | Patency (days) | Pathogenicity |
|---|---|---|---|---|---|---|---|
| *E. acervulina* | Anterior small int. | Ovoid, pg, no mp, no res 12-23x9-17 | Ovoid, Stieda, no res ? | 1 | 4 | ? | + |
| *E. brunetti* | Posterior small int. | Ovoid, pg, no mp, no res 14-34x12-26 | Ellipsoidal, Stieda, res 13x7.5 | 1-2 | 5 | ? | ++ |
| *E. maxima* | Middle small int. | Ovoid, pg, no mp, no res 21-42x16-30 | Ovoid, Stieda, no res 15-19x8-9 | 1.5-2 | 5-6 | A few | + |
| *E. mitis* | Anterior small int. | Spherical, pg, no mp, no res 10-21x9-18 | Ovoid, Stieda, no res 10x6 | 1-2 | 4-5 | 10 | + |
| *E. mivati* | Anterior small int. | Ovoid, pg, mp, no res 11-20x12-17 | Ellipsoidal, Stieda, res 7-12x5-6 | 3 | 4-5 | 6-12 | ++ |
| *E. necatrix* | Middle small int. | Ovoid, pg, no mp, no res 12-29x11-24 | Ovoid, Stieda, no res ? | <1 | 6-7 | 12 | +++ |

| Table 27.IV. Characteristics of some common species of *Eimeria* of the chicken (continuation) | | | | | | | |
|---|---|---|---|---|---|---|---|
| **Specie** | **Location** | **Oocyst (µm)*** | **Sporocyst (µm)*** | **Sporulation (days)** | **Prepatency (days)** | **Patency (days)** | **Pathogenicity** |
| *E. precox* | Anterior small int. | Ovoid, pg, no mp, no res, 20-25x16-20 | Ovoid, Stieda, no res. | 2 | 2.5-4 | 4+ | ? |
| *E. tenella* | Ceca | Ovoid, pg, no mp, no res, 14-31x9-25 | Ovoid, Stieda, no res ? | 1.5-2 | 6 | 5+ | +++ |

(*) pg = polar granule, mp = micropyle, res = residuum, Stieda = Stieda body

### c. Medical importance

Not all coccidia are equally harmful. Some are very pathogenic, others cause mild disease only when they exist in large numbers, and others behave as commensals. Regardless the species, they rarely cause disease when they are present in low numbers; coccidiosis is a disease of confined animals that have the opportunity to accumulate important numbers of parasites. In general, the coccidia are more harmful in young hosts. As a rule, coccidial infections produce strong immunity. A first infection leaves considerable resistance to further clinical episodes and subsequent exposures may elicit resistance to further infections.

Although there are reports of systemic changes in infected hosts,[5] the major pathogenic mechanism of the coccidia is the destruction of hosts cells, especially during the first meront generation. The major clinical manifestations are an intense diarrhea, sometimes bloody, and rapid loss of condition. With species particularly pathogenic (e.g., *E. tenella* in chickens, *E. zuernii* in cattle), severe disease and even death may occur before oocysts appear in the feces.

## THE GENUS *Isospora*

*Isospora* are primarily intestinal parasites of carnivores, pigs, and humans. Their oocysts have been reported from ruminants and fowl but these may be pseudoparasites picked up with their feed.

### a. Identification and classification

In the veterinary practice, the identification of *Isospora* has the same basis as the identification of *Eimeria*. *Isospora*, however, is characterized by the presence of two sporocysts in the mature oocyst, each containing four sporozoites (Figure 27.9). Oocyst containing two sporocysts which, in turn, contain four sporozoites are commonly called ***Isospora*-type.** Table 27.V. presents some characteristics of common *Isospora*.

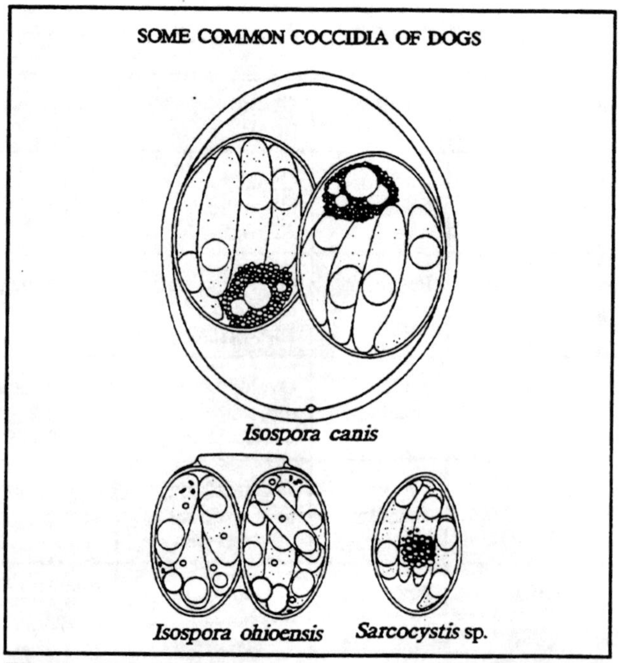


**Figure 27.9.** Some common coccidia of the dog. Oocysts of *I. canis* and *I. ohioensis* and sporocyst of *Sarcocystis* sp.

**Table 27.V. Characteristics of some common species of *Isospora***

| Species | Host | Location | Oocyst (µm)* | Sporocyst (µm)** | Sporulation (days) | Prepatency (days) | Patency (days) | Pathogenicity |
|---|---|---|---|---|---|---|---|---|
| *I. suis* | Pig | Small intestine | Spherical, 17-25x16-21 | Ellipsoidal 13-14x8-11 | 3-5 | 5 | 3-13 | ++ |
| *I. canis* | Dog | Posterior small int. | Ellipsoidal 34-42x23-36 | Ellipsoidal 18-28x15-19 | 2 | 9-11 | 28 | + |
| *I. ohioensis* | Dog | Sm. & lg. intestine | Ellipsoidal 20-27x15-24 | Ellipsoidal 12-19x9-13 | <7 | 3.5-4.5 | 7-35 | none |
| *I. felis* | Cat | Sm. & lg. intestine | Ovoid, 32-53x26-43 | Ellipsoidal 20-27x17-22 | 2+ | 7-10 | 10-20 | + |
| *I. rivolta* | Cat | Sm. & lg. intestine | Ovoid 21-29x18-26 | Ellipsoidal 14-16x10-13 | 1-2 | 4-7 | 66+ | + |
| *I. belli* | Human | Small intestine | Ellipsoidal 20-33x10-19 | Variable, 9-14x7-12 | 5 | ? | ? | + |

(*) With the exception of *I belli* which has all three, the oocysts of these species do not have micropyle, residuum, or polar granule.

### b. Biology

The life cycle of *Isospora* is essentially similar to that of *Eimeria*. The oocysts of some *Isospora* species (*I. canis, I. felis*) are infective for rodents and birds. The sporozoites experience limited multiplication in the mesenteric lymph nodes and. occasionally, other organs of these species which can act as transport hosts of the parasites.

The genus *Cystoisospora* was proposed for these species but it has not had wide reception.

### c. Medical importance

The same criteria discussed for *Eimeria* are applicable to *Isospora* infections. Most of the damage of the infection is related to the destruction of host cells during merogony and gametogony. *Isospora*, however, seems to be less pathogenic than *Eimeria*, many hosts carry the parasite without showing any clinical manifestation.

## THE GENUS *Cryptosporidium*

Different from the other intestinal coccidia, most *Cryptosporidium* are host non-specific parasites. They occur in the intestinal tract but occasionally infect the respiratory apparatus, especially in birds.

### a. Identification and classification

Over 20 species of *Cryptosporidium* have been described but only six are considered valid nowadays. Four of them affect homothermous: *C. parvum* of many mammals (including humans), *C. muris* of mice and cattle, *C. baileyi* of chickens, and *C. meleagridis* of turkeys.

Their identifying characteristics is that the oocysts are very small (1.5-5 µm), pass already sporulated, develop four naked (without sporocysts) sporozoites, and that their microgametes do not have flagella.

### b. Biology

*C. parvum* is the species of more concern to medicine (*C. muris* appears not to be pathogenic for cattle) and the most studied. Upon ingestion of the sporulated oocyst, the sporozoites invade the epithelial cells of the small intestine (and, occasionally, bile ducts and respiratory passages) and lie in a cytoplasmic vacuole just underneath the cellular membrane. Each sporozoite divides into eight 5x1 µm merozoites within the first day. The merozoites leave the host cell and each invades an adjacent cell to produce four merozoites this time. The merozoites do not have a conoid, polar ring, or micropore.

Most of the second generation merozoites develop into gametes that appear already by 48 hors of infection. The 1.5-5 µm, rounded or oval oocysts form soon thereafter and develop the infective sporozoites before leaving the intestine.

### c. Medical importance

Experimental transfers have demonstrated that *C. parvum* is a zoonotic parasite with little host specificity. Actually, some of the first epidemics registered were in veterinary students working with calves. The parasite infects humans, ruminants, pigs, horses, carnivores, rodents, etc. The disease, however, is fairly common only in humans and calves, and affects particularly the very young. It appears that many infected hosts control the infection spontaneously.

In the United States, about 4% of diarrheic human patients have *C. parvum* oocysts in their stools but about 13% of 169 asymptomatic patients undergoing routine bile examination also showed oocysts. Infected people who develop symptoms have a severe watery diarrhea with intestinal cramps and rapid loss of weight that rarely lasts more than 1-3 weeks. In immunocompromised (AIDS) patients, an intractable diarrhea and severe weight loss may lead to death.

Calves appear to be the most susceptible among the domestic animals. In North America, most studies in diarrheic calves have shown that about 25% are passing *C. parvum* oocysts. The affected animals are usually 1-3 weeks of age.

In domestic animals other than calves (pigs, horses, carnivores), clinical cryptosporidiosis has been sporadically reported in immunosuppressed or very young animals.

The pathogenic mechanism of *C. parvum* is unknown. Because little or no tissue damage or reaction is observed, the prevalent opinion is that the parasite must interfere with the biochemistry of absorption at the microvillus level.

## THE GENUS *Toxoplasma*

The only important species in the genus, *Toxoplasma gondii* (from Gr *toxo*= bow, and Lat *plasma*= body) is essentially a parasite of the intestine of felids that can use some 200 species of other vertebrates (including humans and felids) as intermediate hosts.[6]

### a. Identification

As the definitive host, the cat harbors five morphological types of parasites during the merogonic and gametogonic cycles in its intestinal cells, and the oocysts that are discharged in the feces at the end of these cycles.

The description of the forms in the intestinal tissue has been given by Dubey[7] but it is of little use to the veterinary practitioner.

The **oocysts** are passed as 10x12 µm unsporulated oocysts with a thin wall and a zygote that occupies almost all its interior space. In 1-5 days they mature to 11x13 µm sporulated oocysts that contain two 6x8 µm sporocysts without a Stieda body. Each sporocyst encloses four 2x6-8 µm **sporozoites** (Figure 27.10).

Two types of parasites occur in the intermediate hosts: tachyzoites and bradyzoites.

The **tachyzoites** (from Gr *takhus*= swift, *zoon*= animal) are small (6x2 µm, Figure 27.10), crescent-shaped, active parasites that invade any nucleated host cells and divide rapidly by multiple fission into meronts until bursting the cell.

The **bradyzoites** (from Gr *bradus*= slow) are slender, crescent-shaped parasites (7x1.5 µm) that divide slowly and accumulate in the cytoplasm of the host cell. This accumulation distends the host cell that may reach up to 60-100 µm in diameter. The cluster of bradyzoites is surrounded by a thin (<0.5 µm), argentophilic wall of host origin constituting a **tissue cyst**.

The tachyzoites, bradyzoites, and sporozoites have all a similar structure.

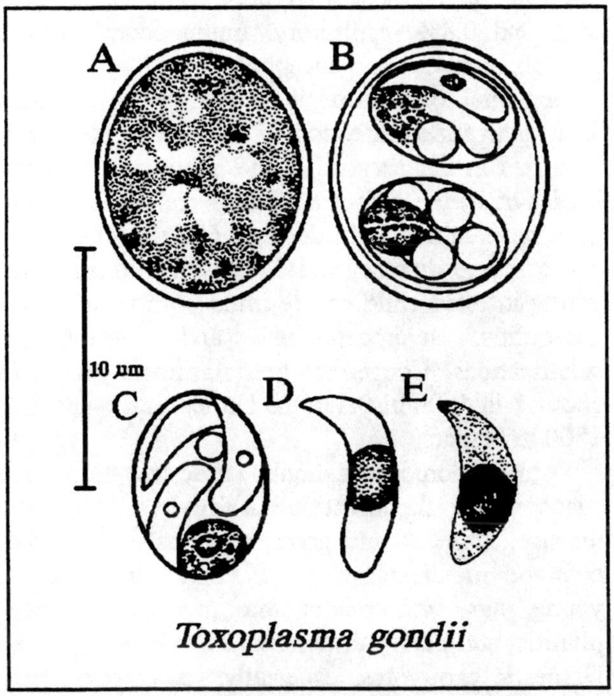


**Figure 27.10.** Immature (A), and mature (B) oocyst, mature sporocyst (C), sporozoite (D), and tachyzoite (E) of *Toxoplasma gondii*.

**b. Biology**

The **intermediate hosts** (over 200 species that include primates, ruminants, pigs, horses, carnivores, rodents, marsupials, insectivores, and many birds) are usually infected by ingestion of bradyzoites in **undercooked meats** (particularly mouton or pork), or **mature oocysts** contaminating their food, water, or hands (Figure 27.11). The parasites turn into tachyzoites, invade epithelial intestinal cells, multiply until the cells rupture, and spread (free or inside parasitized white cells) by the lymph and blood. Most parasites are captured by the lymph nodes and are found in macrophages or monocytes but, in a few cases, they overwhelm the nodes and may invade any other organ. These cycles of invasion, multiplication, rupture, and new invasion of host cells proceed for 1-2 weeks and are the fundamental pathogenic mechanism of toxoplasmosis. During the second week of infection, tachyzoites start being replaced with bradyzoites which soon are the only type of organisms found in the host. Clusters of bradyzoites (cysts) may occur in any organ but are more common in nervous and muscle tissue. The cysts persist for many years, perhaps for the life of the host, and cause no harm. The parasites of cysts that open are probably rapidly disposed of by the immune system.

Toxoplasmosis can also be transmitted **congenitally**. Except in the mouse, congenital transmission occurs only when the mother becomes infected during pregnancy and tachyzoites infect the placenta. Transmission through eggs, transfusions, etc. is theoretically possible but very rare. Transmission by transplants is recognized as important now because the immunosuppressed recipient is often overwhelmed by infections that were asymptomatic in the donor. Probably bradyzoites from ruptured cysts, that would have been destroyed by the donor's immunity, turn into tachyzoites in the immunosuppressed individual.

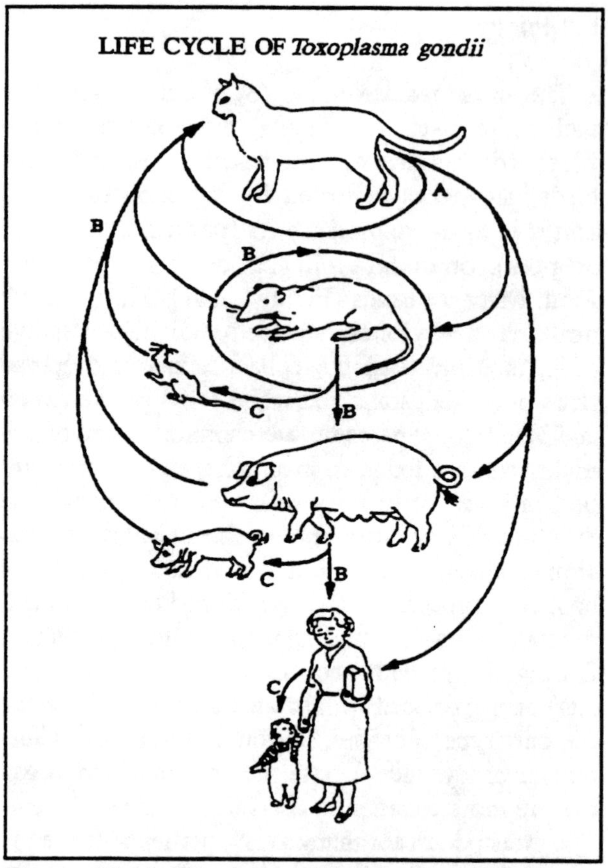


**Figure 27.11.** Life cycle of *Toxoplasma gondii.* Fecal (A), carnivorous (B), and congenital (C) transmission.

The **definitive host** (cats) is usually infected by ingestion of bradyzoites in the flesh of intermediate hosts , or sporozoites in mature oocysts. Tachyzoites are destroyed by the acidity and enzymes of the stomach so they are an unlikely source of oral infection. The bradyzoites or sporozoites penetrate epithelial cells of the cat small intestine and multiply for several generations passing for 5 different morphological types, and ending with the formation of gametes (gametogony). By 3-10 days of infection with cysts, or 19-21 days after infection with oocysts, immature oocysts start being discharged in the feces. Patency last only 1-2 weeks, rarely longer, and, under normal circumstances, may occur only once in the definitive host's life. The cat develops enough immunity to prevent formation of future oocysts but not to eliminate all the parasites.

Subsequent infections with *Isospora felis* or treatment with immunosuppressors may trigger new short episodes of patency.

During the process of intestinal multiplication, parasites often spread to the extraintestinal tissues of the cat and generate an infection comparable to that in intermediate hosts. Remnants of intestinal and tissue parasites remain in the cat maybe for life.

### c. Medical importance

Serological surveys indicate that 16-40% of the people in the United States or Great Britain and 50-80% of those in continental Europe or Latin America are infected with *T. gondii*. The large majority of the cases, however, are asymptomatic. About 90% of the infections with clinical manifestations show only mild fever, prolonged lymphadenopathy, and often myositis, 4% are nervous, 1.4% myocardial, and 0.8% respiratory. Immunocompromised patients often develop encephalitis.

Congenital toxoplasmosis is more severe. It begins as a generalized infection of the fetus but later it localizes in the nervous tissue. About 40% of the babies of acutely infected mothers are born infected, 26% have subclinical infection, 6% a mild disease, 4% a severe disease, and 3% die as neonates. Severely infected children are often born with retinochoroiditis, hydrocephalus, and intracerebral calcifications. Congenital toxoplasmosis occurs in about 1 in 4000 births in the United States and 1 in 1500 in France.

Among domestic animals, cattle and horses are susceptible to the infection but fully resistant to the disease. In sheep and goats, the most evident and common manifestation is abortion. Outbreaks in young pigs, with pneumonia, myocarditis, encephalitis, and placental necrosis have been reported. Domestic carnivores, especially young ones, may develop respiratory and digestive manifestations.

Serological studies have shown that 15-40% of adult cats in the USA are infected with *T. gondii* although only about 1% are passing oocysts at any given time. The intestinal infection of cats rarely produces clinical symptoms.

## THE GENUS *Neospora*

*Neospora canimum* is a coccidia recognized only in 1988.[4] Previously, it was confused with *T. gondii* with which it has many similarities.

### a. Identification

The tachyzoites are ovoid, crescent-shaped, or rounded, 3-7x1-5 μm and found in neural cells, macrophages, fibroblasts, endotheliocytes, myocytes, hepatocytes, and other cells. The bradyzoites are 6-8x1-1.8 μm and found only in nervous tissue forming round or oval cysts of up to 107 μm long. At this moment, differentiation between *N. caninum* and *T. gondii* can be done only with monoclonal antibodies specific to each parasite.

### b. Biology

*N. caninum* has been found in dogs, cattle, sheep, goats, and horses and has been transmitted experimentally to cats, mice, rats, and gerbils. Transplacental infection occurs in domestic carnivores, cattle, sheep, and horses and may take place in successive pregnancies. Experimentally infected dogs and cats did not pass oocysts.

Other details of the life cycle are not known yet.

### c. Medical importance

The major pathogenic mechanism of *N. canimum* appears to be the destruction of nervous and other cells during the multiplication of the tachyzoites.

In dogs, the most severe disease occurs in pups congenitally infected from subclinically infected dams. The disease manifests itself as an ascending paralysis that affects young dogs that otherwise are well alert. The hind limbs are more affected that the front legs but paralysis of the jaw and muscle flaccidity may occur. The patient may survive for months.

In cattle, the mayor manifestation is abortion or an ascending paralysis of the congenitally infected calves. It is estimated that a fourth of all cattle abortions may be due to this parasite.

## THE GENUS *Sarcocystis*

*Sarcocystis* are heteroxenous (with definitive and intermediate hosts) parasites of the intestine of predators (definitive hosts) and the vessels and muscles of preys (intermediate hosts).

### a. Identification and classification

The oocysts of *Sarcocystis* (from Gr *sarx*= flesh, and *kustis*= bladder, cyst) are of medium size (from 15x12 to 20x16 μm, depending on the species) and pass sporulated. Originally, they contain two sporocysts, each with four sporozoites. They have a smooth, thin (<1 μm) wall and lack oocyst residuum or micropyle. The oocyst wall is very thin and the sporocysts often stretch it forming a dumbbell-shaped figure. Many sporocysts actually break the oocyst wall and pass as individual sporocysts in the feces (from 12x8 to 15x10 μm, depending on the species, Figure 27.9). The sporocysts have a residuum but not a Stieda body. As with *Eimeria* and *Isospora*, the morphology of the oocysts or sporocysts often permits species identification.[8] Table 27.VI. lists some characteristics of common species of *Sarcocystis*.

Two generations of **merozoites** occur in the vascular endothelial cells of the intermediate hosts from the second to the seventh week of infection. Several generations of ovoid, non infective parasites (**metrocytes**) occur in cysts in the skeletal muscles (and, occasionally, in the brain) from the eight to the eleventh week of infection. The metrocytes finally divide into conventional, infective **bradyzoites** by the 75th day of infection. There is, however, considerable variation among species, *S, gigantea* or *S. medusiformis* of cat/ sheep may take months or even years before forming infective bradyzoites. The structure of the merozoites and bradyzoites is as in the other coccidia (Figure 27.1) but the metrocytes lack rhoptries and micronemes.

The parasites in the muscle cells lie inside a vacuole and are surrounded by a wall that constitutes a cyst (**sarcocyst**). Depending on their species and age, the sarcocysts may be microscopic or macroscopic. In most species, the wall produces internal septa that divide the parasites into discrete groups. The ultrastructure of the wall has been divided into 24 types that are of taxonomic importance.[5] Exact classification of species of *Sarcocystis* by study of the sarcocysts is not a job for the practitioner.

**b. Biology**

*Sarcocystis* requires an intermediate host for development. The infection of the **intermediate host** (ruminants, pigs, horses, birds) starts with the ingestion of sporulated oocysts or sporocysts and the release of the infective sporozoites. By day 7 of infection, the parasites are seen within endothelial cells of the capillaries, multiplying into a **first generation meront**. By day 19, the merozoites invade new endothelial cells and start multiplying into a **second generation meront**. By day 46, the merozoites of second generation invade the skeletal muscle and start multiplying into some ovoid, non-infective parasites (**metrocytes**). By day 75, the metrocytes have turned into infective **bradyzoites**. The bradyzoites probably live as long as the host. The merozoites and metrocytes of *Sarcocystis* are equivalent to the tachyzoites of **Toxoplasma**, and the multiplication of the metrocytes in the muscles is akin to the merogony.

The infection of the **definitive host** (canids, felids, humans) begins with the ingestion of bradyzoites in the flesh of infected intermediate hosts. The released bradyzoites penetrate cells of the lamina propria of the small intestinal and develop into ovoid, 10-20 µm sexual cells. There is no meront generation in the definitive host. The microgametes fertilize the macrogametes within 24 hours of infection and the zygote develops the infective sporozoites before the oocysts leave the intestine. The beginning of patency depends on the species but usually occurs in the second week of infection.

The definitive host apparently does not develop immunity to the parasite because dogs can be infected repeatedly with *Sarcocystis*.

**c. Medical importance**

Only some species of *Sarcocystis* are pathogenic for the **intermediate host**. Those which have been reported to cause disease are: *S. cruzi* for cattle, *S. tenella* for lambs, *S. capricanis* for goats, and *S. miescheriana* and *S. suihominis* for pigs. They must not be very pathogenic, however, because almost 100% of cattle and sheep are infected with muscle cysts of *Sarcocystis* but the natural disease is rarely reported.

The most evident clinical sign in acute sarcocystiasis of ruminants and pigs is a normocytic, normochromic, primarily hemolytic anemia of unknown cause. The predominant lesions at necropsy are localized mononuclear inflammation, hemorrhages, and necrosis in many organs. This is probably the result of the massive destruction of endothelial cells.

Experimental infections in calves have produced fever, mild to severe anorexia, diarrhea, weight loss, weakness, anemia, muscle twitching, and prostration, depending on the infective dose. Abortion and stillbirths occurred in heavy infections of adult cattle.. As the infection becomes chronic, poor growth, loss of hair on the neck, rump, and tail, and hypersalivation and nasal discharge were noted.

Using pair-fed controls, it was recently shown[9] that *S. cruzi* infections reduce the retention and utilization of nitrogen by calves and depress the production of somatomedin C, a major anabolic hormone. It was speculated that the infection stimulates production of the cytokines, tumor necrosis factor alpha and interleukine 1, which may have a critical participation in the pathogenesis of the infection.

*Sarcocystis* does not seem to be pathogenic for the **definitive host**, except humans. Humans experimentally infected with sarcocysts of *S. hominis* or *S. suihominis* developed vomiting, diarrhea, and respiratory distress. Dogs, cats, and wild carnivores have been infected experimentally with several species of *Sarcocystis* but only a few dogs and coyotes vomited or experienced a brief anorexia.

**Table 27.VI. Characteristics of some common species of *Sarcocystis***

| Species | Hosts | Oocyst (μm)* | Sporocyst (μm)** | Sarcocyst (μm)*** | Prepatency (days) | Patency (days) | Pathogenicity |
|---|---|---|---|---|---|---|---|
| *S. cruzi* | Dog/ cattle | Dumbbell-shaped 19-21x15-18 | Ellipsoidal 13-22x6-15 | 1 cm long, <1 μm wall | 8-33 | 3-70 | calves +++ |
| *S. hirsuta* | Cat/ cattle | Dumbbell-shaped 12-18x11-14 | Ellipsoidal 11-14x7-9 | 1 mm long, 6 μm wall | 7-9+ | 6-17+ | calves + |
| *S. hominis* | Human/ cattle | Dumbbell-shaped 20x15 | Ellipsoidal 14-15x10-11 | ?, 6 μm wall | 9-10 | >42 | calves + human + |
| *S .tenella* | Dog/ sheep | Dumbbell-shaped infrequent | Ellipsoidal 13-16x8-11 | 0.5 mm long, 25 nm wall | 8-17+ | ? | lambs +++ dog + |
| *S. gigantea* | Cat/ sheep | Dumbbell-shaped 15-18x10-14 | Ellipsoidal 10-14x8-10 | 1 cm long, 25 nm | 10-14 | 4-43 | lambs + |
| *S. bertrami* | Dog/ horse | Dumbbell-shaped infrequent | Ellipsoidal 15-16x9-11 | 1 cm long, ? wall | ? | ? | no |
| *S. mie-scheriana* | Dog/ pig | Dumbbell-shaped infrequent | Ellipsoidal 12-18x7-13 | 4 mm long ? wall | 8-9 | ? | pig + |
| *S. sui-hominis* | Human/ pig | Dumbbell-shaped 18-20x12-15 | Ellipsoidal 11-14x1011 | 1.5 mm long, ? wall | 12-14 | 18+ | pig +++ human +++ |

(*) All oocyst in these species lack micropyle, residuum, and polar granule, (**) All sporocysts in these species lack Stieda body but have residuum, (***) All sarcocysts in these species are compartmentalized.

## REFERENCES


1. Levine N.D. 1988. *The Protozoan Phylum Apicomplexa*, 2 vols, CRC Press, Boca Raton, Florida, 203+154 pp.

2. Lindsay, D. S. and Todd, K.S. 1993. Coccidia of mammals. In Kreier, J.P. (ed.), *Parasitic Protozoa*, vol. 4., 2nd ed., Academic Press, San Diego, 89-131.

3. Long, P.L. 1993. Avian coccidiosis. In Kreier, J.P. (ed.), *Parasitic Protozoa*, vol. 4. Acdemic Press, San Diego, 1-88.

4. Sloss M.W., Kemp, R.L. and Zajac, A.M. 1994. *Veterinary Clinical Parasitology*, 6th ed., Iowa St. Univ. Press, Ames, 198 pp.

5. Barriga O.O. and Arnoni, J.V. 1981. Pathophysiology of hepatic coccidiosis in rabbits. Vet. Parasitol. 8:201-210.

6. Dubey J.P. and Beattie C.P. 1988. *Toxoplasmosis of Animals and Man.* CRC Press, Boca Raton, Florida, 220 pp.

7. Dubey, J.P. 1993. *Toxoplasma, Neospora, Sarcocystis,* and other tissue cyst-forming coccidia of humans and animals. In Kreier, J.P. (ed), *Parasitic Protozoa,* 2nd ed., Academic Press, San Diego

8. Dubey J.P., Speer C.A. and Fayer R. 1989. *Sarcocystosis of Animals and Man.* CRC Press, Boca Raton, Florida, 215 pp.

9. Fayer, R. and Elsasser, T.H. 1991. Bovine Sarcocystosis: how parasites negatively affect growth. Parasitol. Today 7:250-255.

# Chapter 28

# THE ORDER PIROPLASMIDA OR PIROPLASMS

The **Piroplasmida** (from Lat *pirum*= pear, and Gr *plasma*= body) are pear-shaped, ovoid, round, or rod-shaped Apicomplexa of the erythrocytes and, sometimes, other blood cells. They need a tick as an intermediate host and biological vector, in which they multiply sexually. There are two genera of veterinary importance: *Babesia* and *Theileria*.

## 1. Morphology

The Piroplasms lack conoids, sporocysts, and oocysts. The cellular membrane of the sporozoites have a single layer as compared to the three-layered cellular membrane of the Eucoccidida and Haemosporida. As compared to the Haemosporida (that form hemozoin), they do not form pigment from the hemoglobin when they parasitize erythrocytes.

*Babesia* have a polar ring and infect only erythrocytes (but see below). The intraerythrocytic forms are pyriform, oval, or round organisms 1.5 to 5 um long. They produce 1, 2, or 4 parasites in each red blood cell, often disposed in V or in tetrads (Figure 28.1).

. *Theileria* lack a polar ring and infect lymphocytes first and erythrocytes later. In the lymphocytes they produce meronts with 13-50 nuclei and in the erythrocytes, 1, 2, or 3 parasites per cell (Figure 28.1). The intraerythrocytic forms are round, ovoid, or rod-shaped organisms commonly less than 1-2 um long, most often isolated but sometimes in pairs or in tetrads (Figure 28.1).

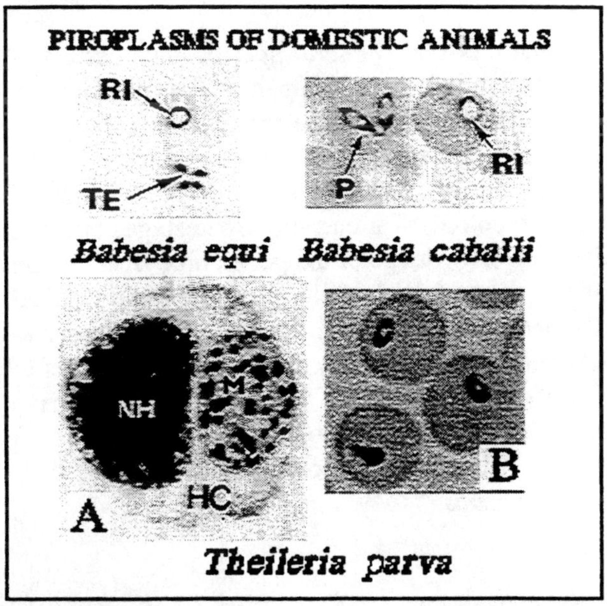


**Figure 28.1.** Some piroplasms of domestic animals. A, lymphocyte with meront; B, erythrocytes with merozoites; HC, host cell cytoplasm; M, meront; NH, nucleus of host cell; P, pyriform stages; RI, ring stages; TE, tetrad stages.

## 2. Classification and identification

*Babesia* can be distinguished from *Theileria* by the characteristics given under Morphology. The more restricted geographic distribution of *Theileria* facilitates the differentiation in many areas.

About 73 species of *Babesia* have been described from diverse mammals but only a little more than a dozen are important parasites of domestic animals. They are often separated in large species (> 2.5 μm long) and small species (≤ 2.5 μm long). Identification of species still relies on observation of the morphology of the intraerythrocytic stages in Giemsa-stained thin blood smears but it demands highly trained personnel. Table 28.I lists some of the species of veterinary importance with some of their identifying characteristics. Antigens specific for each species have not been obtained yet so serology is not reliable to distinguish among species. DNA probes have been developed and genetic markers found, however, which have proved useful for the identification of a few species.

About a dozen *Theileria* species have been described so far, all from ruminants. The most important to veterinary medicine are *T. parva, T. annulata,* and, secondarily, *T. mutans* (Table 28.II). Identification of species relies on observation of the morphology of intraerythrocytic stages but it is difficult. Knowledge of the geographic distribution of the species, and of the pathology and clinical manifestations of the infection is also necessary to formulate a diagnosis. Some successful attempts to identify species (but not strains) by serology have been done recently. Table 28.II list some common species of veterinary importance and some of their characteristics.

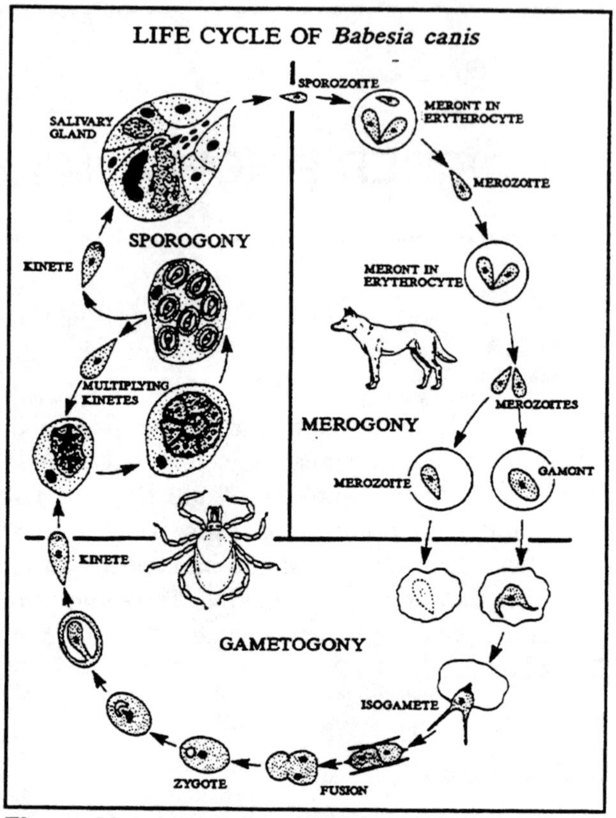


**Figure 28.2.** Life cycle of a typical *Babesia.*

## 3. Biology

For years the piroplasms were distinguished from other Apicomplexa because they were believed not to have a sexual phase of reproduction. Recently Mehlhorn and Schein[1] reviewed the evidence that they actually reproduce sexually in the tick vector.

### a. *Babesia*

*Babesia* are transmitted by a variety of ticks (see Table 28.I). The most important species (*B. bovis* and *B. bigemina*) infect cattle and are transmitted by *Boophilus* ticks.

The sporozoites are injected into the host with the saliva of an infected tick during its blood meal. The parasites contact the erythrocytes with their apical complex and penetrate the cells inside a vacuole. Different from the Eucoccidida and Haemosporida, the Piroplasmida soon leave the parasitophorous vacuole and lie in the cytoplasm of the host cell. Most parasites divide rapidly into two pyriform organisms forming a V shape characteristic of *Babesia*. *B. equi* and *B. microti* sometimes divide also into four parasites forming a Maltese cross. The new parasites soon leave the host cell to invade other red blood cells. Many erythrocytes are destroyed during this process. The cycles of reproduction and invasion continue until the host dies or controls the infection. Some parasites remain inside the host cells as spherical or oval organisms that do not develop any further. The pyriform parasites are asexually multiplying **trophozoites** but the spherical organisms are **gamonts** or precursor sexual cells.

When the parasites are taken by an appropriate tick during its blood meal, the trophozoites degenerate but the gamonts become 4-7 μm, polymorphic **isogametes** (of a same shape) in the tick gut.[2] Formerly, they were known as Stranhlenkörper or ray-bodies. Pairs of gametes fuse and form pear-shaped, 7-8 µm long, motile zygotes (**kinetes**) that enter the hemocele and invade various organs of the tick. Those in organs other than the salivary glands divide asexually and originate new kinetes which, in time, invade new organs. In this process, they may invade the tick oocytes and pass to the next tick generation in the eggs. This **transovarian transmission** (see page 85) has been demonstrated in all *Babesia* except *B. equi* and *B. microti*. Those kinetes that enter the salivary glands develop into 1.5-3.0 µm long, pyriform **sporozoites**. The development of the sporozoites requires some development of the salivary glands that occurs during a blood meal so the infective sporozoites are formed during a meal following that meal where the tick acquired the infection. The first sporozoites appear in the saliva after a few days of feeding (see Table 28.I). Each single salivary alveolus may contain several thousand sporozoites.

Because the sporozoites of *B. equi* and *B. microti* undergo a cycle of multiplication in the lymphocytes (like *Theileria*) before invading the erythrocytes, some experts have proposed to include these two species in the genus *Theileria*.

**b. *Theileria***

*Theileria* are transmitted by a variety of ticks (see Table 28.II). All the vectors are two- or three-host ticks (see page 83) because, different from *Babesia*, *Theileria* are not transmitted accross tick generations.

The sporozoites are injected by an infected tick during its blood meal and they are phagocytized by lymphocytes within a few minutes of inoculation. Each sporozoite starts growing and dividing its nucleus inside the lymphocyte to develop into a meront with 13 to 50 nuclei (formerly called a Koch's body). The infection stimulates the proliferation of the infected cells which divide synchronously with the parasites and cause an enlargement of the affected lymphoid organ. By the second week of infection, the meront forms 1-2 um long pyriform merozoites that burst the lymphocyte and invade the erythrocytes (by the 8th day of infection with *T. annulata* and by the 13th day with *T. parva*). Two forms occur inside the red cells. One form is constituted by coma-shaped parasites, 1-2.5 µm long (**trophozoites**) that multiply into V-shaped pairs or Maltese cross tetrads. This multiplication often causes rupture of the host cell. The other group is formed by spherical or ovoid sexual forms (**gamonts**) that do not multiply.

The above account corresponds to the lymphoproliferative *Theileria* (*T. parva, T. annulata, T. hirci*) which multiply in the lymphoid cells and are the most pathogenic for domestic animals. There is also an hemoproliferative group (*T. mutans, T. sergenti*) which multiplies in the erythrocytes.

When ingested by an appropriate tick with its blood meal, the gamonts develop into 8-12 µm long **isogametes** (formerly known as Stranhlenkörper or ray-bodies) which soon fuse to form a club-shaped, motile, 14-22 µm long zygote (**kinete**).[3] The kinetes enter the hemocele and wait for the development of the salivary glands in the next meal to invade the glands and multiply in them. By the 3th-5th day of attachment to the host, each kinete has formed thousands of ovoid, infective sporozoites, about 1 um in diameter, that start to pass in the saliva. The kinetes of *Theileria* do not invade tissues other than the salivary gland so this genus is not transmitted to the next generation of ticks.

## 3. Medical importance

**a. *Babesia***

For its importance to cattle health, babesiosis has been called "the bovine malaria." As a matter, babesiosis may be worse for cattle than malaria for humans; whereas malaria affects 500 million people, babesiosis is a real risk for 50-70% of the 1.4 billion cattle in the world. Cattle babesiosis exist wherever there are cattle and appropriate tick vectors (see Table 28.I). A combination of babesiosis and anaplasmosis was called "Texas fever" in the United States. It was eradicated by elimination of the vector tick in a campaign that lasted from 1907 to 1942 and cost 500 million dollar in 1988 dollars. Experts have estimated that the return of babesiosis to the United States would caused losses of more than one billion dollar a year to the cattle industry. Every head of cattle infected with *Babesia* represent a loss of $ 7 to $ 20 dollar per year, included the cost of control.

**Bovine babesiosis**. Five species of *Babesia* infect cattle, the most important being *B. bovis* and *B. bigemina*.[4] The disease (particularly by *B. bigemina*) starts with **fever** about 5-8 days after infection, and **parasitemia** appears a couple of days later. In acute cases (uncommon) the animals may die in a few days of **hypotensive shock**. In chronic cases (common), the animals develop increasing parasitemia and **anemia** with **hemoglobinemia. Hemoglobinuria** is common in severe cases. The affected animals become **weak** and stops gaining weight or **lose weight**. They may die, mostly from the anemia, or recover after a few weeks.

*B. bovis*-infected erythrocytes have a tendency to adhere to the endotelial cells of the vessels of the central nervous system and block the circulation. **Nervous symptoms** (agitation, convulsions) rather than anemia are common in these cases.

The fever appears to be caused by parasite and erythrocyte debris released during the destruction of the parasitized cells. The increasing parasitemia results from the invasion and multiplication of parasites in the red blood cells. The anemia is due to mechanical and immune destruction of the cells. The mechanical effect is a direct consequence of the growth of parasites inside them. The immune effect is due to the appearance of neo-antigens on the surface of the parasitized cells (or even adsorbed by non-parasitized cells) as a result of the parasitism. The inmunological effector mechanisms (antibody-mediated lysis, phagocytosis) act on these cells as if they were foreign to the body. The hemoglobinemia and hemoglobunuria is due to the massive destruction of erythrocytes and corresponding release of hemoglobin, and its eventual glomerular filtration. The central nervous system manifestation asre caused by the blockage of local circulation and the corresponding anoxia. *B. bovis*-parasitized eryhtrocytes (as *P. falciparum*-parasitized red blood cells) develop some submicroscopic knobs that have a particular affinity for the endothelium of the deep capillaries. Hypotensive shock in the early infection (before an important immune response had time to develop) is due to the activation of the coagulation-complement-kallikrein cascade by parasitic materials. C3a and C5a from complement activation and kallikrein and bradykinin from the kallikrein system are potent vasodilators and hypotensors. Once macrophage activation starts in the early infection, a generalized non-specific inflammation may contribute to thepathogenicity as evidenced by the presence of acute phase proteins. finally, deposition of antigen-antibody complexes in the tissues may contribute to the shock when antibody responses reach a high level.

Few recovered animals eliminate the parasites totally and they remain resistant only to the specific strain of parasite, and only for a few months. Most animals remain as permanent carriers of low levels of parasites for years or life. These animals, however, develop resistance to the species rather than the local strain of parasite. At the beginning the resistance is rather to the disease than to the infection but it increases with the reexposures. Calves until 9 months of age are relatively resistant to the infection. This is not a general characteristics of the babesioses, however, because the same occurs in colts but the reverse is observed in pups and young rodents.

**Ovine babesiosis** is caused by *B. motasi* or *B. bovis* of Europe, northern Africa, and Asia. Its course is like the anemic babesiosis of bovines but less pathogenic. If oftens presents digestive and respiratory manifestations.

**Equine babesiosis** is caused by *B. equi* or *B. caballi*, both of them present in the United States. Because *B. equi* often forms tetrades along with pairs in the eryhtrocytes, some authorities have created the genus *Nutallia* for this species. This seems an inconsequential biological characteristic, however, to justify a new genus. More important are the reports that, like *Theileria*, *B. equi* is able to form meronts in lymphocytes. As in the classic bovine babesiosis, equine babesiosis is mostly an anemic condition but the pathogenicity of different strains is quite variable.

**Swine babesiosis** is an anemic condition caused by *B. perroncitoi* and B. *trautmanni* in Europe and nothern Africa.

**Canine babesiosis** is caused by *B. canis* in most of the world (including theUnited States and Central and South America) and *B. gibsoni* in Asia and northern Africa. The first produces a clinical pictue like that of *B. bigemina* of cattle but the second rarely presents icterus or hemoglobinuria. The disease is considerably more severe when conbined with *Ehrlichia canis* infection.

**Human babesiosis** caused by cattle or rodent parasites is a rare condition that has been reported especially in splenectomized people.

**b. *Theileria***

The most patogenic *Theileria* are *T. parva*, agent of the **East Coast Fever** of East and Central Africa, and *T. annulata*, agent of the Mediterranean or **Tropical theilerosis** around the Mediterranean sea, India, and southern Russia. In both cases, the severity of the infection is largely dependant on the susceptibility of the host (calves are more resistant than adults), the strain of parasite, and the size of the inoculum.

By the second week of infection, the signs of theilarosis begin with a **hyperplasia of the lymph nodes** that drain the inoculation site. **Fever** appears 1-4 days later and lymp node enlargement spreads throughout the body. In severe infections, inappetence, respiratory distress, diarrhea, and loss of condition develop. The animals finally become recumbent and die. Leukopenia but not anemia is characteristic of *T. parva* whereas anemia but not leukopenia is characteristic of *T. annulata.*[5]

Mild infections may recover after 3-10 days of fever whereas severe disease may cause death during the second week.

The pathophysiology of theileriasis corresponds to the affected cells: lymphocytes in the lymphoproliferative group and erythrocytes in the hemoproliferative group.

*T. parva* infects preferentially T lymphocytes whereas *T. annulata* does not show a clear predilection for particular lymphocytes and also infects macorphages/monocytes. *Theileria* stimulates the proliferation of the parasitized lymphocytes through an IL-2 mechanism so that the host cells divide synchronously with the parasites. The parasitized lymphocytes invade the lymphatic organs replacing the regular cells like a lymphoma and interfering with their normal functions. In the later stages of the disease there is an extensive lympholysis of unknown origin that affects parasitized as well as normal cells. Parasitized cells accumulate in lungs and the gastrointesinal tract; their later destruction contributes to the production of pulmonary edema and gastrointestinal ulcers. Complement is activated in the late disease what may contribute to the production of pulmonary edema. Its causes are unknown, however, since immune complexes have not been detected.

Most animals recovered from theileriosis develop a strong premunition to the infective strain. Low levels of parasites remain in their circulation, however, and they still may be susceptible to other strains of the same species. As an exeption, *T. parva* appears to produce sterile immunity.

**Table 28.I. Characteristics of some common *Babesia* species**

| Species, host | Vector tick | Infective stage | Infection time* | Morphology in eryhtrocyte | Distribution |
|---|---|---|---|---|---|
| *B. bigemina*, cattle | *Boophilus* spp. | Nymphs, adults | 9 days (nymph) 16 days (adult) | 4-5x2 μm, pyriform, acute angle, paired | Worldwide |
| *B. bovis*, cattle | *Boophilus* spp. *Rhipicephalus bursa* | Larvae | 2-3 days (larva) | 2.0x1.5 μm, rounded, obtuse angle, paired | Worldwide |
| *B. major*, cattle | *Haemaphysalis punctata* | Adults | ? | 2.6x1.5μm, like *B. bigemina* | Europe, N-W Africa |
| *B. divergens*, cattle | *Ixodes ricinus* | Lavae | ? | 1.5x1.0 μm, like *B. bovis* | Europe |
| *B. motasi*, sheep & goats | *Rhipicephalus bursa* | Adults | ? | 2.5-4x2.0 μm, acute angle, paired | Europe, Asia, Africa |
| *B. ovis*, sheep & goats | *Rhipiccephalus bursa* | Adults | 3-5 days (adult) | 1.5x1.0 μm, rounded, obtuse angle, paired | Europe, Asia, Africa |
| *B. caballi*, equines | *Hyalomma* spp. *Dermacentor* spp. | Adults | ? | 3.0x2.0 μm, pyriform, acute angle, paired | Worldwide |
| *B. equi*, equines | *Dermacentor* spp. *Hyalomma* spp. *Rhipicephalus* spp. | Nymphs, adults | 3-5 days (adult) | 1.7x2.0 μm, rounded, obtuse angle, pairs or tetrads | Worldwide |
| *B. trautmanni*, pigs | *Rhipicephalus* sp. | ? | ? | 3.5x2.0 μm, narrow and long, acute angle, paired | S. Europe, Africa |
| *B. perroncitoi*, pigs | ? | ? | ? | 0.7x2.0 μm, pleomorphic mostly rounded & single | Sardinia, Sudan, Vietnam |
| *B. canis*, dogs | *Rhipicephalus* sp. *Haemaphysalis* sp. *Dermacentor* sp. | Nymphs, adults | 2-3 days (adult) | 5.0x2.5 μm, pyriform, acute angle, paired | Worldwide |
| *B. gibsoni*, dogs | *Rhipicephalus* sp. *Haemaphysalis* sp. | ? | ? | 1.2x3.2 μm, rounded, pleomorphic. like *E. equi* | Asia, Africa |
| *B. felis*, cats | ? | ? | ? | 1.0x2.5 μm, rounded | Africa |
| *B. herpailuri*, cats | ? | ? | ? | 2.6μm, pyriform, acute angle, paired | Americas |
| *B. microti*, rodents | *Ixodes* spp. | Larvae, nymphs | ? | 1.5-2.0 μm, ameboid, in pairs or tetrads | Europe, America, Laboratory |

(*) Time when sporozoites appear in the tick saliva from moment of attachment.

**Table 28.II. Characteristics of some common *Theileria* species**

| Species, host | Vector tick | Predominant morphology* | Pathogenicity* | Distribution |
|---|---|---|---|---|
| *T. parva*, cattle | *Rhipicephalus* spp. *Hyalomma* spp. | 80% rod-shaped; 1.5-2x0.5-1.0 μm; single | 90-100% mortality | Africa |
| *T. annulata*, cattle | *Hyalomma* spp. | 70% round or oval; 0.5-2.7 μm; single, in pairs or tetrads | 10-90% mortality | S. Europe. Asia, Africa |
| *T. mutans*, cattle | *Amblyomma* spp. *Haemaphysalis* spp. | 55% round or oval; 0.6-2.0 μm; single, in pairs or tetrads | < 1% mortality | Africa, Caribbean |
| *T. velifera*, cattle | *Amblyomma* sp. | Pleomorphic, small rods 1-2 μm long with rectangular veil | None | Africa, Caribbean |
| *T. hirci*, sheep and goats | *Rhipicephalus* sp.? | 80% round; 0.6-2.0 μm; single, in pairs or tetrads | 46-100% mortality | S. Europe, Asia, Africa |
| *T. ovis*, sheep and goats | *Rhipicephalus* sp. *Haemaphysalis* spp.? | Like *T. hirci* but sparser | None | Asia, Africa |

(*) Most *Theileria* are pleomorphic. This is the percentage and characteristics of the predominant forms.
(**) Expressed as reported mortality of untreated hosts.

## REFERENCES


1. Mehlhorn H & Schein E. 1985. The Piroplasms: life cycle and sexual stages. Adv. Parasit. 23:37-103.

2. Kakoma, I. and Mehlhorn, H. 1994. *Babesia* of domestic animals. In Kreier, J.P. (ed.), *Parasitic Protozoa*, 2nd. ed., Academic Press, San Diego, 141-216.

3. Mehlhorn, H., Schein, E. and Ahmed, J.S. 1994. *Theileria*, in Kreier, J.P. (ed.), *Parasitic Protozoa*, 2nd. ed., Academic Press, San Diego, 217-304.

4. Purnell, R.E. 1981. Babesiosis in various hosts. In Ristic, M. and Kreier, J.P. (eds.), *Babesiosis*, Academic Press, New York, 25-63.

5. Barnett, S.F. 1968. Theileriasis, In Weinman, D. and Ristic, M. (eds.), *Infectious Blood Diseases of Man and Animals*, Academic Press, New York, 269-328.

# APPENDIX 1

# THE IMMUNOLOGY OF PARASITIC INFECTIONS

### Characteristics of the anti-parasite immunity

Simple observation suggests that immunity to viral and bacterial infections is different from the immunity to parasitic infections. Whereas most viroses and bacterioses are acute events that rapidly kill the host or are terminated by immunity, most parasitoses are chronic. Actually, the immune system responds identically to identical stimuli with disregard of the nature of the pathogen itself. The immunological differences between viral or bacterial (prokaryote) infections and parasitic (eukaryote) infections depend on:

1) the nature of the corresponding antigens,
2) their mode of presentation, or
3) the ability of the pathogens to modulate or escape immunity.

A number of characteristics of the parasites may explain their apparent inefficiency to. trigger immune responses and their reduced susceptibility to immunity (see also 4. Evasion of host immunity by parasites, below).

**a. Antigenic complexity**. Parasites generally produce more, and chemically more complex antigens than viruses or bacteria. The antigens resulting from the metabolism of the parasite are called **metabolic antigens**, excretion-secretion (ES) products, or exo-antigens. They are commonly enzymes or catabolites generated by the living, thriving parasites. They also release body components which are called **somatic antigens**, structural antigens, or endo-antigens. These are commonly released only upon dead and degradation of the parasites. Many parasites also possess antigens widely distributed in nature **(heterophile antigens)**. Finally, parasites may also alter host proteins during the infection so that they become antigenic **(host-derived antigens).** Of all these materials, only the metabolic antigens are likely to contain substances essential to the living parasite. Immune neutralization of these substances probably is lethal to the parasite but these antigens must compete with all the other antigens for the attention of the immune system. Because metabolic antigens are usually less concentrated and chemically more similar to the host's materials (this is, less immunogenic) than the other antigens, they are rarely successful in the competition.

**b. Physiologic complexity**. Because parasites possess a more complex physiology than viruses and bacteria, they have more alternatives to elude the action of immunity. For example, nematodes may have different versions of a same enzyme **(isozymes)**. If antibodies are produced against one version, the parasite may restrict its production in favor of the other versions that are not affected by immunity.

**c. Structural complexity**. Because of their size and structural complexity, parasites are less susceptible to immune effects that would be successful against viruses or bacteria. For example, macrophages can only gnaw at the external cuticle or tegument of helminths, and the parasite can probably repair the damage as fast as it is inflicted. Even if a metabolic enzyme (released by dead parasites, for example) induces the production of neutralizing antibodies, these antibodies may not have the opportunity to reach the enzyme in the tissues of the *living* parasite. If a nematode ingested macrophages or antibodies, they may be digested before having a chance to act against the parasite.

**d. Biological complexity**. Nematodes enter their host as infective larvae (usually L3s) and proceed to develop into L4s, juveniles, and adults. Each of these stages has a characteristic biochemistry and distinctive antigens. By the time the immune system reacts to the corresponding antigens, the parasite may have molted to the next stage and not be susceptible to that immune response any more. In the case of the platyhelminths, these worms have such a rapid turn-over of their tegument that any antibody or macrophage attached to their tegument will be released into the circulation before they have the time to cause permanent damage.

**e. Location.** Many parasites are located in the intestinal lumen where complement is inactive and IgM, IgG, macrophages, and other effector cells are scarce. Others are located inside cells *(Toxoplasma, Trichinella)* , or in the brain *(Cysticercus cellulosae, Babesia bovis, Plasmodium falciparum)* which are beyond the reach of immunity.

**f. Antigen presentation.** As explained above, parasites produce many antigens at the same time which stimulates antigenic competition. Because the antigens responsible for protection are comparatively little antigenic (otherwise the parasites would be eliminated consistently), the corresponding responses are commonly averted in favor of stronger, non-protective antigens.

Also, production of antigens in the mucosal lumens triggers the preferential production of IgA antibodies. These antibodies do not activate complement or stimulate phagocytosis which are some of the major mechanisms to dispose of parasites. IgA antibodies act by occupying the receptors on viruses or bacteria that are necessary for these microorganism to attach to host cells and invade the host. Because many parasites enter the host tissues by mechanic or enzymatic means (without the need for receptors), IgA antibodies are ineffective to prevent parasite invasion by these organisms.

**g. Hypobiosis.** Many parasites can enter in hypobiosis during infection (larvae of *Toxocara, Ancylostoma, Strongyloides, Trichinella,* gastrointestinal nematodes of ruminants, *Toxoplasma* and *Trypanosoma cruzi* in chronic infections). Because of the diminished metabolism during this phase, antigen production is minimal and any immune response that acts on metabolic pathways would be much less effective.

## RELEVANCE OF IMMUNOLOGY TO PARASITOLOGY

Immune responses are automatic responses to appropriate stimuli. They do no discriminate about the final result of the reaction. An immune reaction may be lethal to the invading organism (**protective immunity**), harmful to the host (**hypersensitivity** or allergy), or indifferent to either (**irrelevant immunity**). Most of the immune reactions to parasites that we see nowadays are irrelevant. They may be used, however, to detect the presence of the parasite in a host (**immune diagnosis**). Many of the strong protective reactions must have been eliminated during evolution: either they were effective enough to exterminate the parasite, or the parasite evolved to attenuate the reaction or its consequences. Similarly, antiparasite reactions that caused severe damage to the host must have been purged during evolution. There is still a number of circumstances, however, in which the pathogenesis of the parasite is mediated by hypersensitive responses of the host.

There are 5 areas of immunology that are of particular relevance to parasitic infections:

1) Diagnosis
2) Pathology
3) Protection,
4) Evasion of host immunity
5) Epidemiology

## 1. DIAGNOSIS

Diagnosis of parasitic infections is commonly performed by recovering parasitic elements (eggs, cysts, or larvae) from host excretions or tissues (feces, urine, bronchial washings, blood). These **direct methods** are simple and accurate procedures that should be preferred whenever it is possible. There are occasions, however, in which immunological exams are more convenient:

**a. Detection of inaccessible parasites.** Parasites located in the nervous system (e.g., cysticerci, *Toxoplasma*). liver (hydatid cyst), muscles (e.g., *Trichinella),* or other tissues (*Toxocara*) are largely inaccessible to direct methods but could be revealed by appropriate immunological tests.

**b. Detection of prepatent infections.** In some cases the parasite causes disease before reaching adulthood and releasing eggs or larvae (e.g., ostertagiasis, fascioliasis *hepatica*, pneumonia due to ascarides, visceral, ocular, and cutaneous larva migrans). Immunological tests can identify the presence of the parasite in these cases.

**c. Detection of chronic infections.** In many chronic infections the number of parasitic elements is too small to be found easily by direct diagnostic methods (e.g., malaria, Chagas' disease, strongyloidosis, genital trichomoniasis). Diagnosis of the infection may be important, nevertheless, because the infected individual is a source of infection for others. Immunological tests can facilitate greatly the identification of the chronic carrier.

**d. Improvement of direct methods.** In some cases the direct methods are little efficient (e.g., strongyloidosis, biopsy for trichinelliasis or toxocariasis, canine echinococcosis, amoebiasis), or require considerable expertise and a long time (e.g., canine echinococcosis, malaria, amoebiasis, genital trichomoniasis). In these cases, the immunological tests can avoid these inconveniences.

**e. Epidemiological surveys.** Epidemiological surveys consists of the examination of samples of a large number of individuals to verify the proportion of infected hosts. This may be such a task with inefficient direct methods as to become nearly impossible, but a rather simple operation with immunologic tests. For example, a well trained technician may examine 28 malaria samples in a day by microscopic examination, but 500 by serological tests.

**f. Detection of parasitic load.** The severity of a parasitic infection often depends on the number of parasites in the host. Few direct methods are accurate in detecting parasitic load. Immunological dosage of parasite antigens in the circulation of the host, however, can provide a reasonable estimate of the number of parasites. This is a largely experimental technique yet but it is being used successfully with canine dirofilariasis and is being tested with swine trichinelliasis.

**g. Detection of resistance.** A veterinarian would welcome information about the resistance of a herd or flock to a certain parasite before committing funds and efforts to the prevention of the infection. Investigation of responses to specific antigens that are known to afford protection against the parasite would supply this information. Unfortunately, we do not know enough about protective antigens or reactions in parasitic diseases to apply this method yet. Currently, it is only applicable to ruminant dictyocaulosis. Because we know that dictyocaulosis induces immune resistance after a single infection, any immunological test that verifies that the animals have been infected with *Dictyocaulus* would imply that they developed resistant to reinfections.

The immune diagnosis of parasitic infections is considerably more advanced for human parasitoses than for veterinary parasitoses which only reflects the efforts applied by, and the research funds granted to, the respective professionals. Nevertheless, parasite immune diagnosis is still plagued by cross-reactions (remember the heterophile antigens?) and requires abundant research to select the appropriate antigens.

## 2. PATHOLOGY

Immune reactions that are harmful to the individual are conventionally called **hypersensitivities** or allergies. Although research in this area has been limited, there is a number of cases in which the damage produced by the parasitic infection is actually the result of the immune response mounted by the host against the parasite. We will review a few examples.

**Hypersensitivity type 1.** This hypersensitivity is mediated by IgE antibodies bound to mast cells or basophils. When the antibodies combine with their specific antigen, they trigger the release of vaso-active amines from the cells. This phenomenon is the responsible for the ascarid pneumonia in sensitized animals, some of the systemic manifestations of filarial infections and trichinosis, possible for the digestive symptoms in intestinal nematodiases, some of the symptoms of ectoparasitoses, and the reactions to bee stings. In a these cases, a first contact with the parasite antigens induces the formation of IgE antibodies which attach to the cells. Upon subsequent contacts, these antigens combine with the pre-existing IgE antibodies on mast cells o basophils and release the vaso-active amines.

**Hypersensitivity type II.** This is mediated by the presence of IgM or IgG antibodies on the cell that will be damaged. The antibodies either activate C' which destroys the cell membranes, or opsonize the cells which are phagocytized subsequently. This phenomenon is partially responsible for the anemia that occurs in malaria. babesiosis, and leishmaniasis, and possibly for the myocarditis of Chagas' disease. In the anemias, parasite antigens are expressed on the surface of parasitized cells, or adsorbed from the circulation by normal erythrocytes. The corresponding IgM or lgG antibodies combine with these cells and active the C' or stimulate phagocytosis. In Chagas' disease it is believed that the parasitism of the heart or autonomic nervous ganglia modifies myocardial or nervous proteins enough to be recognize as foreign materials by the immune system.

**Hypersensitivity type III.** It is mediated by an excess of antigen that binds circulating IgG antibodies. The immune complexes so formed precipitate in the tissues and activate C' which destroys cellular membranes in the neighborhood. This mechanism is the responsible for the kidney pathology in human malaria, canine dirofilariasis, schistosomiasis, and trypanosomiases, the cerebral pathology in malaria, the systemic manifestations of babesiosis, larval cestodiases, and possibly trichinosis. In all these cases, the early infection provides the antigens that stimulate antibody formation. The persistence of the parasite and its antigens in the circulation provides later the conditions for the formation of precipitating immune complexes.

**Hypersensitivity type IV**. This is a cell-mediated immunity that harms the host's tissues. It is the responsible for the pathology of schistosomiasis, migratory nematode larvae, leishmaniasis, the heart lesions of Chagas' disease, and some lesions by ectoparasites.

## 3. IMMUNE PROTECTION

The host commonly opposes the parasitic infection by non-specific mechanisms of natural resistance first (innate mechanical, physiological, or biochemical barriers, and non-specific mechanisms like the acute phase response). The acute phase response is particularly important because it sets the stage for the immune response that will come subsequently. If these mechanisms fail to remove the parasite, the specific immune response takes over.

In regard to **natural resistance**, all the mechanisms applicable to viral and bacterial infections also operate against parasitic infections, although not necessarily with the same efficiency. Two mechanisms, however, are characteristic of parasitic infections: absence of host's signals and absence of host's structures.

**a. Absence of host's signals**. The infective stage of the parasite that penetrates a host requires a specific set of biochemical conditions ("signals") to trigger its further development. Lack of the *exact* signals in the *exact* proportions will prevent the establishment of the parasite. This is why the ruminant nematode, *Haemonchus contortus*, does not infect non-ruminants hosts. In a few cases, an abnormal host may provide the signals necessary for invasion and nutrition, but not the subsequent signals for growth and development. In these cases, the parasite remains in the abnormal host as a preadult stage, a larva migrans in the case of *Toxocara canis* in humans, for example.

**b. Absence of host's structures**. Some parasites require specific structures for invasion or for their metabolism. For example, *Plasmodium knowlesi* of humans penetrates the erythrocytes by attachment to a glycoprotein receptor that is part of the Duffy blood group. Duffy negative persons (who lack this protein), therefore, are insusceptible to *knowlesi* malaria. Also, *P. falciparum* metabolizes the (normal) A hemoglobin with very specific enzymes. The S hemoglobin (of the sickle cell anemia) is not degraded by these enzymes. People with sickle cell anemia, therefore, do not support the life of the parasite.

In regard to **acquired immunity**, there are three general mechanisms by which the host may protect itself from the parasite:

**a. By attacking the parasite structures.** For example, trypanosomas, plasmodia, and babesia are destroyed by phagocytosis; several helminths are destroyed by enzymes of neutrophils, eosinophils, or plasma cells; trypanosomas, larval cestodes, and hematophagous arthropods may be destroyed by C'; migratory nematode larvae may be destroyed by lymphokines or cytotoxic cells. In all these cases the effect of the immunity is directed against the parasite of its tissues.

**b. By affecting the parasite physiology.** For example, neutralization of essential enzymes may kill *Ascaris, Ancylostoma,* and other nematodes; antibodies may occupy parasite receptors that are essential to the first contact with the host before invasion (malaria, schistosomes). In all these cases, the immune defensive mechanism is directed against the physiology of the parasite rather than against its structures.

**c. By modification of the parasite environment**. For example, the expulsion of many gastrointestinal nematodes is mediated by an allergic reaction that does not affect the parasite itself but changes the biochemical constants of the parasite habitat so drastically that the parasite cannot live there anymore. Also, the defense against some hematophagous ectoparasites consists of a sustained vasoconstriction that prevents them from feeding. In these cases, the immune attack is against the environment of the parasite rather than against its structures or physiology.

The complexity of the physiology, biology, and antigenic composition of parasites prevented for many years the production of modern anti-parasite vaccines. Recent advances in immunology and molecular biology, however, have open possibilities that may result in important progress in the near future.[1]

## 4. EVASION OF HOST IMMUNITY BY PARASITES

Parasites preceded immunity for more than 400 million years. Attending to the inception of immunity from the beginning, they had ample opportunity to adapt to the peculiarities of the immune response, take advantage of every possible loophole for survival, and pass these characteristics to their offspring. Those that adapted are the parasites of today, those that faded were lost in the paleontologic register. I believe that evasion of host immunity is the counterpart of, and inseparable from, protective immunity to parasites.

There are a number of mechanisms by which parasites can evade host's immunity. Here we will discuss the most common of them.[2]

**a. Seclusion in immunoprivileged sites**. Immunoprivileged sites are those places of the body that are beyond the reach of the immune system (inside the cells, inner eye, brain, fetus, etc). Parasites in these locations are little affected by immunity and can developed freely.

**b. Imitation of host antigens**. In virtually every case known, the antigens responsible for eliciting anti-parasite protection are little immunogenic. It has been hypothesized that the host and its parasites are affected by a phenomenon of convergent evolution in which their proteins tend to become similar. As a result, the host does not recognize readily the parasitic antigens as foreign substances.

Dineen[3] speculated that weak parasite antigens may help the parasite regulate its own population: few parasites would produce little antigen which would be ignored by the host; many parasites (which may endanger the life of the host and, consequently, that of the parasites) would produce enough antigen to elicit a protective reaction that would eliminate the parasites until they would fall below the threshold to stimulate protective immunity. A similar strategy used by some parasites (e.g., *Schistosoma,* larvae of *Taenia taeniaeformis,* some African trypanosomas) is the adsorption of host materials on their own body coverings to disguise their presence to the immune system.

**c. Production of soluble antigens.** Some parasites (e.g., blood and tissue protozoa, *Schistosoma, Dirofilaria)* produce large amounts of antigens that are found in the circulation or tissues of the host. There is some evidence that these antigens (if they are not inducers of protection) may divert the immune system from reacting to the protection-inducing antigens, or (if they are inducers of protection) may pre-empty antibodies or effector cells by reacting with them away from the parasite. A variety of this strategy is the production by the hydatid cysts of substances that activate the complement before it reaches the cysts.

**d. Antigenic variation**. Some parasites (e.g., African trypanosomas and malaria parasites) have the ability to change the major protection-inducing antigen in the course of an infection. After a wave of parasites exhibiting an antigen with a particular specificity is wiped out by the immune system, a new wave expressing an antigen with a different specificity arises.

**e. Modulation of host responses**. Many parasites have demonstrated the capacity to depress (or selectively enhance) host immunity. We know now that humoral and cell-mediated immunity are mutually exclusive to some extend. A parasite may stimulate the non-protective type of response to protect itself from the type of response that may kill it. Since immune depression by parasites is often non specific, it may aggravate or facilitate intercurrent diseases. It has been demonstrated that parasites may use immune enhancement of specific immune responses to eliminate competing species.

**f. Evasion of effector mechanisms**. Some parasites simply evade the immune mechanisms that may kill them. *Toxoplasma gondii*, for example, forms its own vacuole inside the macrophages that, different from the normal vacuole, does not fuse with the lysosomes that are loaded with enzymes that can degrade the parasite. *Babesia* spp. starts in the regular vacuole but escape to the cytoplasm of the macrophage before the vacuole fuses with the lysosomes.

**g. Metabolic inhibition**. Many parasites are able to enter in hypobiosis in the course of an infection. Hypobiosis means that the parasite produces less antigens, and is less susceptible to any effect that depends on competition for metabolic pathways.

**h. Host unresponsiveness.** It has been recently demonstrated that not all hosts have the class II MHC proteins to produce the conjugate with the parasite antigens that is necessary to start the immune response. This means that some hosts are genetically unable to produce a protective response to that parasite. We still do not know the extend or significant of this phenomenon but those animals probably keep spreading the infection.

## 5. EPIDEMIOLOGY

There is a number of ways how immunity may affect the epidemiology of parasitic infections. For example, the reaction of the intestinal mucosa to *Oesophagostomum* larvae not only generates pathology but also spreads the maturation and oviposition of the parasites in time, and assures that the pastures will remain contaminated throughout the season of inclement weather. Immunity to *Toxocara canis* allows the larvae to remain hypobiotic in the tissues of the bitch until late pregnancy. At that time, the larvae are re-activated and pass to the offspring in uterus. Because it is the best studied, we will discuss the effect of immunity to the gastrointestinal nematodes of sheep on the transmission of the infection.

Upon infection with many nematodes, particularly the gastrointestinal nematodes of the ruminants (GINR), a proportion of the infective larvae matures to adults immediately whereas other remain hypobiotic in the intestinal mucosa (**larval arrest**). In some cases, the production of hypobiotic larvae is due to host immunity (e.g., *Haemonchus)*, and in others to a pre-conditioning of the infective larvae by cold weather before infection (e.g., *Ostertagia)*. Because most infections with GINR are acquired in the fall (see below), the adult parasites live for only a few weeks or a couple of months, and the adult sheep finally develop immunity to the adult worms, sheep go through winter with few adult parasites and many hypobiotic larvae in their gut. The relaxation of immunity that occurs during lactation (in early spring), however, permits:

a) the maturation of the arrested larvae,
b)an increase of fecundity of the few adult parasites still present in the intestine, and
c) the immediate maturation of the few infective larvae remaining in the pastures after the winter that are picked up by the animals in spring.

As a consequence, during spring there is an increase of adult parasites in the gut (because of the maturation of the arrested larvae), and a marked increase of the eggs passed in the feces (because of increase fertility) during the second month after parturition. This increase of egg output is called **lactational rise** or spring rise.

Because the resistance of the animals is re-stimulated by this enhanced infection, most of the adults parasites are expelled from the gut after a couple of weeks (**parasite expulsion**). Although the parasite load of the ewes and the number of eggs passed become low again, the pastures were contaminated during the best season (with optimal temperature and humidity) to assure the development of the eggs and the formation of infective larvae.

These larvae are picked up by the lambs of the new generation which start developing light infections (because pasture contamination is not massive yet and they still eat little grass) and contributing with their own eggs to the pasture contamination. Toward the middle of the summer the infection of the lambs has become substantial and their contribution to pasture contamination is important. The heat of the summer, however, kills some eggs and larvae and inhibits the development of the remaining so eggs and pre-infective larvae accumulate in the pastures.

When the moderate temperatures and rains of fall arrive, these eggs and larvae mature rapidly and cause massive contamination of the pastures with infective larvae. Because the grown lambs eat a lot of grass at this time and have not developed strong immunity yet, many acquire heavy infections and show clinical symptoms. Those which survive get rid of the adult parasites after a couple of months by a combination of immunity and natural dead of old parasites. They do contain, however, arrested larvae picked up during the fall. The cold of the winter kills most of the infective larvae in the pastures so infections cease by this time. Lack of new infections and the negligible production of antigen by the arrested larvae allows immunity to wane slowly during the winter to initiate a new cycle of lactational rise in the spring (see accompanying figure).

With modifications, the same sequence of events is observed with most farm animals.

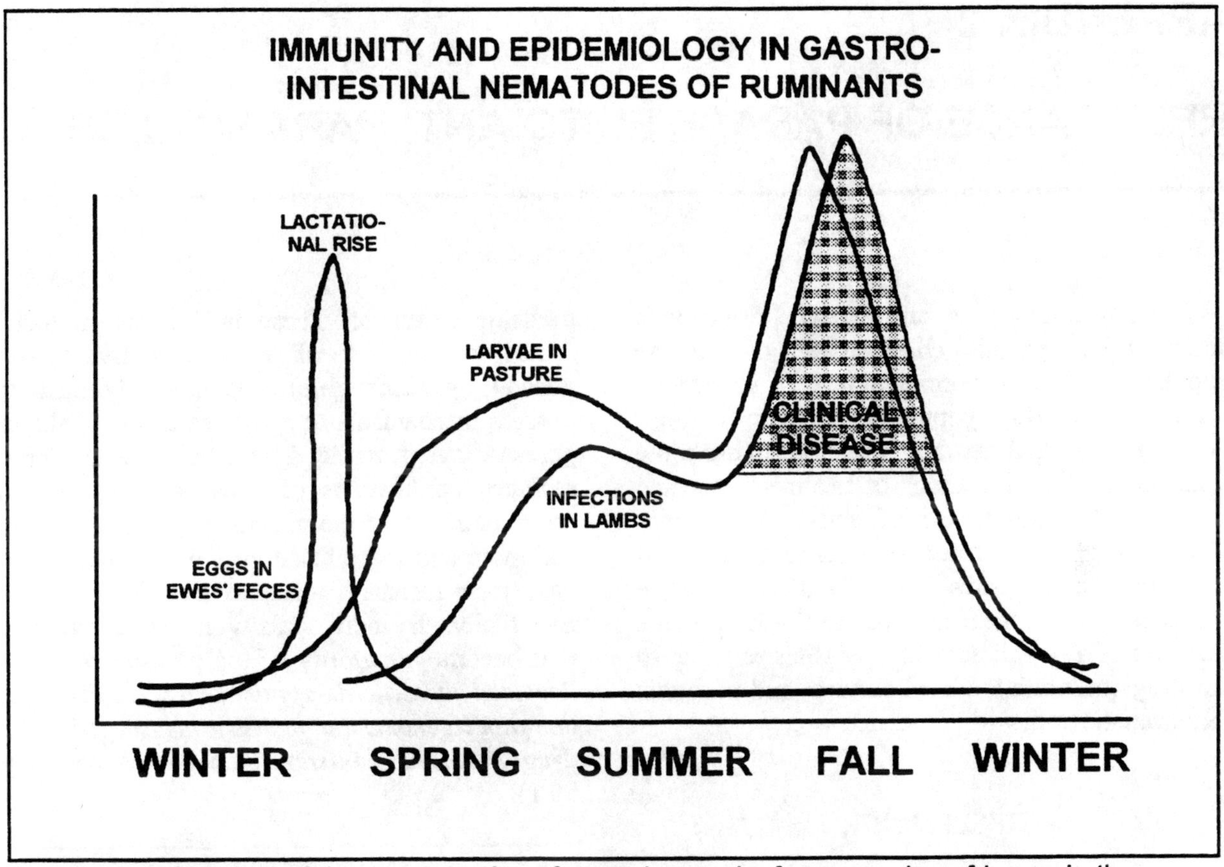


**Figure 29.1**. Changes of the concentration of eggs in ewes's feces, number of larvae in the pasture, and severity of the infection in lambs, with the seasons and host immunity.

## REFERENCES

1. Barriga, O.O. 1994. A review on vaccination against protozoa and arthropods of veterinary importance. Vet. Parasitol. 55:29-55.

2. Barriga, O.O. 1984. Immunomodulation by nematodes. A review. Vet. Parasitol. 14:299-320.

3. Dineen, J.K. 1963. Immunological aspects of parasitism. Nature 197:268-269.

# APPENDIX 2

# RESISTANCE OF PARASITES TO ANTI-PARASITIC DRUGS

The susceptibility to anti-parasitic drugs is a heterogeneous genetic characteristic of parasite populations. Due to normal biological variability, some members of the population are more susceptible to the effect of the drug while others are more resistant. For considerations of treatment cost and host toxicity, the dosage of anti-parasitic compounds is generally fixed at a concentration that kills *almost* all parasites. Typically, a very effective anti-parasitic treatment is lethal to 90-99% of the parasites of a population. The parasites resistant to the drug concentration used survive, and pass this characteristic to their descendence.

## RESISTANCE

**Drug resistance** exists in a population when the population contains a greater proportion (frequency) of individuals able to tolerate doses of the drug than a normal population. The **normal** (or susceptible) **population** is a natural population of the same species which has not been subjected to selection by the anti-parasitic drug being tested. The **degree of resistance** to a given anti-parasitic agent is measured as the ratio of the concentration that kills 50% ($LD_{50}$) of the resistant population (R) to the concentration that kills 50% of the susceptible population (S). A resistance (or resistance ratio) of 2 means that the drug must be twice as concentrated to obtain in the resistant population the same effect as in the normal population. Resistance ratios of 2 to 2000 have been reported.

### Generation of resistance

From the discussion above it follows that a few particularly resistant parasites survive each anti-parasitic treatment. These individuals are not affected by the dose of parasiticide that kills the general (= susceptible) population because they possess mechanisms to elude the action of the anti-parasitic agent at the dose administered. Through repeated applications of a parasiticide, more and more members of the general population are killed and more and more resistant individuals are left to pass their resistant genes to the next generation. Eventually, the individuals with the resistance trait will become a majority of the parasite population. *Repeated parasiticide application selects a population with a genome that makes it insusceptible to the drug at the administered concentration* (Figure 30.1).

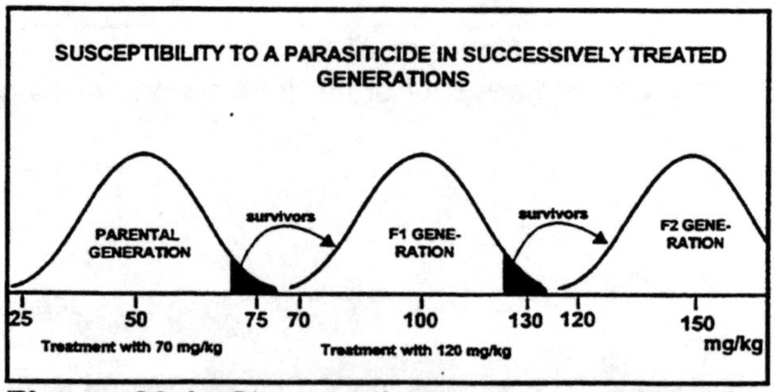


**Figure 30.1.** Changes in the susceptibility of a parasite to a drug following successive treatments.

Normal populations contain a few individuals with alleles that code for minor biochemical departures from the population biochemistry (e.g., isozymes with less affinity for a substrate) and very rare individuals with alleles that code for drastic departures (e.g. an enzyme that does not exist in the normal population). The action of parasiticides with short time of action (such as anthelmintics) can be counteracted by the proportion of parasites with minor biochemical changes. Also, the high efficiency of the modern anthelmintics kills all or a large proportion of the susceptible worms with a single application. Because no susceptible genome is left to dilute the resistant genes, these alleles accumulate in the surviving population. For these reasons, resistance of nematodes to anthelmintics is commonly a polygenic trait.

On the other hand, avoidance of the action of persistent parasiticides (such as insecticides) requires the drastic biochemical changes codified by the very rare alleles. For this reason, resistance of arthropods to insecticides commonly depends on a single gene.[1]

Single gen resistance is usually quite strong (because it depends on drastic biochemical changes), and develops rapidly. In this case an individual parasite is either susceptible (genotype s/s) or resistant (R/s or R/R) so changes in the frequency of a single allele in the population generate a resistant subpopulation. Polygenic resistance, on the contrary, is weaker (because it depends on the accumulation of minor biochemical changes), and develops more slowly. In this case a large number of levels of susceptibility or resistance may occur, from homozygous susceptible to homozygous resistant. It may even occur that changes in the frequency of several genes are necessary before resistance is manifested phenotypically in a population.

**Current status of the problem**

Development of resistance of parasites to parasiticides has been known for a long time. It was reported in protozoa (*Plasmodium falciparum* against quinine) in 1910, in arthropods (*Boophilus* sp. against sodium arsenite) in 1938, and in nematodes (sheep trichostrongylids against phenothiazine) in 1954.

Among the **protozoa** of humans, the problem has increased gradually. Resistance of *P. falciparum* now includes several other drugs, chloroquine (the most important anti-malaria drug nowadays) among them. Cases of *Trichomonas vaginalis* resistant to metronidazole and of *Giardia intestinalis* resistant to metronidazole and furazolidone have been reported. Because of the manner in which they are used, the anti-coccidials of veterinary importance were among the first to cause extensive resistance: in a study of *Eimeria tenella* isolates done in the mid 1970s it was found that 27% of 198 were resistant to amprolium, 62% of 72 to buquinolate, and 41% of 201 to decoquinate.[2]

Among the **nematodes**, by 1987 resistance had extended to *Haemonchus, Ostertagia,* and *Trichostrongylus* of sheep and goats against the benzimidazoles[a] and the levamisole/morantel group, *Nematodirus* of sheep and goats against benzimidazoles, small strongyles and *Strongylus vulgaris* of horses against benzimidazoles, and *Ostertagia* of cattle to levamisole and *Trichostrongylus* axei of cattle to oxfendazole.[3] More recently, resistance of *Oesophagostomum* spp. to levamisole, and of *H. contortus* to ivermectin have been reported.[4]

Among the **arthropods** of veterinary importance, by 1986 resistance had been reported for about 170 species which included 14 ticks, 2 mites, 6 sucking lice, 2 biting lice, 130 diptera, 4 hemiptera, and 8 fleas, and involved to different extent DDT, cyclodienes, organophosphates, carbamates, pyrethroids, and others.[5,6,7,8]

**Drug resistance in arthropods and nematodes**

Arthropod resistance to insecticides (and acaricides) has developed more rapidly and through larger geographic areas than nematode resistance to anthelmintics. The former has extended all over the world whereas the latter has remained largely localized in Australia-New Zealand, North America, Great Britain, and parts of continental Europe. The following reasons may explain these differences:

**1. Spatial mobility**. Whereas most arthropods have their own means of transportation, helminths move only with their hosts. This restricts the spread of resistant helminths and interferes with the contribution of their genetic material to neighboring

---

[a] Thiabendazole, cambendazole, parbendazole, albendazole, oxibendazole, mebendazole, fenbendazole, and oxfendazole.

susceptible populations. Mobility may be an important element in the generation of resistance as judged by the much greater number of flying diptera that developed resistance as compared with non-flying arthropods.

**2. Restricted selection**. Only the population of parasites that becomes in contact with the anti-parasitic drug is selected for resistance. It has been estimated that only 3-5% of the population of *H. contortus* is present in the sheep during outbreaks that call for treatment. The remaining of the population is present in the pastures as eggs or larvae so it does not get selected. Among arthropods, on the contrary, the entire population of permanent ectoparasites (mites, lice) is on the host during treatment, or a large part of the population of temporary ectoparasites (ticks, fleas, true bugs, flies, mosquitoes) visit the host while the insecticide is still active. Also, with many arthropods (flies, mosquitoes) insecticides are applied to the environment which assures the contact of the drug with a large proportion of the arthropod population.

**3. Pharmacokinetics of anthelmintics and insecticides**. Most anthelmintics persist in the host at active levels for less than 24 hours. As a consequence, resistant nematodes enjoy a survival advantage for only a brief period, and mildly resistant worms may counteract the effect of the drug with temporary physiologic mechanisms (such as reduction of energy demands, use of energy reserves, switching to alternative pathways). In contrast, the longer-lasting insecticides provide a prolonged survival advantage to resistant arthropods, and demand a robust mechanism for survival.

**4. Genetic nature of the resistance**. For the reasons explained above, resistance to insecticides is often single gene-dependent whereas resistance to anthelmintics is commonly polygenic. As discussed before, single gene resistance develops more rapidly than polygenic resistance.

**5. Detection of resistance.** Whereas the removal of only 50% of the internal helminths may be regarded as a clinical success (and resistance go unnoticed), persistence of half the population of external arthropods is clearly visible and readily noticed.

## MECHANISMS OF RESISTANCE

There is a number of mechanisms by which parasites may become resistant to the action of anti-parasitic agents but only 3 have been verified so far: reduced penetration, detoxication, and insensitivity of the action site. In most cases, resistance against an anti-parasitic agent is a complex phenomenon that involves more than one mechanism in the same or different parasite species.

### 1. Reduced penetration

This is a rather uncommon mechanism studied particularly in the housefly and *Boophilus* ticks. The *pen* gene of the housefly codes for unidentified modifications of the fly cuticle that reduces the penetration of carbaryl, DDT, and dieldrin insecticides. A pyrethroid-resistant strain of *B. microplus* also showed reduced penetration of some pyrethroid isomers.

### 2. Detoxification

A well known example is the presence of DDTase (DDT-dehydrochlorinase) which is present only in DDT-resistance insects. This enzyme transforms DDT into the less toxic component, DDE. Resistance to organophosphates also depends on several detoxifying mechanisms, one involves the presence of phosphatases and carboxylesterases in resistant insects that degrade the insecticides into non-toxic compounds. Resistance to carbamates and pyrethrins depends mainly on oxidative degradation of the active molecules.

### 3. Insensitivity of the action site

Organophosphate and carbamate insecticides act mainly by inhibition of the arthropod acetylcholinesterase (AChE). Arthropods resistant to these insecticides possess a different AChE which is much less susceptible to inhibition by organo-phosphates or carbamates (and is often less active to transform its substrate, acetylcholine).

A recessive *kdr* gene (for *k*nock*d*own *r*esistance) that avoids the initial knockdown characteristic of DDTase resistance has been identified in flies resistant to DDT. The existing evidence suggests that the product of this gene reduces the sensitivity of nervous cells to DDT. The *kdr* gene confers cross-resistance to pyrethrins and methoxychlor, whereas DDTase does not.

Resistance to the benzimidazole anthelmintics belongs to this category.[9] The benzimidazoles act by inhibition of the polymerization of tubulin and inhibition of the fumarate reductase. These two actions are known to be related but their exact relation is unknown. Tubulin is a soluble protein that polymerizes to form the microtubular framework of the cell. Fumarate reductase is a mitochondrial enzyme that converts fumarate to succinate, a major anaerobic energy-producing pathway. The tubulin of benzimidazole-resistant nematodes is chemically different and binds considerably less benzimidazole compounds that the tubulin of susceptible nematodes.

## RECOMMENDATIONS TO PREVENT OR DELAY DRUG-RESISTANCE

The first 6 items are commonly recommended for the use of private practitioners. The others may be better fit for industry or extensive campaigns.

**1. Frequency of treatment**

Because selection for resistance occurs only while the parasite population is in contact with the anti-parasitic agent, frequent treatments will select more parasites and accelerate the development of resistance. Among nematodes, the maximum selection pressure will occurs when the frequency of treatments coincide with the prepatent period of the parasite. In this case, the susceptible nematodes will be killed before oviposition and only the descendence of the resistant parasites will accumulate in the environment for future infections. Sparing treatments will delay the development of resistance.

**2. Dosage of anti-parasitic agent**

Sub-optimal doses will leave a larger proportion of drug-resistant parasites alive to contribute their resistant genome to the next generation (Figure 30.1). Sub-optimal dosage is common when the doses are calculated on the basis of the average weight of the animals (rather than on the weight of the heaviest animals) or when the farmers cut down the doses to save money. Use of the highest dose compatible with cost and toxicity will kill the greatest proportion of parasites and will leave only a small number of resistant organisms for future infections.

**3. Spectrum of the anti-parasitic agent**

Wide spectrum parasiticides are commonly very effective against the primary parasite species for which they were formulated but less effective against secondary species. In this case, the drug will leave alive a large proportion of the secondary parasites to contribute their resistant genome to future infections. If the circumstances permit, it is better to use narrow spectrum parasiticides to eliminate only the intended parasite to the largest extent possible..

**4. Pasture management**

The population of parasites (e.g., gastrointestinal nematodes) of a farm exists as parasitic stages in the gut of the infected animals and as free living stages in the pastures. Their proportions vary along the seasons or with management: whereas the parasitic population is relatively greater during droughts or when the stock is moved to clean pastures, the free living population is proportionally greater during spring (see Figure 29.1) or in pastures subjected to continuous grazing. Only the parasitic stages are selected for resistance during treatment. The descendence of these resistant parasites is diluted more or less among the free living (susceptible) stages in the pasture when they leave their host.

Treating animals and moving them to a clean pasture makes sense to reduce pasture contamination but all the larvae in the pasture will be descendants from the drug-resistant parasites and, therefore, resistant themselves. From the viewpoint of resistance, this will be appropriate only when the conditions of the pasture (drought, cold weather) are such that they do not permit the development of the eggs. An alternative to minimize contamination *and* drug resistance is to treat the animals at the beginning of the lactational rise to avoid contamination of the pasture and excessive infection of the new animals, and rest the pasture during winter to let the resistant eggs and larvae die off.

**5. Alternation of parasiticides.**

Experience has shown that parasites develop side-resistance, this is, cross-resistance against all the anti-parasitic agents with a same mechanism of action (e. g., the benzimidazoles, levamisole/morantel, organophosphates). Alternate use of parasiticides within a same group is equivalent to the repeated use of the same compound. If anti-parasitic agents are alternated, they should belong to groups with different mechanisms of action, and be changed not sooner than yearly. This assumes that the susceptible parasites are biotically more fit than the susceptible parasites and will slowly replace them if the selecting parasiticide is absent. Although the predominance of susceptible parasites in the undisturbed nature suggests that the susceptible parasites are more fit, this has not probed to be true in every case

**6. Total management control.**

The most common methods of parasite control are: **timed treatment**, in which the animals are treated at the best time to prevent heavy build-up of infections; **integrated control**, in which timed treatments are combined with adequate changes of pastures, and; **total management control**, which uses every possible means to control parasitism (treatment, pasture rotation, mixed grazing, age management, etc.). Total management control reduces the use of parasiticides and discourages the selection of resistant parasites.

**7. Production of new parasiticides**

The production of a new anthelmintic, from discovery to marketing, takes 6-8 years and about $ 30 million. This is the reason why only 4 chemical classes of anthelmintics have been produced in the last 30 years (benzimidazoles, levamisole, morantel, and avermectins). With an expected commercial life constantly shortened by the development of drug resistance, significant efforts to produce new parasiticides appear to be an unlikely prospect.

**8. Manipulation of parasiticide structure**

It has been proposed that slight structural modification of a parasiticide to which resistance has developed might make it toxic again. The wide prevalence of side-resistance suggests that this is a groundless hope.

**9. Pharmacokinetics manipulation**

Modifications that will prolong the time of activity of anthelmintics in the host may overcome the rather fragile polygenic anthelmintic resistance. Because the nematodes are little mobile, a nematode population is usually restricted to a single farm so its genetic pool is expected to be too small to contain genes for single gene resistance. However, this is a theoretical consideration, single gene resistant still might became widespread in these circumstances.

**10. New formulations**

New formulations of insecticides to deposit more insecticide on treated animals or increase cuticle penetration in arthropods would raise the effective level of active substance and kill a greater proportion of parasites.

**11. Mixtures of parasiticides**

Although administration of mixtures of parasiticides is often recommended, only the use of parasiticides with different modes of action or detoxication pathways is expected to produce some delay in the development of resistance.

**12. Synergism or additives**

The addition of compounds that counteract the mechanism of resistance (e.g., oxidase inhibitors for carbamates, esterase inhibitors for organophosphates) may turn a parasiticide to which resistance developed into an active compound again. However, these compounds may be expensive, toxic, difficult to formulate, and, in some cases, parasites have developed resistance to the combination parasiticide-additive.

**13. Physiological parasiticides**

Important research is being conducted on the use of analogues or inhibitors of physiologic regulators (growth, juveniles, or molting hormones, pheromones) for the control of parasitism. Because genes that inhibit these functions would be incompatible with life, resistant genes must not exist in nature.

**14. Alternatives to the use of parasiticides**

Investigation of vaccines against parasites is being pursued enthusiastically at present and attempts at selecting hosts genetically resistant to parasites are being renewed. The historic results of these investigations are not very encouraging but the recent advances in immunology and molecular biology have opened a number of viable possibilities.

Chemical control is, and probably will be for some time, an essential component of parasite control. In turn, drug resistance is probably an inevitable consequence of chemical control. Currently we are in a race to see whether alternative means will be available before chemical control becomes obsolete. In the meanwhile, it is judicious to regard parasiticide sensitivity as a natural resource that must be preserved at all cost.

## REFERENCES

1. Le Jambre, L.F. 1985. Genetic aspects of anthelmintic resistance in nematodes. In Anderson, N. and Waller, P.J. (eds.), *Resistance in nematodes to anthelmintic drugs*. CSIRO Division Animal Health, Glebe, N.S.W., Australia, 97-106.

2. Chapman, H.D. 1982. Anticoccidial drug resistance. In Long, P.L. (ed.), *The Biology of the Coccidia,* University Park Press, Baltimore, 429-452.

3. Waller, P.J. 1987. Anthelmintic resistance and the future for roundworm control. Vet. Parasit. 25:177-191.

4. Prichard, R. K. 1990. Anthelmintic resistance in nematodes: extent, recent understanding and future directions for control and research. Intern. J. Parasitol. 20:515-423.

5. Georghiou, G.P. and Mellon, R.B. 1983. Pesticide resistance in time and space. In Georghiou, G.P and Saito, T. (eds.), *Pest Resistance to Pesticides*, Plenum Press, N.Y. 1-46.

6. Nolan, J. and Schnitzerling, H.J. 1986. Drug resistance in arthropod parasites. In Campbell, W.C. and Rew, R.S. (eds.), *Chemotherapy of Parasitic Diseases*, Plenum Press, N.Y., 603-620.

7. Solomon, K. R. 1983. Acaricide resistance in ticks. Adv. Vet. Sci. Comp. Med. 27:273-296.

8. Nolan, J. 1990. Acaricide resistance in single and multi-host ticks and strategies for control. Parassitol. 32:145-153.

9. Roos, M. H. 1990. The molecular nature of benzimidazole resistance in helminths. Parasitol. Today 6:125-127

# APPENDIX 3

# PATHOPHYSIOLOGICAL CHARTS

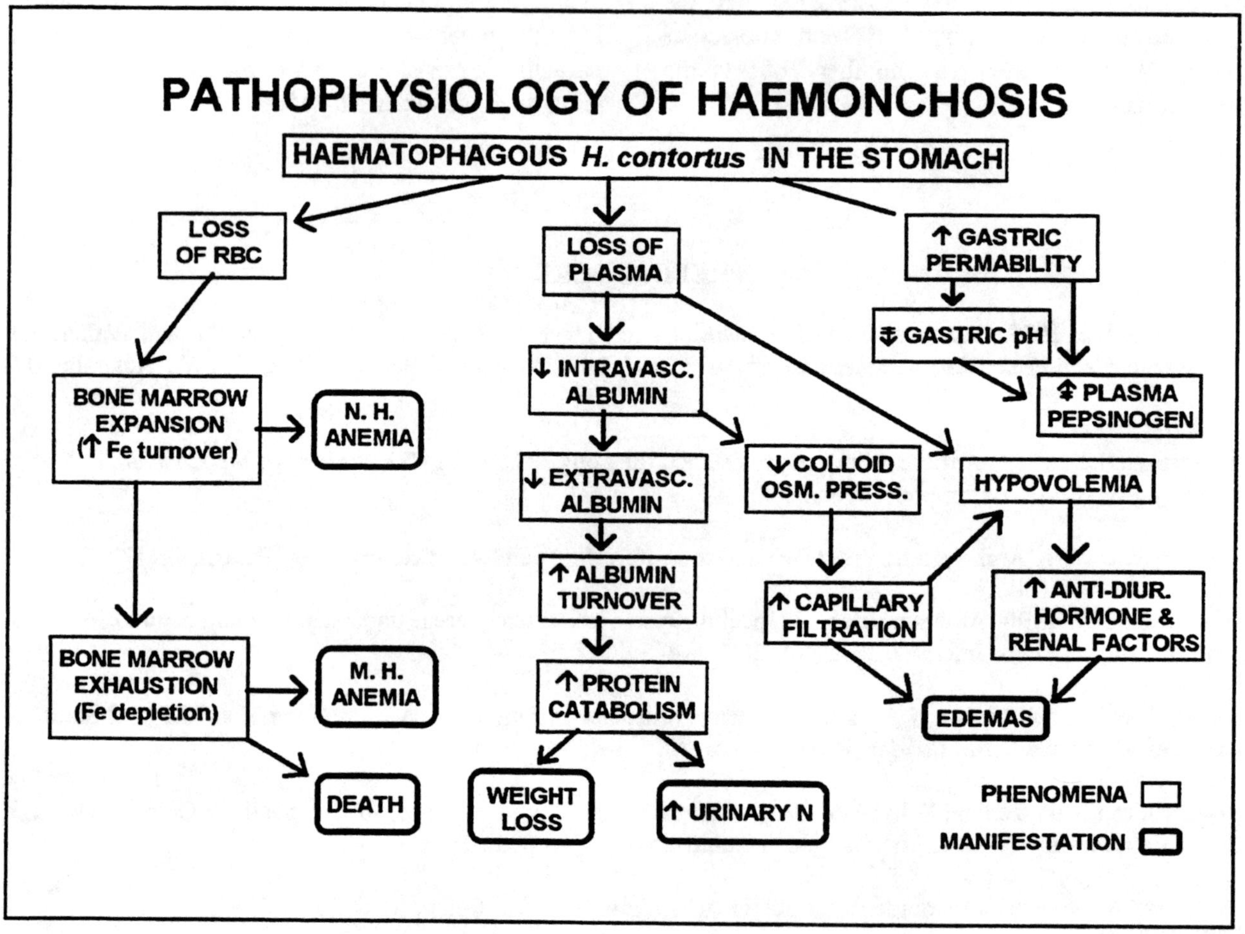

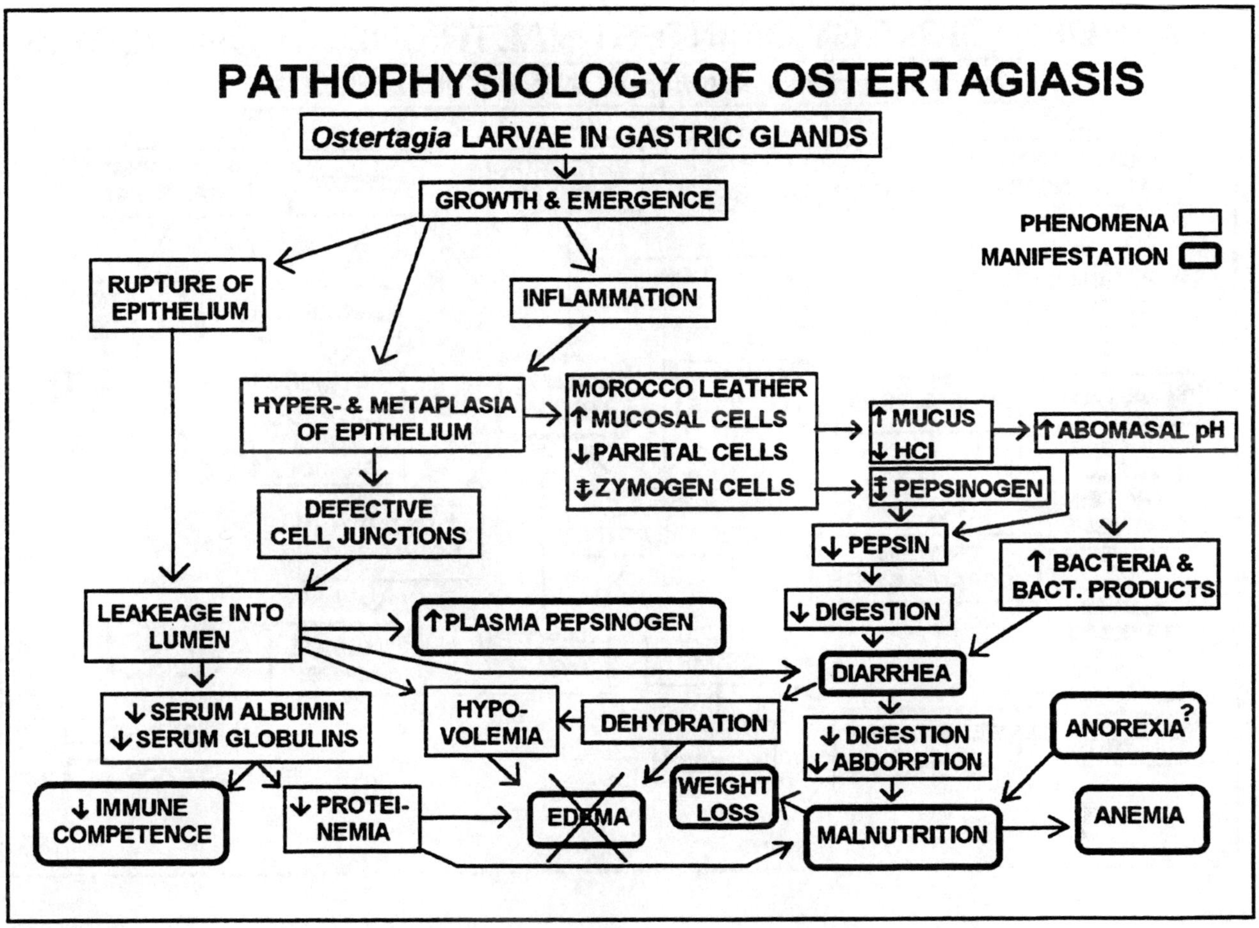
PATHOPHYSIOLOGY OF OSTERTAGIASIS
Ostertagia LARVAE IN GASTRIC GLANDS
GROWTH & EMERGENCE
PHENOMENA
MANIFESTATION
RUPTURE OF EPITHELIUM
INFLAMMATION
HYPER- & METAPLASIA OF EPITHELIUM
MOROCCO LEATHER
↑ MUCOSAL CELLS
↓ PARIETAL CELLS
↓ ZYMOGEN CELLS
↑ MUCUS
↓ HCl
↑ ABOMASAL pH
↓ PEPSINOGEN
DEFECTIVE CELL JUNCTIONS
↓ PEPSIN
↑ BACTERIA & BACT. PRODUCTS
LEAKEAGE INTO LUMEN
↑ PLASMA PEPSINOGEN
↓ DIGESTION
DIARRHEA
↓ SERUM ALBUMIN
↓ SERUM GLOBULINS
HYPO-VOLEMIA
DEHYDRATION
↓ DIGESTION
↓ ABDORPTION
ANOREXIA?
↓ IMMUNE COMPETENCE
↓ PROTEI-NEMIA
EDEMA
WEIGHT LOSS
MALNUTRITION
ANEMIA

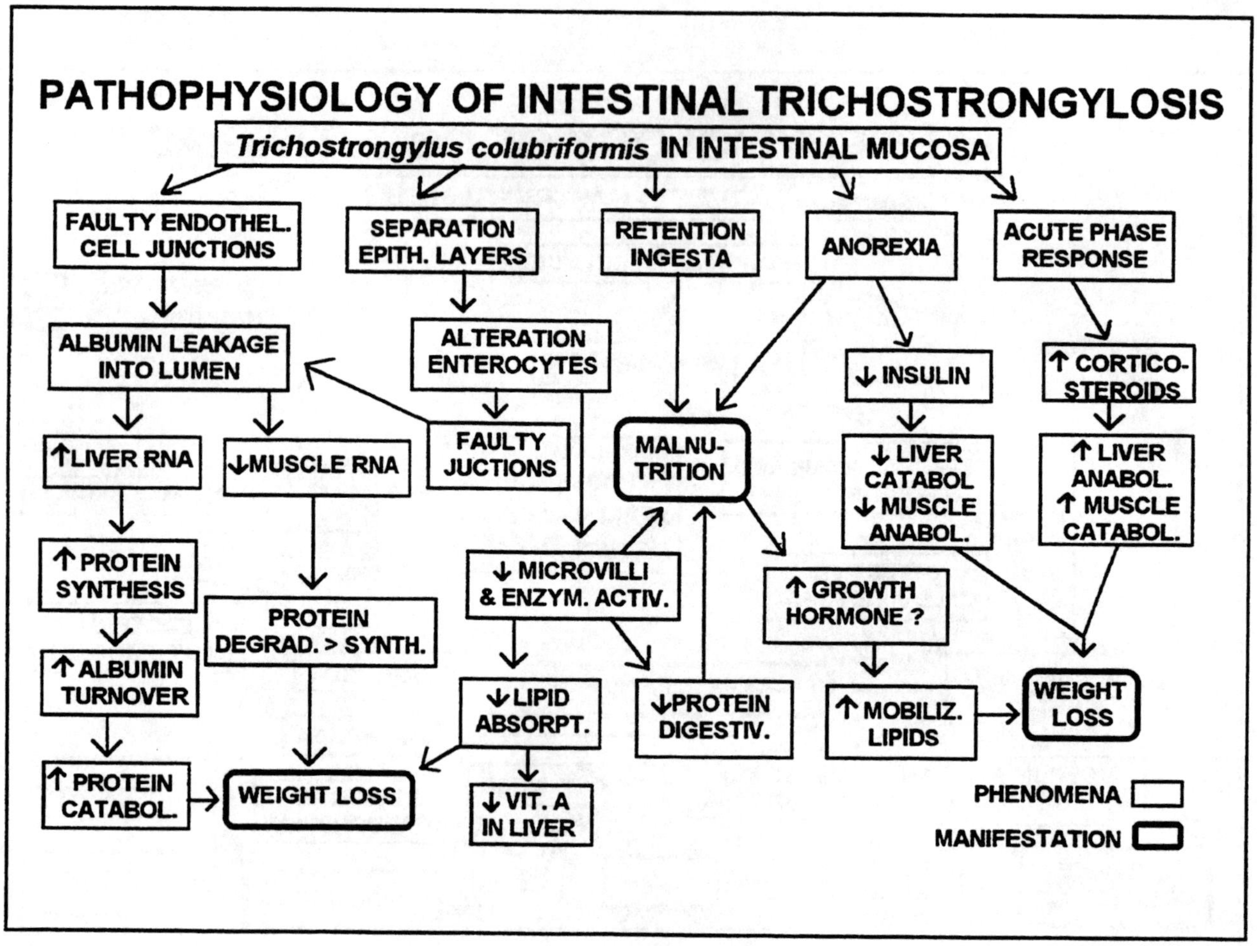
PATHOPHYSIOLOGY OF INTESTINAL TRICHOSTRONGYLOSIS
*Trichostrongylus colubriformis* IN INTESTINAL MUCOSA
FAULTY ENDOTHEL. CELL JUNCTIONS
SEPARATION EPITH. LAYERS
RETENTION INGESTA
ANOREXIA
ACUTE PHASE RESPONSE
ALBUMIN LEAKAGE INTO LUMEN
ALTERATION ENTEROCYTES
↓ INSULIN
↑ CORTICO-STEROIDS
↑LIVER RNA
↓MUSCLE RNA
FAULTY JUCTIONS
MALNU-TRITION
↓ LIVER CATABOL ↓ MUSCLE ANABOL.
↑ LIVER ANABOL. ↑ MUSCLE CATABOL.
↑ PROTEIN SYNTHESIS
↓ MICROVILLI & ENZYM. ACTIV.
↑ GROWTH HORMONE ?
PROTEIN DEGRAD. > SYNTH.
↑ ALBUMIN TURNOVER
↓LIPID ABSORPT.
↓PROTEIN DIGESTIV.
↑ MOBILIZ. LIPIDS
WEIGHT LOSS
↑ PROTEIN CATABOL.
WEIGHT LOSS
↓ VIT. A IN LIVER
PHENOMENA
MANIFESTATION

# PATHOPHYSIOLOGY OF CANINE DIROFILARIASIS

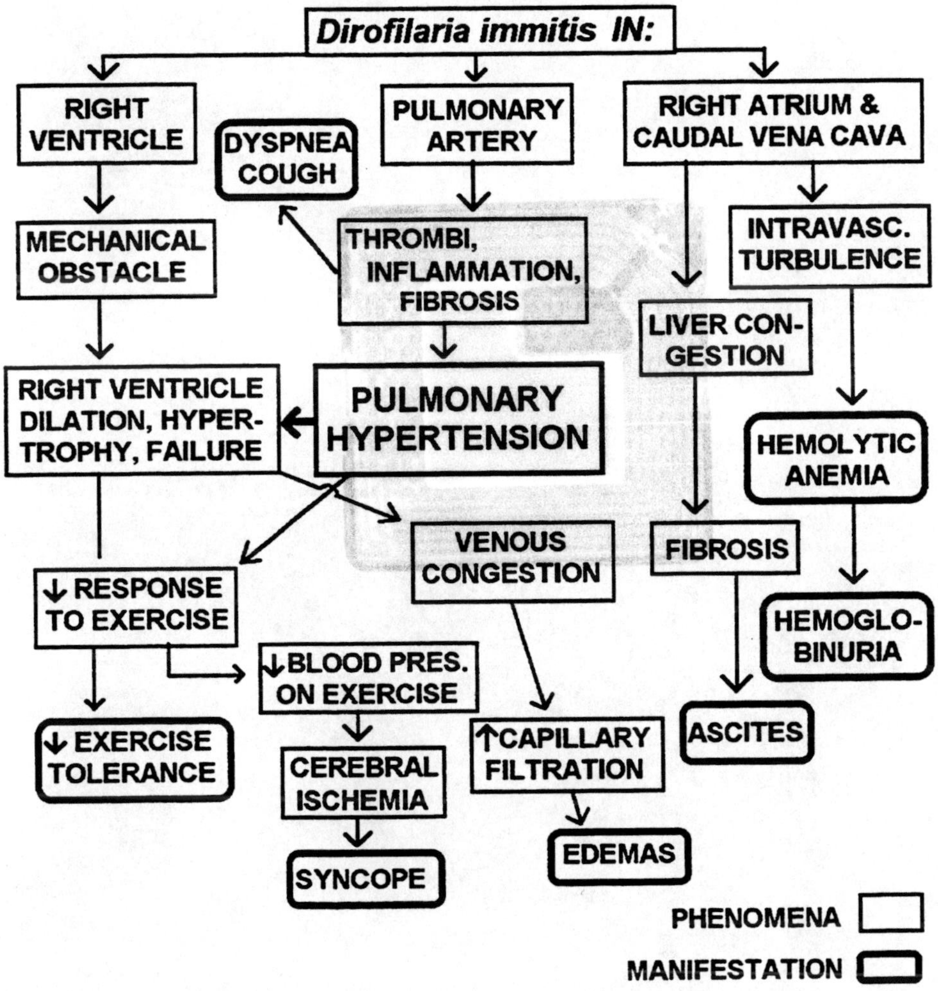